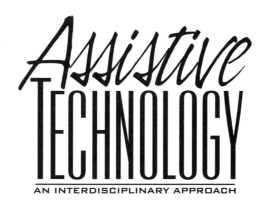

Assistive
TECHNOLOGY

AN INTERDISCIPLINARY APPROACH

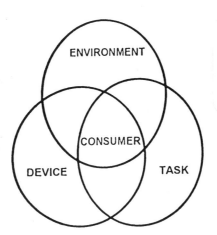

D1387753

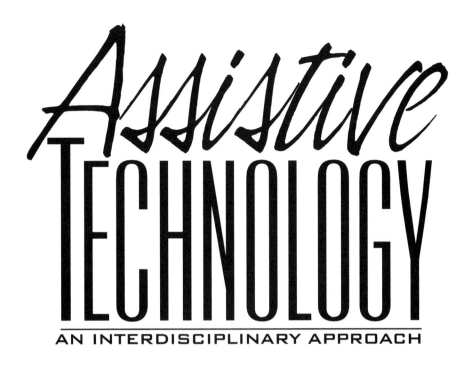

Assistive TECHNOLOGY
AN INTERDISCIPLINARY APPROACH

BEVERLY K. BAIN, Ed.D., O.T.R., F.A.O.T.A.
Assistive Technology Project Coordinator and
Adjunct Associate Professor
Department of Occupational Therapy
New York University
New York, New York

DAWN LEGER, Ph.D.
Associate Research Scientist
Department of Occupational Therapy
New York University
New York, New York

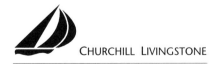

CHURCHILL LIVINGSTONE

New York, Edinburgh, London, Madrid, Melbourne, San Francisco, Tokyo

Library of Congress Cataloging-in-Publication Data

Assistive technology : an interdisciplinary approach / [edited by]
  Beverly K. Bain, Dawn Leger.
      p.   cm.
    Includes bibliographical references and index.
    ISBN 0-443-07552-2 (alk. paper)
    1. Rehabilitation technology. 2. Self-help devices for the
disabled.   I. Bain, Beverly K. II. Leger, Dawn
    [DNLM: 1. Self-Help Devices. 2. Technology Transfer.
  3. Rehabilitation—instrumentation.   WB 320 A8479 1997]
  RM950.A87   1997
  617'.03—dc21
  DNLM/DLC
  for Library of Congress   97-8215
                                                                      CIP

© **Churchill Livingstone Inc. 1997**

Distributed in the United Kingdom by Churchill Livingstone, Robert Stevenson
House, 1–3 Baxter's Place, Leith Walk, Edinburgh EH1 3AF, and by associated companies, branches, and representatives throughout the world.

Medical knowledge is constantly changing. As new information becomes available,
changes in treatment, procedures, equipment and the use of drugs become necessary. The editors/authors/contributors and the publishers have, as far as it is possible, taken care to ensure that the information given in this text is accurate and up
to date. However, readers are strongly advised to confirm that the information,
especially with regard to drug usage, complies with the latest legislation and standards of practice.

The Publishers have made every effort to trace the copyright holders for borrowed
material. If they have inadvertently overlooked any, they will be pleased to make
the necessary arrangements at the first opportunity.

Acquisitions Editor: *Carol Bader*
Production Editor: *Elizabeth A. Lipp*
Production Supervisor: *Kathleen R. Smith*
Desktop Coordinator: *Kathy-Jo Dunayer*
Cover Design: *Jeannette Jacobs*
Illustrator: *Robert Corren*
Photographer: *Tony Velez*

Printed in the United States of America

First published in 1997   7   6   5   4   3   2   1

Contributors

Beverly K. Bain, Ed.D., O.T.R., F.A.O.T.A.
Assistive Technology Project Coordinator and Adjunct Associate Professor, Department of Occupational Therapy, New York University, New York, New York

Adrienne F. Bergen, P.T.
Seating and Wheeled Mobility Specialist, Dynamic Medical Equipment, Westbury, New York

Cristina Mickley Burwell, M.A.
Lecturer, Department of Occupational Therapy, Boston University; Consultant, Human Factors Engineering, GTE, Boston, Massachussetts

Amy G. Dell, Ph.D.
Associate Professor, Department of Special Education, The College of New Jersey, Trenton, New Jersey

Julie S. DeMicco, M.A., O.T.R./L.
Occupational Therapist, YAI/NYL Gramercy School, New York, New York

Ruth Dickey, M.A., O.T.R./L.
Instructor, Clinical Occupational Therapy, Columbia University Faculty of Medicine; Supervisor, Occupational Therapy, Rusk Institute of Rehabilitation, New York University Medical Center; Formerly Director, TEAMS Lab, Rehabilitation Medicine Department, Mt. Sinai Hospital, New York, New York

Kenneth F. Dooley, M.S., C.R.C., N.C.C.
Vocational Rehabilitation Counselor, Program Monitoring Specialist, Vocation and Educational Services for Individuals with Disabilities (VESID), New York, New York

Manny Halpern, M.A., C.P.E.
Adjunct Assistant Professor, Department of Occupational Therapy, Program of Ergonomics and Biomechanics, New York University; Ergonomics Coordinator, Occupational and Industrial Orthopaedic Center, Hospital for Joint Diseases, New York, New York

Jeff Harten, M.S.
Director, Industrial Medicine, Kessler Institute for Rehabilitation East, East Orange, New Jersey

Deena Garrison Jones, O.T.R., C.D.R.S.
Outpatient Senior Therapist, Certified Driver Rehabilitation Specialist and Adaptive Driving Coordinator, Woodrow Wilson Rehabilitation Center, Fishersville, Virginia

Barbara A. Kollodge, O.T.R./L., A.T.P.
Supervisor, Assistive Technology Unit, Rusk Institute of Rehabilitation/New York University Medical Center, New York, New York

Donna W. Kozberg, M.B.A., M.F.A., M.R.C.
President and Chief Executive Officer, LIFT, Inc., Mountainside, New Jersey

Dawn Leger, Ph.D.
Associate Research Scientist, Department of Occupational Therapy, New York University, New York, New York

Rita Marie Levey, M.A., O.T.R./L.
Occupational Therapist, Department of Occupational Therapy, Saint Charles Rehabilitation Center, Albertson, New York

Hildy S. Lipner, MA, C.C.C./S.L.P.
Adjunct Clinical Assistant Professor, Department of Speech and Language Pathology and Audiology, New York University, New York, New York; Chief Communication Disorders/Audiology, Institute for Child Development, Hackensack University Medical Center, Hackensack, New Jersey

Jane Miller, M.A., O.T.R.
Instructor, Department of Occupational Therapy, New York University, New York, New York; Consultant, Private Practice, Pittstown, New Jersey

Richard W. Nead Jr., B.A.
Adaptive Driving Instructor, Kessler Institute for Rehabilitation, West Orange, New Jersey

Lori Petruccelli-Safer, L.P.T.A., M.A., O.T.R./L.
Hand Therapist, Department of Physical Therapy, Bayonne Hospital; Home Care Therapist, Bayonne Visiting Nurse Association, Bayonne, New Jersey

Patricia A. Ryan, M.Ed.
Senior Research Scientist, Director, Upward Bound Program, The Metropolitan Center for Urban Education, New York University, New York, New York

Linda Stern, M.A., O.T.R./L., M.B.A.
Occupational Therapist and Case Manager, Transitions of Long Island, Manhasset, New York

Gail Tishcoff, M.A., O.T.R./L.
Clinical Supervisor, Department of Occupational Therapy and Physical Therapy, The Shield Institute Adult Day Treatment Center, Bayside, New York

Barry A. Wolf, M.Ed., O.T.R./L.
Clinical Manager, Back-to-Work Program, JFK Johnson Rehabilitation Institute, JFK Medical Center, Edison, New Jersey

Foreword

Assistive technology (AT) has become increasingly integrated into rehabilitation services in the past 15 years. Although recognition of the value of AT has grown, there is still considerable confusion about how it can be most effectively applied to obtain successful outcomes. *Assistive Technology: An Interdisciplinary Approach* will help clarify roles, provide a perspective on systematic evaluations, and increase awareness of how AT fits into a broad range of professional disability services.

The editors, Drs. Beverly Bain and Dawn Leger, emphasize that four elements need to be considered in any AT service: the consumer, the task to be performed, the environment where the task is to be accomplished, and the assistive devices that can facilitate this activity. This may seem like basic common sense, but it has all too frequently been overlooked. *Assistive Technology: An Interdisciplinary Approach* is written for rehabilitation service providers who are not necessarily AT specialists and may enable them to disseminate this concept among rehabilitation professionals and consumers with disabilities.

Technology solutions and services in training and employment environments play a large part in rehabilitation services. It is encouraging to see how the authors relate worksite issues to other environments rather than the other way around. Too often in the past, books have stressed in-home technology solutions and then tried to stretch them to the worksite, often with minimal success. Given the rapid changes in telecommunications–computer–television convergence, in the near future we may all require almost business level communications capacity at home in order to be competitive and to be integrated into our communities. It makes sense to think about linking environments and the ways that AT needs are met.

Given the breadth of AT and its applications, it is difficult to imagine anything but the interdisciplinary approach emphasized here. AT service providers work in a variety of settings (e.g., hospitals, rehabilitation centers, schools, workplaces, and independent living centers) and have emerged from a broad spectrum of practical and professional preparation experiences. This book will help professionals understand the wide range of technological applications and the range of skills that are needed to effectively use technology in all the environments a consumer needs it in without overwhelming them with the details only an AT specialist provider needs to master.

AT (tools), personal assistance services (cooperation), and adaptive or compensatory strategies (techniques) are three critical elements of any individual's support system. Support systems need to work in a wide range of environments, and they change over time. AT needs to work within the context of a support system and the other people, tools, and techniques that need to function effectively together. When people with disabilities develop support systems, they often figure things out on their own, something professionals sometimes forget. By the time individuals with disabilities start looking for AT and AT services, they have usually run through a lot of options for addressing the identified goal and tasks. The consumer's experience is an integral part of professional services, and a fundamental reason why the consumer must be an integral part of the professional team. Every consumer should be considered an expert on addressing and identifying his or her own life goals and tasks for independent living. When an individual with a disability seeks direct professional intervention, it is vital that an appropriate service delivery program be available. Qualified practitioners should function as team members, in a coordinated manner that is efficient, systematic, and results in an outcome satisfactory to the consumer. Drs. Bain and Leger have years of experience in developing AT services that meet these objectives and in this book share their cumulative knowledge with you.

Alexandra Enders, O.T.R./L.
President Elect
Rehabilitation Engineering and Assistive
Technology Society of North America

viii

Foreword

Preface

When the first graduate assistive technology (AT) course was taught at New York University in 1985, there were two textbooks available; one was highly technical and the other was a resource book. As three graduate courses were developed, it was necessary to design teaching materials to supplement lectures, demonstrations, and hands-on laboratory experiences. All courses were taught by a variety of experts in the field of rehabilitation, including occupational therapists, physical therapists, rehabilitation counselors, speech pathologists, special educators, rehabilitation engineers, vendors, and more importantly, users of AT. In the last four years, these three courses have developed into the basis for an advanced master's degree program in occupational therapy with a specialty in AT. Courses have been taught to a variety of professionals, always with the emphasis on interdisciplinary collaboration.

It was early recognized that AT devices and services could be utilized by a systems approach, not by simply matching each new device to each new consumer. Through discussions at professional meetings and work in the field, it became apparent that for AT services to be effective and for AT devices to be fully used and not abandoned, the environment where the devices were to be used must be a vital component of the technology system. Individuals with disabilities are participants in school, work, and community activities, and each of those environments presents different challenges that must be addressed by the AT team, as well as the consideration of the home setting. The input of the consumer as an active participant in the AT team ensures that the team focuses on increasing independence and addresses the preferences and goals of the AT consumer. The evaluation must then include an evaluation of the consumer, the tasks he or she wishes to accomplish, the environments where these tasks would be done, and the devices that might be used. All four elements are part of a synergistic system, where the sum of the parts working together is greater than their value alone. All of these elements must be considered together, and the removal of one component can have a negative impact on the consumer, who must also be an active participant in the total rehabilitation process.

Assistive Technology: An Interdisciplinary Approach was first conceived as a manual for interdisciplinary teams, developed with the support of a grant from the U.S. Department of Education Rehabilitation Services Administration and with the guidance of an interdisciplinary advisory board of consumers and professionals. As interest and demand grew, professional art and photography were added as were additional chapters designed to reach a broader audience. The culmination of many years of research and teaching assistive technology, this book is inspired by and dedicated to people with disabilities and those who work in the area of assistive technology. The recognition of these key concepts—the "synergy" among the four elements (consumer, task, environment, and device), and the holistic approach to rehabilitation—will greatly improve outcomes for individuals with disabilities, and consequently for society as a whole.

Beverly K. Bain, Ed.D., O.T.R., F.A.O.T.A.
Dawn Leger, Ph.D.

X

Preface

Acknowledgments

First, we wish to thank the U.S. Department of Education Rehabilitation Services Administration, for supporting the courses and later, the specialized advanced master's degree program in occupational therapy at New York University, with four grants from 1984 to 1996. We give special thanks to Mrs. Willene DeMond, regional training coordinator. With these training grants, we were able to educate assistive technology providers from many disciplines and develop the material included in this book.

Thanks also to the many contributors who spent time and effort to write, rewrite, and discuss the concepts in this book; Dr. Deborah R. Labovitz, chair of the Department of Occupational Therapy at NYU and project director of the RSA grants, for her encouragement; the interdisciplinary advisory committee, many of whom provided chapters and editorial assistance, for their guidance and enthusiasm; Charles Sprague and the administration of the School of Education at NYU, for continued support; and the helpful staff in the Department of Occupational Therapy, especially Tako Nishiyama and Elizabeth Jackson.

No AT book would be complete without the many illustrations and photographs that enhance the written material. We applaud the fine work of the artist, Mr. Robert Correa, recently deceased, and the photographer, Mr. Tony Velez. Special thanks to Barbara A. Kollodge, for allowing us to transform into a photography studio the Assistive Technology Lab at the Rusk Institute of Rehabilitative Medicine, New York University Medical Center. Our contacts at Churchill Livingstone—Carol Bader (Editor, Allied Health) and Elizabeth Lipp (Production Editor)—have been extremely supportive, and we appreciate their efforts.

Thanks especially to the many consumers who taught us so much, and especially Craig Fabian, an extraordinary man who published our first manual from his wheelchair with an adapted computer system. And finally, we appreciate the support of our family and friends, who were behind us from the concept to the final product.

Contents

xiv

Contents

BEVERLY K. BAIN
KENNETH F. DOOLEY
DAWN LEGER

Assistive Technology

AN INTERDISCIPLINARY APPROACH

In most cases, especially in the workplace, technology becomes the great equalizer and provides the person with a disability a level playing field on which to compete.
—Mary B. Radabough[1]

This interdisciplinary book is written for rehabilitation service providers who have a limited knowledge of assistive technology (AT). It presents a systems approach to using AT in the rehabilitation process to return an injured employee to work, to enable a severely disabled individual to attend school or to become employed, or to assist an individual with a progressive disease or an elderly person to remain on the job and independent at home for an extended period of time. Emphasis is placed on principles, concepts, and methods that have proved useful to consumers, that have enhanced the effectiveness of service providers, and that should assist the health care professional in using these devices and approaches to increase both the functioning and the independence of individuals with disabilities. Issues discussed include defining the AT system, who can benefit from using it, how AT is useful, where and when it can be used effectively, and how to determine whether high or low technology best serves the purpose. The focus of this book is the achievement of the optimal level of functioning, independence, and quality of life for persons with disabilities. What is presented is equally applicable to the selection and use of AT for independence at home, school, work, and in the community.

Today, medical science enables many people to survive conditions that previously were fatal and others with severe disabilities to live longer. The application of AT may assist these individuals to improve their quality of life at home, in the workplace, and in the community. In addition, several laws, including the Technology Related Assistance for Individuals with Disabilities Act (TRAID),[2,3] the Americans with Disabilities Act (ADA),[4] the Individuals with Disabilities Education Act (IDEA),[5] and the Rehabilitation Act of 1973[6] as amended (Rehabilitation Act),[7–9] mandate a consideration of AT.

To provide appropriate services to people with disabilities, it is increasingly necessary for rehabilitation professionals to develop their skills in this rapidly changing field. For the individual with a disability who may require and use these services and devices, a better level of understanding and knowledge about AT will be helpful for their active collaboration in the decision-making process, in making more informed and more satisfactory choices, and for avoidance of technology abandonment.

DEFINITIONS

As defined in the 1992 revision of the Rehabilitation Act, *rehabilitation technology* is "the systematic application of technologies, engineering methodologies, or scientific principles to meet the needs of and address the barriers confronted by individuals with disabilities in areas which include education, rehabilitation, employment, transportation, independent living, and recreation."[9] This term includes the subjects of rehabilitation engineering, assistive technology devices, and assistive technology services.

The terms *assistive technology device* and *assistive technology service* are defined by the TRAID act,[2] and these definitions are incorporated into the 1992 amendments of the Rehabilitation Act.[9] As defined, an assistive technology device (ATD) is "any item, piece of equipment, or product system, whether acquired commercially off the shelf, modified, or customized, that is used to increase, maintain, or improve functional capabilities of individuals with disabilities." An AT service is "any service that directly assists an individual with a disability with the selection, acquisition, or use of an assistive technology device." The definition lists a variety of specific services that are included.[9]

LEGISLATIVE MANDATES

In the United States, laws are continuously being refined and amended. It is the responsibility of the rehabilitation specialist to keep abreast of legislative changes and to inform consumers about relevant changes and opportunities. Since the passage of the ADA in 1990,[4] a concerted effort is underway on the part of employers, persons with disabilities, and their advocates to define reasonable accommodations. The ADA is designed to facilitate the opportunity for thousands of persons with disabilities to obtain and retain employment, to use public transportation and other facilities, and to become more productive members of the community. The ADA is essentially a "civil rights act" for persons with disabilities. Much of what has been mandated by the ADA must be negotiated through the courts, and individuals with disabilities must take an active role in defining the terms of their participation in the community and workplace.

Laws exist that delineate the responsibility of school districts to provide services, including AT, to preschool and school-aged children, and institutions of higher education.[10-12] The passage of the Tech Act in 1988 (also known as TRIAD) mandated the availability of AT devices and services to persons with disabilities.[2] This broad-based act provides technology services for the entire life span of a person with a disability and therefore covers education and employment as well as other social service provisions. IDEA[5] extended the provision of the Tech Act to the local level, stipulating that the devices and services should enhance the educational opportunities of children with disabilities. In 1992, the Tech Act was reauthorized.[2] It requires states to specify the manner in which they will provide ATD and AT services, how their plans meet specified objectives, and the activities of rehabilitation engineering centers for research and development. Table 1-1 contains highlights of the important legislation concerning AT that has been passed since 1973.

Table 1-1. Legislation for Assistive Technology in the United States, 1973–1994

Legislation	Purpose
Rehabilitation Act of 1973 (PL 93–112)	Provides rehabilitation services to all eligible individuals regardless of disability
Rehabilitation Act Amendments of 1978 (PL 95–602)	Establishes National Institute of Disability and Rehabilitation Research, increases funding for rehabilitation engineering research
Rehabilitation Act Amendments of 1986 (PL 99–506)	Adds rehabilitation engineering to mandated services that states must provide
Rehabilitation Act Amendments of 1992 (PL 102–569)	Redefines AT services, extends state mandate for rehabilitation technology services
Education for All Handicapped Children Act of 1975 (PL 94–142)	Provides free appropriate education for every child with a disability; AT not required but suggested by mandate to use "supplementary aids" if needed
Education of the Handicapped Act Amendments of 1986 (PL 99–457)	Adds provisions regarding use of technology; mandated design and adaptation of technology for teaching students with disabilities. Priority to train personnel in special education technology
Developmental Disabilities Assistance & Bill of Rights Act Amendments of 1987 (PL 100–146)	Adds AT as priority for funding. AT to strengthen legislative goals for independence, productivity, and integration
Technology-Related Assistance for Individuals with Disabilities Act (TRIAD) of 1988 (PL 100–407)	Provides increased access to ATDs and AT services
Technology-Related Assistance for Individuals with Disabilities Act (TRIAD) of 1994 (PL 103–218)	Establishes greater role for advocacy services and consumer responsive activities
Americans with Disabilities Act (ADA) of 1990 (PL 101–336)	Integrates AT as a civil right of all persons with disabilities
Individuals with Disabilities Education Act (IDEA) of 1990 (PL 101–476)	Mandates provision of AT to every child with need, research and development of AT, and AT for transition to work

Legal and social service policies vary widely throughout the world. Most industrialized nations provide some services and protections for persons with disabilities, but other developing nations may not have the resources or expertise about ATDs. The Rehabilitation Engineering and Assistive Technology Society of North America (RESNA) is an interdisciplinary organization based in Washington, DC, that also has international influence. At their annual meeting, participants come from all over the world, from Hong Kong to Australia, to share their findings and make important connections with other researchers, engineers, and therapists. The group provides a forum for the exchange of information through publications and meetings. Professional special interest groups explore new research areas and assist in the development of guidelines for practice in many disciplines.

BAIN ASSISTIVE TECHNOLOGY SYSTEM

In this book, AT is part of a synergistic system of four integrated components: the consumer, the task, the device, and the environment.[13] The organizing principle is the purpose or task to be achieved, and the degree to which the purpose or task is accomplished is a measure of the success, or failure, of the system.

The Bain Assistive Technology System (BATS) is illustrated in Figure 1-1, in which the consumer is shown as the focus of the other three elements, all forming an integrated interlocking whole. As one is concentrating on any of the elements, it may be moved into the focal position, with the other three elements arrayed about it to maintain the integrated wholeness of the system. Neglect of any of the elements puts the entire effort in danger of failure or reduced effectiveness and may lead to abandonment of the ATD.

ATDs and AT services, like technology itself, are being developed at such a rapid rate that it is not possible for any one person or discipline to

Figure 1-1. The Bain Assistive Technology System (BATS).

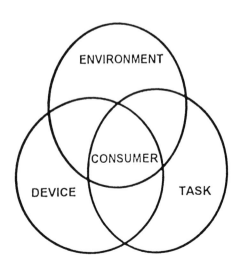

keep current in all areas. It is a shared concern of all people interested in rehabilitation. Each person brings a perspective and type of expertise stemming from his or her background, training, and experience. It will therefore be stressed throughout this book that the collaboration, communication, and coordination of effort by a rehabilitation team working with a person with a disability is essential for effective service delivery. The members of such a team may vary from time to time, from problem to problem, from one individual to another, and over the life span of the same individual. Because finding qualified team members may be difficult, suggested readings and resources for consultation are included at the end of each chapter. It is of critical importance that the consumer with the disability is actively involved in directing the team efforts, as the ultimate arbiter of the success or failure of AT.

The application of AT is complicated because there is not one device for every user, each user has individual needs, and the environments where these devices are used vary from time to time. A problem-solving approach is required, and throughout this book, guidelines are presented to assist the reader. The salient concept to remember is that because there are so many variables, it is unlikely for there to be only one solution to the problem(s). The best solution can only be made by considering the individual's needs, all possible devices, and all environments where the individual will use the devices.

This book is written by an interdisciplinary team of professionals and people who use AT. We do not endorse any products, manufacturers, or suppliers of ATDs. Throughout the book, products that were effective in specific situations are mentioned for purposes of illustration only. We neither endorse nor promote any particular manufacturer or product, and we emphasize that the prescription, adaptation, and use of ATDs must be performed by a professional, with the input and advocacy of the consumer and/or caregiver. Furthermore, although every effort has been made to provide the most up-to-date information in this book, the reader should be aware that new developments in devices and methodology are made every day. The reader should also know that research and field testing for many products may not be available. Nevertheless, it has been our experience that when the BATS approach outlined in this book is used, it facilitates the making of effective decisions and it encourages the long-term use of AT by the consumer with a disability.

For clarification, several words frequently used by both persons with disabilities and AT professionals need to be defined as they are referred to in this book; *patient, client, consumer, user*, and *caregiver* or *careprovider*. AT services are primarily delivered in nontraditional medical models: therefore, the person who applies or interacts with the equipment is referred to as a user or consumer, not as a patient or client. In some cases, the term *user* denotes a person who interacts with the equipment or receives services, whereas a consumer could be the person or agency that purchases the equipment or services for the person with a disability. In this book, the terms *user* and *consumer* may be used interchangeably. The words *caregiver* and *careprovider* also need clarification. A caregiver is a family member, friend, or attendant who gives "exceptional personal and supportive care" to the person with the disability, whereas a careprovider could be an insurance company, professional, or attendant who provides basic care. In this book, we refer to the caregiver as a member of the rehabilitation team.

The distinction between "high" and "low" technology also varies among disciplines, some even adapting the term *lite* technology to avoid the possibility of value judgments implicit in the word *low*. In this book, low technology is used to describe nonelectronic devices; high technology involves electronic or electric equipment. This simple distinction is made throughout the text, recognizing that some "low-tech" materials are, in fact, very sophisticated.

The BATS is presented in more detail in Chapter 2; that chapter also discusses how AT, as an integral part of the competent practice of rehabilitation, has assumed greater importance in recent years as better technology has become available, as persons with disabilities have demanded it, and finally as the law has come to require it. Chapter 3 discusses how each part of the BATS must be meticulously evaluated to prepare an appropriate assessment of the total system. A sample assessment instrument is included. Chapter 5 gives a basic nontechnical overview of electronics necessary to understand and work with ATDs. Chapter 6 includes a section on switches and a set of switch selection guidelines. The following section includes chapters on how *telecommunications* and *augmentative and alternative communication (AAC) aids* encourage personal interaction in the home, at school, at work, and in the community; how *environmental control units* (ECUs) increase the independence of people with disabilities; how *computers* provide opportunities for people with disabilities to compete in school and in the workplace; and how various *mobility aids* enable the person with a disability to travel and function in society. Section 8 presents an overview of *ergonomics* relevant to home or work site modifications, the prevention and amelioration of *cumulative trauma disorders*, and a brief chapter on *occupational rehabilitation* programs. The chapters in Section 9 deal with service delivery: the manner in which technology can enhance the possibilities for employment and accessible living arrangements for persons with disabilities. Chapter 26 describes a model for service delivery of AT. According to Phillips, "The potential of assistive technology to enhance the functioning and independence of persons with disabilities is well recognized. Although technology has benefitted many people, there are numerous reports of dissatisfaction and disuse of technology."[14] Throughout the book, we stress the important role of the consumer in the application of AT.[15]

It is the intent of this book to present useful and effective approaches to using AT in a rapidly changing world. New information about cumulative trauma disorders, for example, highlights the need for the technology team to keep up to date on research findings. A study suggests that persons using wheelchairs may have a greater disposition to developing upper extremity injuries, including carpal tunnel syndrome.[16] Without proper follow-up, many consumers may suffer needlessly from injuries that result from their use of a wheelchair. We strongly advocate that success can only be reached through cooperation and collaboration of all parties— the person with a disability, the caregiver, and the allied health professional—in each step of the process, from initial screening to assessment, selection, training, implementation, and follow-up.

REFERENCES

1. Radabough MB: Speech at RESNA Conference, Washington, DC, June, 1990

2. Technology-Related Assistance for Individuals with Disabilities Act of 1988. PL 100–407, Title 29, U.S.C. 2201 et seq: U.S. Statutes at Large, 102, 1044–1065, August 19, 1988

3. Technology-Related Assistance for Individuals with Disabilities Act of 1994. PL 103–218, Title 29, U.S.C. 2201 et seq: U.S. Statutes at Large, 108, 50–97, March 9, 1994

4. Americans with Disabilities Act (ADA) of 1990. PL 101–336, Title 42 U.S.C. 12101 et seq: U.S. Statutes at Large, 104, 327–378, July 26, 1990

5. Individuals with Disabilities Education Act (IDEA) of 1990. PL 101–476, Title 20, U.S.C. 1400 et seq: U.S. Statutes at Large, 104, 1103–1151, October 30, 1990

6. Rehabilitation Act of 1973. PL 93–112, Title 29, U.S.C. 701 et seq: U.S. Statutes at Large, 87, 355–394, September 26, 1973

7. Rehabilitation, Comprehensive Services, and Developmental Disabilities Amendments of 1978. PL 95–602, Title 29, U.S.C. 701 et seq: U.S. Statutes at Large, 92, 2955–3017, November 6, 1978

8. Rehabilitation Act Amendments of 1986. PL 99–506, Title 29, U.S.C. 701 et seq: U.S. Statutes at Large, 100, 1807–1846, October 21, 1986

9. Rehabilitation Act Amendments of 1992. PL 102–569, Title 29, U.S.C. 701 et seq: U.S. Statutes at Large, 100, 4344–4488, October 29, 1992

10. Developmental Disabilities Assistance and Bill of Rights Act Amendments of 1987. PL 100–146, Title 42, U.S.C. 6000 et seq: U.S. Statutes at Large, 101, 840–859, October 29, 1987

11. Education for All Handicapped Children Act of 1975. PL 94–142, Title 20, U.S.C. 1401 et seq: U.S. Statutes at Large, 89r, 773–796, August 23, 1977

12. Education of the Handicapped Act Amendments of 1986. PL 99–457, Title 20, U.S.C. 1400 et seq: U.S. Statutes at Large, 100, 1145–1177, October 8, 1986

13. Bain BK: Steps in a problem solving evaluation for assistive technology. AJOT Technology Special Interest Section Newsletter 5(2):1–3, 1995

14. Phillips B: Technology abandonment from the consumer point of view. NARIC Q 3:3–11, 1992

15. Batavia A, Hammer G: Toward the development of consumer-based criteria for the evaluation of assistive devices. J Rehabil Res Dev 27:425, 1990

16. Boninger ML, Robertson RN, Wolff M, Cooper RA: Upper limb nerve entrapments in elite wheelchair racers. Am J Phys Med Rehabil 75(3):170–276, 1996

Rationale for Using Assistive Technology in Rehabilitation

There are many philosophic tenets in the rehabilitation of persons with disabilities. Some of the salient ones include (1) every person is a valuable member of society; (2) persons with disabilities must be recognized for their total capabilities, and they must be active participants in all phases of their rehabilitation; (3) rehabilitation of persons with disabilities is a complex process that can best be accomplished by a collaboration between the interdisciplinary team and the person with a disability and the family or caregivers; (4) environmental conditions must be considered in the rehabilitation process, for they can increase or hinder the functional abilities of persons with disabilities; and (5) adaptive devices can be used to compensate for most impairments and thereby enhance the function and independence of most persons with disabilities.[1–6]

PHILOSOPHY

The philosophy of rehabilitation has evolved from policies of protection and productivity of the "handicapped person" to the focus on rights, advocacy, and empowerment of individuals who happen to have disabilities. This evolution can be demonstrated by comparing the 1947 National Council on Rehabilitation definition, "rehabilitation is the restoration of the handicapped to the fullest physical, mental, social, vocational and economic usefulness of which they are capable," with the 1990 definition of rehabilitation as "a holistic and integrated program of medical, physical, psychosocial, and vocational interventions that empower a [person with a disability] to achieve a personally fulfilling, socially meaningful, and functionally effective interaction with the world."[1]

Rehabilitation that is enhanced by the use of assistive technology (AT) must be based on the generic tenets of rehabilitation. In the Rehabilitation Act as amended, the term *rehabilitation technology* includes assistive technology devices (ATD), AT services, and rehabilitation engineering.[7,8] Members of a rehabilitation team need to be cognizant that ATDs are tools to enable persons with disabilities to reach their goals, ATDs can be used in the total process of delivering rehabilitation services, and frequently, technology devices need to be modified or built by rehabilitation engineers. For any device to be an effective tool in the rehabilitation process, it must be carefully evaluated and monitored considering the consumer's abilities and goals, all the environments in which the device will be used, and the specific task the consumer wants to accomplish.

TECHNOLOGY SYSTEM

I posit that rehabilitation using AT is a process driven by a synergistic system consisting of four integrated and interdependent parts: (1) the person who needs to accomplish a task to maximize his or her function, (2) the task(s) that need to be accomplished, (3) the technological device(s) that will best assist the person to accomplish the task(s), and (4) all the environments in which the person needs to accomplish the task(s). In this book, the Bain Assistive Technology System (BATS) is presented as a means to deliver services to persons with disabilities.[9] Rehabilitation AT can be considered an extension of a person's abilities that enables him or her to live, learn, work, and play with a greater degree of independence and to reach a higher quality of life when all parts of the system work together. This technology system is *synergistic* in that each part is enhanced by the combined interaction of each other part, resulting in the total effect being greater than the effect of each individual part. For example, the human body can be viewed as a synergistic system. When a muscle is overtaxed, the body will compensate by drawing power from the surrounding muscles, which when working together produce the desired effect. Thus in the synergistic BATS, all the elements taken together produce a stronger effect. We can imagine a case in which a severely involved person needs a powered wheelchair and lives on the second floor of a walk-up apartment building. An effective AT means of mobility—a powered wheelchair—prescribed in the clinic is of no value in this case, until a solution is reached that considers the environment in which the AT will be used that addresses the entire mobility problem in relation to the obstacle presented by a flight of stairs.

Chapter 1 defined ATDs and AT services. This chapter discusses the rationale of who can benefit from AT, how they can use ATDs, and why when applied appropriately, both ATDs and AT services can expand the rehabilitation process.

A major principle of a rehabilitative approach is the commitment "to the restoration of the disabled to a life that is purposeful and satisfying, one that allows each individual the opportunity to function ... as a member of society with the capabilities to meet the responsibilities of that society."[3] This should be the intention for using AT.

WHO CAN BENEFIT FROM ASSISTIVE TECHNOLOGY

There are thousands of examples of persons who can benefit from AT, and here are some reasons why.

- Beth is a 5-year-old who is scheduled to enter kindergarten in the fall, but she is unable to communicate verbally with anyone, except through hand and facial gestures.
- Harold was critically injured playing sports in high school, and as a result, both of his legs are paralyzed.
- Burt, a 52-year-old accountant, has hands so badly disabled by arthritis that he has difficulty holding a pen.
- Mrs. Cory lives alone and uses a walker to get around her apartment. Her right hand is virtually nonfunctional.

Today, through the use of ATDs and AT services, these individuals can all reach higher levels of independence and life satisfaction. Their problems can be alleviated or solved by using recently developed ATDs.

- Beth can learn to use an augmentative and alternative communication (AAC) aid so everyone will be able to understand what she wants to say.
- Harold can go to any sporting event in a van adapted for his powered wheelchair.
- Burt can be trained in the use of a personal computer that will allow him to perform accounting tasks and prepare reports with a minimum of physical effort.
- Mrs. Cory can call for assistance or turn on lights or appliances using a special remote control that she carries in her pocket.

HOW ASSISTIVE TECHNOLOGY
CAN ENHANCE CAPABILITIES

Through the use of technological devices, many activities that can improve the quality of life become possible with a minimum amount of learning and physical effort. The use of appropriate AT could afford all persons with disabilities, regardless of age or physical challenge, to have more control over themselves and their environments and to have greater freedom of movement, exploration, and participation alongside their peers at home, school, and work and in the community.[10] ATDs can promote independence and a greater quality of life by

- Increasing safety by enabling a person to remotely turn on lights rather than having to walk or wheel into a dark house
- Using an answering machine rather than risking a fall while attempting to answer the telephone

- Providing a means to summon assistance in case of an emergency
- Reminding a person to take medication or do a medical procedure through preset lights, chimes, bells, or computer signals

Many new technological advances can save time and energy for persons as they prepare for work or school, travel via public or private transportation, interact in modified accessible classrooms and workplaces (including electric doors, adjustable chairs and tables, robots, etc.), move with ease about their environment, and communicate with others by electronic rather than manual means. Furthermore, after a full day of work or school, these persons can relax and enjoy their leisure time by remotely controlling television, video cassette recorder, or radio equipment; playing computer games; socializing on a hands-free phone; or going to special sports or musical events in accessible environments. Each of these activities serves to increase the self-esteem and self-confidence of persons who may do things the same as others or do things a little differently or to enable persons with disabilities to obtain an education or a job, compete in the workplace, participate in community activities, and contribute to society.

SCHOOL

A nonverbal child in school can use an AAC aid to communicate in class and with other children on the playground. If a student with poor manipulative skills is unable to write clearly and quickly, he or she can use a computer to prepare homework assignments and to take tests. Many school environments have been adapted to accommodate wheelchairs, and powered wheelchairs can help a student to be mobile and keep up with peers when changing classes. Modified cars, buses, or vans can enable students who use wheelchairs to attend schools and colleges rather than be isolated in home-based educational programs. Students with visual impairments or learning disabilities can listen to books on tape or computer using special ATDs. Computer databases and the internet can expand the educational, leisure, and research abilities of everyone, including persons with disabilities. Furthermore, with the advances in telecommunications, high school, vocational, and college courses can be learned from home computer access.

WORKPLACE

In the workplace, due to the prolific development of time-saving and cost-efficient devices for the general public, the person with a disability has a vastly expanded potential for employment and job selection. For example, persons with visual or manipulative impairments can use voice-activated computers and telephones; persons with hearing impairments can use telephone amplification or telecommunication devices; persons with physical limitations can use standing wheelchairs or scooters with powered seats that adjust to higher work stations; and the whole area of telecommunication and teleconferencing today makes it possible for people with any disability to work at home rather than cope with inaccessible transportation and work sites.

WHAT MAKES THE SYSTEM EFFECTIVE

The use of devices is only part of the rehabilitation process; the other major factor is the people who render AT services. For AT to be effective, an interdisciplinary team effort is required with the consumer and caregiver(s) as central members in each step of the process. If consumers are to continue to benefit from the devices and services, they must need and want them, participate in their selection, and learn how to use and maintain each device. If the interdisciplinary team members are to be effective, they must

- Carefully evaluate the consumer's abilities and needs
- Be knowledgeable of high- and low-technology solutions
- Analyze the task that is to be accomplished
- Train the consumer in the use and maintenance of all devices in all the various environments in which the consumer will need to use them
- Reevaluate the consumer, the ATD, the environments, and the tasks as changes occur
- Assist in finding and securing funding for the acquisition of ATDs and services
- Locate supplies and professional experts
- Network with rehabilitation professionals and AT users
- Contribute to the quality and development of new devices

The basic reason for using any ATD is to be able to accomplish a task and, when possible, to do so in a more effective and efficient manner. Approaches as to how to accomplish this goal may vary according to the professional background, skills, and aptitudes of the team members, but the process should remain constant for screening the consumer who can benefit from AT, analyzing the tasks to be performed, selecting the most appropriate device, training the consumer in the use and maintenance of the ATD, and following up on the functional use of the device in all environments.

CONCEPTS AND PRINCIPLES

The rationale for using an ATD to enhance a consumer's function is based on several concepts and principles. For example, occupational therapists work with what are known as "frames of reference." These are guidelines for practice that provide directions for assisting individuals in problem identification and problem remediation in relation to a specified element of the profession's domain of concern.[11] In working with a person with a disability, an occupational therapist may use a rehabilitation and/or a biomechanical frame of reference. The biomechanical frame of reference is the therapeutic base for using a powered scooter when traveling long distances, for using a remote control device to activate appliances, and for using a computer. By reducing the energy expended for these activities, consumers can increase their endurance for other activities of daily living and/or leisure activities. When consumers use AT to increase their function, they also conserve the energy of the caregiver.

The rationale for intervention in the rehabilitative frame of reference is to "compensate for disability by learning to live with one's capabilities in all aspects of life, adapt the environment to obtain independence."[4] The biomechanical frame of reference seeks to "reduce deficits through a direct cause and effect treatment process—exercise and activity."[4] For example, a person who has a spinal cord injury with minimal manipulative skill may need an environmental control unit (ECU) to operate the phone or turn on lights, may need a powered wheelchair to become mobile, may learn to use a computer for written communication or a possible vocational goal, and may need adaptations in their home, school, and work environments. Additionally, the therapeutic process may include many other purposeful activities and an exercise program.

In the area of technology rehabilitation practice, it is my opinion that the theoretical foundation is based on

1. The rehabilitative approach of compensation and accommodation of each part of the AT system
2. The biomechanical model; specifically, the work simplification/energy conservation principle
3. Theories of learning and motivation
4. The acquisitional frame of reference[12]

To increase the user's functional manipulative abilities based on the rehabilitation principles of compensation, a mouthstick or wrist cuff could be used or a computer and/or ECU could be used. Accommodation could include raising desk and table legs with blocks to accommodate the height of a wheelchair, or an ergonomically designed work station or robot could be used. Ramps, kneeling buses, and electric door openers can be used to accommodate persons who need to use wheelchairs at home, school, or work. Mrs. Cory can increase her functional abilities and independence by modifying the way she performs a task, the environment in which she needs to do the task, and the ATDs that can be used to assist in the accomplishment of the task. To illustrate, she can use a microwave oven placed on a low counter to prepare her meals. She can change her infrequently used dining room into a bedroom, eliminating the need to climb the stairs. And finally, she can use an emergency call button or an ECU for assistance.

The biomechanical principle of work simplification/energy conservation can apply in Burt's case. He can be taught to save himself the stress and long hours of grasping a pencil or pen by using instead the numerical keypad and accounting software in a personal computer. The adapted computer will then also simplify the writing of reports as he uses it for word processing. The major learning theories include classical conditioning, operant conditioning, and social imitational conditioning. For example, when teaching a person to use an ATD, the therapist may use one learning theory or a combination, such as when an AAC aid is prescribed for a nonverbal person who then randomly presses various keys. If that person accidently strikes a useful key and hears the device speak the word *music* and if the person strikes the key again and the response is repeated, the person has learned through operant conditioning that pressing a designated key gives a definite response. That person can further learn, through operant conditioning "shaping," to strike a series of keys (receiving positive reinforcement each time), learning to express the desire to hear music, as the synthesized voice says, "I want to hear the radio." Furthermore, this person may learn through social imitation that the preferred way to ask for anything is to use the AAC aid, rather than pounding on the table or making grunting noises. All these learning models can help Beth in kindergarten, where she can use an AAC aid to convey the important messages locked in her head that she was unable to communicate through speech.

In Harold's case, the acquisitional frame of reference provides an example of theoretical background relevant to technology. The acquisitional frame of reference "provides a structure for linking learning theories, the reality aspect of purposeful activities, and the process of acquiring specific skills needed for successful interaction in the environment."[12] Devices such as "stove minders" that signal when a pot is boiling or automatically turn off the stove at a preset time can be considered adaptive equipment or "low technology." Environmental modifications include advances in tool design, such as electric door openers, adapted one-hand computer keyboards and wrist rests, and electric lifts for powered scooters or wheelchairs. Harold can learn to interact successfully in his environment by learning to use a powered wheelchair and an adapted van to solve his mobility problem. Additionally, technology can enhance Harold's quality of life if he is able to learn to use a computer in preparation for possible employment.

SUMMARY

This chapter has presented major philosophic tenets of rehabilitation and has cited examples of *how* and *why* AT, when applied appropriately, can definitely enhance the process. An effective means to gain this objective is to use the BATS, a holistic synergistic system for evaluating consumers, technology, and the environments in which a task will be performed. Persons with disabilities can benefit physically, psychosocially, and vocationally when they are contributing members of the interdisciplinary rehabilitation team. The objectives of using AT must be based on sound concepts and principles that include accommodation and compensation solutions, energy conservation methods, and learning theories. However, we must also be cognizant that technology is not the "be all and end all" of rehabilitation. Additionally, complicated high technology is not always the only and the best solution but frequently can be used in conjunction with simple "low-tech" adaptive aids. Furthermore, the ATD used for one person may not be the best for another person with a similar problem; each person, each task, every environment, and various devices must be evaluated and reevaluated over time. Most assistive devices are not luxuries but rather are necessary equipment that assist individuals to function more independently, increase their self-esteem, improve their quality of life, and foster their participation in all aspects of society.

REFERENCES

1. Banja JD: Rehabilitation and empowerment. Arch Phy Med Rehabil 71:614–615, 1990

2. Dutton R, Levy L, Simon C: Current basis for theory and philosophy of occupational therapy. pp. 58–91. In Hopkins H, Smith H (eds): Willard and Spackman's Occupational Therapy. 8th Ed. Lippincott-Raven, Philadelphia, 1993

3. Licht S: Rehabilitation and Medicine. Waverly Press, Baltimore, 1968

4. Pedretti LW: Occupational Therapy Practice Skills for Physical Dysfunction. 3rd Ed. CV Mosby, St. Louis, 1990

5. Trombly CA (ed): Occupational Therapy for Physical Dysfunction. 3rd Ed. Williams & Wilkins, Baltimore, 1989

6. Wright B: Physical Disabilities: A Psychological Approach. 2nd Ed. Harper & Row, New York, 1983

7. Rehabilitation Act Amendments of 1986. PL 99–506, Title 29, U.S.C. 701 et seq: U.S. Statutes at Large, 100, 1807–1846, October 21, 1986

8. Rehabilitation Act Amendments of 1992. PL 102–569, Title 29, U.S.C. 701 et seq: U.S. Statutes at Large, 100, 4344–4488, October 29, 1992

9. Bain BK: Steps in a problem solving evaluation for assistive technology. AJOT Technology Special Interest Section Newsletter. 5(2):1–3, 1995

10. Rubin SE, Roessler RT: Foundations of the Vocational Rehabilitation Process. (3rd Ed.) PRO-ED, Austin, TX, 1987

11. Mosey AC: Applied Scientific Inquiry in the Health Professions: An Epistemological Orientation. 2nd Ed. American Occupational Therapy Association, Rockville, MD, 1996

12. Mosey AC: Psychological Components of Occupational Therapy. Lippincott-Raven, Philadelphia, 1986

CHAPTER 3

Evaluation

Robert lies motionless while two paramedics evaluate his vital signs in preparation for transferring him to an acute hospital where he will be further examined and evaluated by medical personnel to determine the extent of the injuries sustained in an automobile accident just a few minutes before. These evaluations will be the beginning of many evaluations Robert will receive in the next few years as he progresses from an acute hospital, to a rehabilitation center, to a prevocational/vocational or educational program, and finally to a job interview. Some of the assistive technology (AT) evaluations he might receive within the first few days could be a respiration evaluation to determine if he needs a ventilator and a switch activation method to call for assistance. Once he has been medically stabilized in the acute hospital, Robert could be evaluated for a simple environmental control system that would enable him to control his bed position, use the telephone, and turn on his television or radio. After a month, barring any complications, he may be transferred to a rehabilitation center where he could have several evaluations for AT, including a powered wheelchair, seating and positioning, a more complex environmental control system, computer access, prevocational exploration, and home accessibility. Once he is discharged from the rehabilitation center, he may receive additional AT evaluations in driver training, computer skills, and/or vocational exploration. All these evaluations could be performed by interdisciplinary team members in different environments to assist Robert in tasks he will need to accomplish to live a productive independent life and eventually return to work or school.

With the proliferation of available assistive technology devices (ATDs), it is now necessary to systematically consider possible options to determine which will best meet a consumer's needs and abilities. Recent advances in the integration of access systems require a holistic problem-solving approach when selecting any one device. In today's "high-tech" world, many powered wheelchair systems can be integrated with environmental control units (ECUs), augmentative and alternative communication (AAC) aids, and computers. Because the cost of devices and the fees for professional services are escalating, both "high" and "low" technology devices must be carefully evaluated by the consumer, professionals, and third-party payors. In most cases, a device is purchased only once and may cost thousands of dollars. The "trial-and-error" method is fatiguing for the user and time-consuming for the professional. It is, therefore, prudent for the rehabilitation team, before recommending the purchase of any device, to thoroughly evaluate each part of the system according to the Bain Assistive Technology System, considering (1) the user's needs and abilities, (2) the tasks he or she wishes to accomplish, (3) all possible environments in which the consumer will use the ATDs, and (4) a variety of possible devices that can successfully perform the desired task(s). Too often, the user is forced to accommodate to the technology rather than vice versa, because a partial evaluation was performed or no evaluation was done before the selection of the ATDs.

An evaluation is not valid without the full cooperation and participation of the consumer for whom the device is intended. Members of the rehabilitation team must be cognizant of the following:

1. The valuable contributions that the consumer and caregiver have to offer to the assessment process
2. If the assistive device is to be used to its full potential for as long as the consumer can benefit from using it, then the consumer MUST have a major role in the process
3. Assessment is a continual process that requires changes to meet the changing needs and abilities of the consumer, changes in the environment, and changes in ATDs

Research cited elsewhere in this chapter illustrates the significance of these factors.[1]

This chapter presents some guidelines for a systematic and complete assessment, then specific seating and positioning criteria are outlined in Chapter 4. Appendix 3-1 includes an assessment instrument I have developed,[2] and Appendix 3-2 and 3-3 include samples of two other assessment forms.[3,4]

DEFINITIONS

An evaluation refers to a composite picture of the technology system, and an assessment refers to the instrument or means of gathering data from specific testing procedures. An evaluation is the sum of the results of all assessment procedures, such as (1) review of medical, work, and social records; (2) interviews with the consumer and caregiver(s); (3) observations of the consumer performing various activities and observations of various methods of performing the same tasks by other individuals; (4) evaluations and testing with standard and nonstandardized instruments; and (5) checklists or inventories. The Minnesota Rate of Manipulation Test (American Guidance Service, Circle Pines, MN) is a standardized test that can be used to assess visual-motor perception as part of the evaluation of a consumer's ability to use a computer. The consumer's computer ability might also be assessed by using a nonstandardized performance test (e.g., having the consumer actually perform the task of word processing at a computer). Checklists or inventories are usually paper-and-pencil tests; however, several computerized inventories are being developed. In addition, a computerized assessment instrument is available to evaluate consumer performance in activities of daily living, including work performance.[5] There are two general AT assessments,[3,4] but it is more common to use separate evaluations for different purposes. For example, there are evaluations for positioning, powered wheelchairs, driver training, augmentative communication devices,[6] ECUs,[7] occupational rehabilitation, and computers.[8]

WHO SHOULD PERFORM THE ASSESSMENT?

A comprehensive assessment should be carried out by a variety of team members to ensure its objectivity and authenticity. Evaluations should be administered by qualified members of the team who have professional qualifications or by consulting specialists. Some professional organizations are requiring competency examinations for certification as a specialist in technology. In some cases, a complicated seating and positioning evaluation requires a professional with expertise in seating and positioning, and the team may request the assistance of a consultant. Many teams may not be fortunate enough to include a full-time ergonomist whose services would enhance the adaptation of a work environment; therefore when a technical need arises, one is consulted. Other examples might be in cases in which an individual has multiple disabilities, such as hearing or visual impairment complicated by physical disabilities. Because this area of rehabilitation is so complex, it is essential that the team constantly network with consultants in a variety of fields, including biomedical, electrical, or mechanical engineers; computer hardware and software developers; and "garage geniuses" who have developed many practical devices.

The composition of the assessment team will vary according to such factors as the service delivery system (e.g., public or private institutions), consumer's needs and abilities, geographic location, funding, and support systems that are available. Most teams will include the consumer and caregivers; a physician who may need to authorize the assessment services and purchase of equipment; occupational therapists and/or physical therapists who may perform many sensorimotor, physical, psychosocial, and cognitive evaluations; rehabilitation counselors who will assess the job and match the consumer abilities; insurance case workers who might follow the consumer through each step in the rehabilitation process; rehabilitation engineers who may develop or customize equipment; language or speech pathologists; social workers who may need to find funding and work with the caregivers; and vendors who are knowledgeable about equipment. Other team members might include special educators, mobility trainers, computer experts, psychiatrists, and driving trainers.

Frequently, one professional may be responsible for two or more areas. For example, an occupational therapist may assess the consumer to determine the best control site to use for accessing a switch, then work with a physical therapist and vendor to assess the appropriate wheelchair, and then assess the workplace with a vocational counselor. Because the development of rehabilitation technology teams has emerged so recently, many professionals were not educated in this specialized area; however, in the past five years there has been a noticeable increase in the number of workshops, seminars, conferences, and in-service training courses available to consumers and professionals. According to a survey of 100 randomly selected spinal cord injury treatment centers certified by the Commission on Accreditation of Rehabilitation Facilities, a diverse group of health care professionals are involved in the assessment of AT for this population (Fig. 3-1).[9]

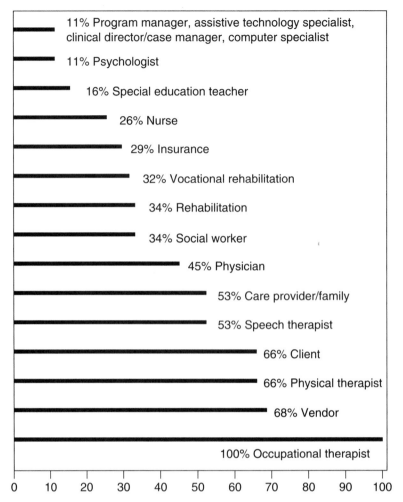

Figure 3-1. Results of a survey of 100 randomly selected spinal cord injury treatment centers certified by the Commission on Accreditation of Rehabilitation Facilities, showing percentage of team members who participated in assessing consumers for ATDs.

WHAT IS THE PURPOSE OF A SYSTEMATIC EVALUATION?

Before the selection of the appropriate device(s) for a person with a disability to use in many environments to accomplish many tasks, a systematic evaluation MUST be completed by the technology rehabilitation team that focuses on the consumer's needs and abilities. With the rapid advances in technology, there is an ever-growing number of devices available; some are complex and expensive, some are simple and off-the-shelf, but no one device is best for every individual, nor will every person who has a particular physical disability need the same equipment. Each part of the system MUST be assessed by a cooperative and collaborative team. Some basic reasons for completing a systematic assessment include

- To identify the needs, goals, and desires of the consumer
- To identify the problem areas and prioritize the primary and secondary areas
- To evaluate the functional abilities of the consumer
- To evaluate various devices for function, availability, safety, and affordability
- To determine the environments in which each device will be used
- To determine what funding is available
- To establish a baseline for monitoring the rehabilitation plan
- To create a schedule for equipment maintenance by qualified service personnel
- To ensure that all areas of the system are constantly being reevaluated and records are kept

A systemic problem-solving approach should increase the possibility that all parts of the technology system are considered, and it has been my experience that this is necessary to increase the likelihood that the device will be fully used. In the survey of facilities for individuals with spinal cord injuries, over 24 specific areas were considered in the assessment for AT (Fig. 3-2). Other results from this survey indicated that 63 percent of the respondents included the consumer as part of the assessment team and 49 percent indicated that caregivers and/or family members were also included.[9]

STEPS IN A PROBLEM-SOLVING APPROACH TO EVALUATION

To facilitate the assessment process, I have developed the following nine steps[10] that should be followed in the given sequence when possible. However, steps may need to be modified according to the service delivery system; the qualifications and availability of the rehabilitation technology team members; and the medical, social, and/or employment status of the consumer. See Table 3-1 for details.

STEP 1

IDENTIFICATION OF THE TASKS

▶ The first step involves the identification of the tasks that the consumer wishes to accomplish, such as manipulation, communication, and mobility. This information is gathered by an occupational therapist who interviews the consumer, family members, and caregivers, then reviews the records and observes the consumer as he or she performs various functional activities. Other individuals who may collaborate with the consumer, caregiver, and occupational therapist may be physical therapists, rehabilitation engineers, and speech therapists.

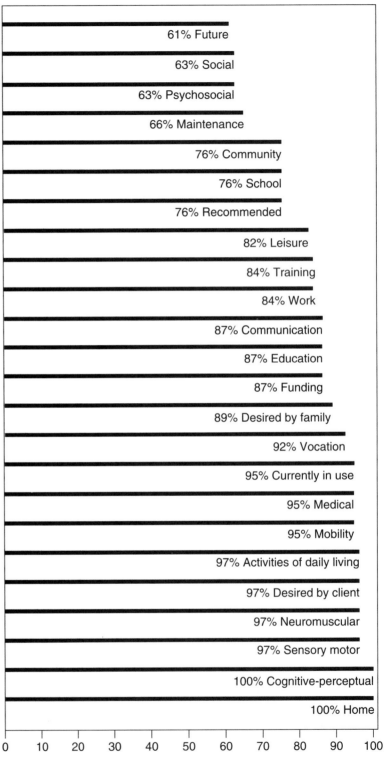

Figure 3-2. Twenty-four specific areas considered by health care professionals in the assessment protocol for AT.

Table 3-1. Steps in a Problem-Solving Approach to the Assessment of Consumers for Assistive Technology Devices (ATDs)

Steps	Part of System	Problem	Action

1	Task	Identify the tasks the consumer needs to accomplish with the ATD
		  Communication
		  Mobility
		  Environmental controls
		  Computer adaptation
		  Switch interface
			Review records
			
			Interview consumers, caretakers, and family
			
			Observation

2	Consumer/user	Identify the consumer's abilities in lying, sitting, and standing positions	Formal testing
			  Motor
			  Manual muscle testing, reflexes, range of motion
			  Coordination
			  Endurance
			  Sensory
			  Psychosocial
			  Cognitive
			  Social
			Interview
			Observation

3	ATD	Based on steps 1 and 2, identify possible devices	Characteristics
			  Input, processing, output, display
			  Commercial availability
			  Safety and reliability
			  Practicality
			  Affordability

4	Environment	Present and future:
		  Bed/chair
		  Home
		  School/work
		  Community
			Interview
			Observation
			On-site visits

5	All	Trial period	Try various devices in a variety of environments
6	ATD	Selection	Order, adapt, or fabricate
7	Consumer/user	Application	Train in use and maintenance
8	All	Documentation	Record in all intra- and interdepartmental files
9	All	Reevaluation	Periodically consumer, ATD, environment, and task(s)

STEP 2

IDENTIFICATION OF THE CONSUMER'S ABILITIES

▶ One of the first areas to be evaluated MUST be the consumer's seating and positioning. Creating a dynamic seating environment is critical to the successful application of any technologic device. It is necessary to evaluate the consumer in various positions (lying, sitting, and standing) in which the task(s) are likely to be performed. The occupational therapist must also evaluate the physical, psychosocial, and cognitive abilities of the consumer. This is accomplished using standard and nonstandard motor tests, manual muscle testing, active range of motion, coordination, endurance, reflexes, and sensorimotor integration. Nontraditional access methods may be considered, including use of the head, tongue, or breath to control the ATD. Psychosocial factors must be taken into consideration as well, to ensure the future acceptance and use of the ATD. Cognitive abilities—following directions, sequencing, comprehending output—should be considered, especially for computers and AAC aids. The therapist may need to observe the client in other settings, such as work, home, or school, to assess the physical environment and the manner in which the consumer interacts in different settings with different people (e.g., peers, therapists, teachers).

STEP 3

IDENTIFICATION OF POSSIBLE ASSISTIVE TECHNOLOGY DEVICES

▶ The team should determine what ATD(s) would be appropriate based on the consumer's needs, goals, and abilities, considering (1) the input method, or how the device will be activated; (2) the processing, or how the device will process information from the switch; (3) the output, or what results are needed; and (4) the feedback, or display that informs the user that the device is operating and that the task is in progress. There are many kinds of input devices (switches), output, and feedback. For example, the various types of switches or input devices include infrared, sonic (voice or ultrasound), radio frequency, and electronic. Some methods of input can be combined, and different switches can be used in different environments. Switches are discussed in greater detail in Chapter 6. The output or results of switch activation can include everything from moving a powered wheelchair to illuminating a light bulb. Some alternative kinds of feedback can be present as well. Feedback is usually auditory, visual, or proprioceptive, and the therapist must take care to consider the functional abilities and needs of the individual consumer.

STEP 4

IDENTIFICATION OF ALL PRESENT AND FUTURE ENVIRONMENTS

▶ It is important to consider all the environment(s) in which the AT will be used. Some devices (e.g., ECUs and AAC aids) will be used in bed, in a wheelchair, in school or the workplace, and in the community. Architectural and electronic barriers should be taken into consideration when evaluating any ATD, and two factors must be considered: changes in the physical climate (weather, noise, light) and changes in the psychosocial climate (family and community acceptance of the ATD). The technology team should work with all other health professionals and caregivers while assessing the physical and psychosocial environment of the consumer. Note that steps 3 and 4 can be reversed, as some therapists prefer to evaluate the environment before looking at ATDs.

STEP 5

EVALUATION OF THE INTERFACE BETWEEN THE CONSUMER AND THE ATD

▶ Based on the evaluations of the task, the consumer, the ATD(s), and the environments, various ATDs should be tried by the consumer. The technology team can start with off-the-shelf equipment and progress to specialty devices as required for the consumer to perform the desired task. (Most vendors and manufacturers of ATDs will lend equipment to rehabilitation teams on a trial basis.) For the technology system to enhance the abilities of the consumer, it must be integrated with all other equipment that is used by the consumer, in all possible environments in which the desired task is to be performed. The technology team must carefully scrutinize the written materials and the ATD itself and network with other therapists, consumers, and vendors to make the best choice for the needs of this consumer. This is a time-consuming process but one that will guarantee that the client's abilities will increase, that the devices will be used, and that the system is cost-effective.

STEP 6

SELECTION OF ATD BY ALL TEAM MEMBERS
▶ After completing all the above steps, and in particular achieving a good match between the consumer and an ATD, the technology team should confer and make a final decision about the selection and acquisition of an ATD. Determine where the ATD can be obtained or if it will need to be adapted or if it will need to be fabricated. (Be sure that the supplier and/or manufacturer is well established and will provide maintenance.) Remember, if a commercial ATD is altered in any way, its warranty is no longer valid.

STEP 7

TRAINING THE CONSUMER TO USE AND MAINTAIN THE ATD
▶ Determine who will train the consumer to use and care for the ATD and how much time will be required for training. (Too often funding for equipment is available but no funding has been allocated for training services.) Frequently, a consumer is given a piece of equipment without any written instructions on its care, maintenance, or contact person in the event of a problem.

STEP 8

DOCUMENTATION OF THE EVALUATION PROCESS
▶ After completing a comprehensive evaluation, a written report should be prepared and distributed to the consumer, the caregiver, the third-party payor, and the rehabilitation team files. The team should document each step of the assessment in all intra- and interdepartmental files. (Photographs or videos are also a valuable means of documentation.)

STEP 9

PERIODIC REEVALUATION OF ALL PARTS OF THE AT SYSTEM
▶ Aside from the usual wear and tear of regular use, changes can occur at many levels of the AT system, prompting the need for periodic reevaluation. The needs and abilities of the consumer may also change, as can the environments in which the ATD is used (from school-based to the workplace). And finally, new advances in technology occur daily, resulting in smaller, less expensive, and more advanced equipment to accomplish certain functions. For example, the power and features of personal computers have grown immensely in the past 10 years, whereas the price and size of the same has diminished exponentially. Periodic reevaluation of the AT needs of the consumer is a must.

CONCLUSION

At times, the evaluation process may need to be changed. Steps can be abbreviated (but never omitted) because of time constraints, the demands of the service delivery system, or the shortage or lack of knowledgeable personnel. A successful result—increasing the functional abilities, independence, and quality of life of the consumer—depends on the performance of a complete and careful evaluation. The best results come with the application of a thorough AT evaluation that takes into consideration the synergistic relationship between the four elements of the system: the consumer, the task, the environment, and the device.

REFERENCES

1. Phillips B: Technology abandonment from the consumer point of view. NARIC Q 3:3–11, 1992

2. Bain BK: The assessment of clients for technological assistive devices. pp. 55–59. In: American Occupational Therapy Association: Technology Review '89: Perspectives on Occupational Therapy Practice. American Occupational Therapy Association, Rockville, MD, 1989

3. Scherer MJ: Matching Person and Technology (MPT) model and assessment instruments. In: Assistive Technology Device Predisposition Assessment. Author, Rochester, NY, 1991

4. Williams BW, Stemack G, Wolfe S, Stanger C: Lifespace Access Profile: Assistive Technology Planning for Individuals with Severe or Multiple Disabilities. Author, Sebastopol, CA, 1993

5. Smith R: OT Fact (software). American Occupational Therapy Association, Rockville, MD, 1990

6. Fishman I: Electronic Communication Aids. College-Hill Press, Boston, 1987

7. Bain BK: Technology. pp. 333–337. In Hopkins H, Smith H (eds): Willard and Spackman's Occupational Therapy. 8th Ed. Lippincott-Raven, Philadelphia, 1993

8. Anson D: Finding your way in the maze of computer access technology. Am Occup Ther 48(2):121–129, 1994

9. Bain BK, Block L, Strehlow A: Survey report on the assessment of individuals with spinal cord injuries for assistive technology. Technol Disability 5:289–294, 1996

10. Bain BK: Steps in a problem solving evaluation for assistive technology. AJOT Technology Special Interest Section Newsletter. 5(2):1–3, 1995

SUGGESTED READINGS

American Occupational Therapy Association: Position paper: occupational therapy and assistive technology. Am J Occup Ther 45:1076, 1991

Angelo J, Smith RO: The critical role of occupational therapy in augmentative communication services. pp. 49–54. In: American Occupational Therapy

Association: Technology Review '89: Perspectives on Occupational Therapy Practice. AOTA, Rockville, MD, 1989

Batavia A, Hammer G: Toward the development of consumer-based criteria for the evaluation of assistive devices. J Rehabil Res Dev 27:425–435, 1990

Enders A, Hall M: Assistive Technology Sourcebook. RESNA Press, Washington, DC, 1990

Hammel JM, Van der Loos M: A vocational assessment model for use of robotics technology. pp. 327–328. In: Proceedings of the 13th Annual RESNA Conference, Washington, DC, 1990

Lee K, Thomas DJ: Control of Computer-Based Technology for People with Physical Disabilities: An Assessment Manual. University of Toronto Press, Toronto, Ontario, 1989

Mann WC, Lane JP: Assistive Technology for Persons with Disabilities. 2nd Ed. American Occupational Therapy Association, Rockville, MD, 1995

Smith R: Technological approaches to performance enhancement. pp. 747–785. In Christiansen C, Baum C (eds): Occupational Therapy: Improving Human Performance Deficits. Slack, Thorofare, NJ, 1991

Van Laere M, Duyvejonck R: Environmental control and social integration of a high-lesion tetraplegic patient: case report. Paraplegia 24:322–325, 1986

*Assistive Technology Devices Assessment**

Instructions: Please complete all sections using this key:
NA = non-applicable; X = denotes problem area;
WFL = within functional limits; WNL = within normal limits.
WE = With Equipment
NFE = Needs further evaluation

BACKGROUND INFORMATION

Name _____ Date _____ Age ___ Sex ___ Phone _____

Height ___ Weight ___ Diagnosis _____

Major functional problem areas: Communication ____ Mobility ____ Computers _____

  Environmental control ____ Other _____

Associated problems: Seizures ____ Vision ____ Hearing ____ Respiration _____

  Other _____

Rehab members working with client: O.T. ____ Rehab Counselor ____ P.T. _____

  Speech/ Language Pathologists _____ Rehab Engineers _____ Psychologists _____

  Others _____

Vocational/ Educational levels _____

Avocational interests: _____

Consumer's goals: _____

ENVIRONMENTS (living and/ or working):

PRESENT: In patient ____ Out-patient ____ Day program ____ Rehab center _____

  Apartment ____ House ____ Group home ____ School ____ Work _____

PROJECTED Living: _____

  Projected School/ Work: _____

HUMAN RESOURCES IN PROJECTED ENVIRONMENT:

  Attendant _____ Number of hours per day _____ Services required _____

  _____

  Family ____ Relationship/Ages _____

  Services Required _____

  Homemaker services _____ Number of hours per day _____ Services required _____

  _____

*Copyright 1989 BK Bain. Revised 1995.

EVALUATIONS:

PHYSICAL/ MOTOR

Bed Position: WNL _____ WFL _____ Poor _____

Sitting tolerance: hours per day: in bed _____ in wheelchair _____

Sitting balance: (no support) Good _____ Fair _____ Poor _____

(with support) WNL _____ WFL _____ Poor _____

Type of support _____

Functional motions key: WNL--WFL--Poor--No function

	STRENGTH		ROM		ENDURANCE	COORDINATION	
	R	L	R	L	(TIME)	GROSS	FINE
HEAD							
EYES							
NECK							
TONGUE							
SHOULDER							
ELBOW							
FOREARM							
WRIST							
HAND							
THUMB							
KNEE							
FOOT							

MUSCLE TONE _____

_____

OPTIMAL BODY PART and motion for control/ accessing equipment (two or more).

1. _____ 2. _____

MOTIVATION to use adaptive devices for: (High-Moderate-Low)

Communication _____ Mobility _____ Environmental controls _____

Computers _____ Play/ Leisure _____ Educational _____ Vocational _____

Other _____

PERCEPTION: (WNL - WFL - NFE - NA)

Visual _____ Auditory _____ Spatial Relations _____

Lateral Neglect _____ Touch _____ Other _____

Specify Equipment Needs _____

COGNITIVE: (WNL - WFL - NFE - NA)

Attention _____ Sequencing _____ Memory _____

Long Term _____ Short Term _____

Other _____

SOCIAL INTERACTION: (High--Moderate-Low)

Peers _____ Staff _____ Family _____ Others _____

| **ASSISTIVE TECHNOLOGY DEVICES CURRENTLY IN USE** |

Be specific. List by name and supplier

Communications _____

Environmental control systems _____

Mobility _____

Computer _____

Other _____

| **PROPOSED PLAN** |

1. What assistive technology devices does the consumer believe he/ she needs?

2. What does the rehab team recommend for the consumer's immediate needs?

3. What are the family's/agencies' long-term plans for this consumer?

4. The evaluators' recommendations to include:

-effectiveness_____

- portability _____

- integration with other devices _____

-precautions in using equipment _____

- training required_____

-available funding _____

- comments _____

_____

_____

_____

What further evaluations are needed: _____

_____

_____

_____

Evaluator _____ Date _____

Scherer Assessment Form*

FORM A: Use Once Per Person

THE ASSISTIVE TECHNOLOGY DEVICE PREDISPOSITION ASSESSMENT - C

Name_____   Date_____

Desired Outcome(s) _____

1. How are your current capabilities in the following areas? Circle the best response for each.

		Good		Average		Poor
a.	Vision	5	4	3	2	1
b.	Hearing	5	4	3	2	1
c.	Speech	5	4	3	2	1
d.	Upper extremity control	5	4	3	2	1
e.	Lower extremity control	5	4	3	2	1
f.	Mobility	5	4	3	2	1
g.	Dexterity	5	4	3	2	1
h.	Learning speed	5	4	3	2	1
i.	Physical strength / stamina	5	4	3	2	1

Put a minus sign (-) beside any of the above that you believe are or will be deteriorating over time.
Then put a plus sign (+) beside any you believe are or will be improving over time.

2. How satisfied are you with what you have achieved in the following areas? Please circle the best response for each.

		Very Satisfied		Satisfied		Not Satisfied
a.	Independent living skills / activities of daily living	5	4	3	2	1
b.	Communication skills	5	4	3	2	1
c.	Physical comfort and well-being	5	4	3	2	1
d.	Overall health	5	4	3	2	1
e.	Social and recreational involvement	5	4	3	2	1
f.	Ability to go where desired	5	4	3	2	1
g.	Educational attainment	5	4	3	2	1
h.	Employment status / potential	5	4	3	2	1
i.	Emotional well-being	5	4	3	2	1

Put a plus sign (+) beside the one(s) you most want to improve over time.

3. How do you feel about your disability?

		Strongly Agree		Neutral		Strongly Disagree
a.	It limits what I want to do.	5	4	3	2	1
b.	My life would be different if I didn't have my disability.	5	4	3	2	1

(Form continues.)

*Copyright 1991 M.J. Scherer and B.G. McKee. Revised 1993, 1994.

(continued)

4. Please check all the statements below that describe you.

❑ encouraged by family	❑ have little privacy	❑ encouraged by friends
❑ encouraged by therapists	❑ curious and excited about new things	❑ am cooperative
❑ find technology interesting	❑ am self-disciplined	❑ prefer a quiet life
❑ am a calm person	❑ want / need to go to school or work	❑ often feel isolated and alone
❑ feel insecure	❑ am patient and easy going	❑ have many things I want to accomplish
❑ am often discouraged	❑ do what my therapist(s) tell me to do	❑ not sure who I am now
❑ am satisfied with my life	❑ am resourceful	❑ want more independence
❑ like to be alone	❑ like having a challenge	❑ have a good self image
❑ am often angry	❑ have made friends with my therapist(s)	❑ feel the general public accepts me
❑ am often depressed	❑ am responsible and reliable	❑ believe my therapist(s) knows what is best for me
❑ accomplish what I set out to do	❑ often feel frustrated	❑ am determined to meet my goals

FORM B: Use For Each Technology

THE ASSISTIVE TECHNOLOGY DEVICE PREDISPOSITION ASSESSMENT - C

Name_____   Date_____

Device / System _____

	This definitely applies to me		This is neutral for me		This does not apply to me
1. I can use this device with little or no assistance from others	5	4	3	2	1
2. I have the funding to get this device	5	4	3	2	1
3. I will benefit from using this device	5	4	3	2	1
4. This device will help me achieve a goal I have	5	4	3	2	1
5. I will feel proud using this device around my family	5	4	3	2	1
6. I will feel proud using this device around my friends	5	4	3	2	1
7. I will feel proud using this device at school or work	5	4	3	2	1
8. I will feel proud using this device out in public	5	4	3	2	1
9. This device will improve my quality of life	5	4	3	2	1
10. This device will *not* change how I usually go about doing things	5	4	3	2	1

Totals: A _____   T _____   D _____   PA _____

Lifespace Access Profile Excerpts*

Name _____

Birth Date _____ Age _____   Date _____

Current Service Sites:

Home _____   Community _____

School _____   Therapy _____

Work _____   Other _____

Assessment and Planning Team

List parents, care and service providers.

Check the box beside each person providing input into this assessment.

❑ Parents_____   ❑ Teacher/Trainer_____

❑ Care Providers_____   ❑ Teaching Assistant _____

❑ Siblings/Relatives_____   ❑ Development Spec._____

❑ Speech & Lang Spec._____   ❑ Psychologist _____

❑ Occupational 'Ther._____   ❑ Vision Hand Spec._____

❑ Physical Therapist_____   ❑ Deaf/H.O.H. Spec._____

❑ Adapt P. E. Spec._____   ❑ Nurse_____

❑ Recreational Ther. _____   ❑ Physician _____

❑ Dev. Scr. Case Coord. _____   ❑ Technology Specialist _____

❑ Social Worker_____   ❑ Vocational Specialist _____

❑ Behavior Specialist _____   ❑ _____

Team Coordinator _____

Was the individual included as an active   ❑ Yes
member of the Assessment and Planning Team?   ❑ No

> **Note:** Refer to the *Lifespace Access Profile* manual for detailed instructions
> on completing each section of this protocol.

Assessment and Program Planning Questions and Goals

1. What do team members want to learn from this assessment? What questions do team members have about the person's resources, abilities, and needs?

SWITCH ACCESS SITES

Primary Switch Access Site
Circle the body site the person can control and use most easily.
Indicate the person's work space and range of motion for this site.

Secondary Switch Access Site
Circle the body site which may provide secondary switch access.
Indicate the person's work space and range of motion for this site.

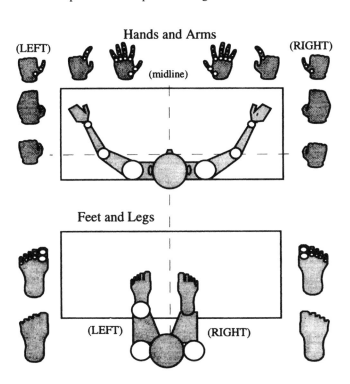

Hands and Arms

(LEFT)   (midline)   (RIGHT)

Feet and Legs

(LEFT)   (RIGHT)

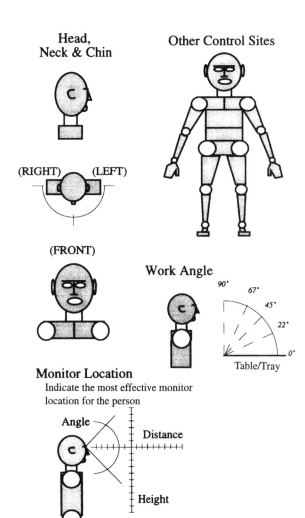

Head,
Neck & Chin

Other Control Sites

(RIGHT)   (LEFT)

(FRONT)

Work Angle

90° 67° 45° 22° 0°

Table/Tray

Monitor Location
Indicate the most effective monitor
location for the person

Angle

Distance

Height

CHAPTER 4

Assessment for the Seated Environment

Over the years, a great deal of research and experimentation has been done regarding the manner by which individuals interface with their work at home, in the school, or in the workplace.[1,2] Studies have centered on room temperature, lighting, chairs, and working surfaces. An entire industry has emerged as ergonomists and designers create better environments for workers, hoping for maximum performance with minimum work-related disability. Chairs that provide proper back support, work surfaces that minimize fatigue, and computer keyboards designed to minimize stress injuries are only a few examples of the technology offered to able-bodied workers.[3] Students, workers, and persons with disabilities have a great need for proper work environments. Chairs and working surfaces that are not properly designed for the user can rob a disabled person of function and possibly interfere with his or her ability to learn and become gainfully employed. Many consumers with disabilities require some type of enabling technology (simple or complex) to succeed in a school or work environment.

Supplying assistive technology (AT) should be consumer centered, based on a clearly identified need, and supported by a thorough assessment including simulation and product trials when needed. The AT team should follow the guidelines in the Bain Assistive Technology System (BATS) described in Chapters 2 and 3, in which the focus is on the performance of a task, and the evaluation includes the consumer, the environment, and the assistive technology device (ATD).[4] Because sitting provides a person with a good base of support from which to produce controlled movements,[3,5–7] most technology is used by consumers in a seated position. Before beginning to assess the consumers' need for additional AT, it is imperative that they be provided with a properly designed seated environment from which they can function comfortably to their greatest potential.

SIX STEPS

Creating a dynamic seating environment involves six steps: identification, assessment, goal setting, intervention, supply, and support. These are described in detail below and in the guidelines presented in Appendix 4-1.

STEP 1

IDENTIFICATION

▶ The process begins when a need is identified by someone. This can be the consumer, caregiver, family member, clinician, educator, or vocational counselor. Usually, someone notices that there is a task that the consumer wants to perform but cannot. The identifier assumes that something can be done to assist the consumer and begins to ask questions, seeking a solution. The consumer may be referred to a professional to begin the problem-solving process. At this point, information is gathered about the task, the consumer, and the environment in which the task will be performed. The AT specialist must evaluate the entire situation and the expectations of everyone involved (consumer, caregiver or significant others, counselors, clinicians, teachers, employer). Does everyone believe there is a problem? It is very important that everyone is very honest from the beginning. People often come into the process with a hidden agenda that can present significant obstacles for the success of any intervention. Some team members (including the consumer) may not be convinced that there is a problem. Some team members recognize the problem but may have unrealistic goals, and when these hidden goals are not met, the "wishing" members are often so disappointed that they cannot see the other benefits of the system and may become depressed or angry.[1] It is important that clinical team members do not override the consumer with their "professional opinions."[8] The consumer is often the best judge of what he or she needs.

STEP 2

ASSESSMENT

▶ Once problems are clearly identified that interfere with the accomplishment of a desired task (instability, extraneous movements, limited range of motion, discomfort, limited endurance) and the expectations are clearly stated, a thorough assessment should be done. To do a complete seating assessment, the team must have access to full psychosocial and perceptual cognitive assessments done by other clinical and educational professionals. The team must be thoroughly informed about the consumer's medical and surgical history and plans, neurologic status, skeletal factors, sensory status, functional status, postural abilities, and communication level. If the AT system will be used in more than one setting, the team will need information about the home, educational, work, and recreational environments, along with the method the consumer will use to transport the seating system. Funding sources should be identified so that the team is aware of possible problems and advanced planning can begin.

Observation The team should observe the consumer at his or her present level of performance while engaged in the designated task(s). A list should be generated beginning with what the consumer is trying to do and what is interfering with his or her performance. This should also include interventions presently used, interventions tried unsuccessfully in the past, and interventions that have produced some successes but do not seem to work totally. With the consumer's permission, clinicians should use a hands-on approach to determine factors that might be limiting the performance of tasks. These include the influence of gravity, limited active and passive range of motion, limited strength, limited control, difficulties with motor planning, pain or discomfort, and respiratory compromise.

Attempts can be made at this point to influence performance using the examiner's hands to provide support, produce small positional changes, and change the home, school, or work environment if necessary. Continuous dialogue between the team members (including the consumer) will provide insight into the nature of the problems presented. Everything should be documented during this process.

Physical Evaluation The next step is a thorough physical evaluation by appropriate team members, usually an occupational therapist and physical therapist. The consumer should be placed supine on a mat for a complete evaluation of available passive range of motion and a skin inspection. This evaluation, with gravity eliminated, offers the clinicians an opportunity to determine the consumer's available range for optimal joint and spinal alignment. It also affords an opportunity to judge tone, discomfort, response to touch, and the influence that movement of one body part has on other body parts.[1,9]

Supine evaluation takes place with the consumer in a supine position (Fig. 4-1A); the team should stabilize the spine in the most neutral position possible (with a slight lumbar curve if available) and then record available range of motion for sitting and other hip movements (be sure to describe any compensations, including the effect on spinal alignment).

At this time, the examiner should measure the underthigh length and the distance from popliteal fossa to heel (Fig. 4-1B). This information is critical for creating a properly fitted, stable sitting base.

Seated evaluation is done once the supine evaluation is recorded. He or she should be placed in supported sitting on a firm surface with a thin top to allow the knees to flex, eliminating the pull of the hamstrings. One examiner should be in front of the consumer (kneeling on the floor with hands on the consumer's pelvis usually works best) and one behind (Fig. 4-2A). The kneeling examiner can evaluate pelvic alignment and mobility by using a hands-on approach on the pelvis, with the consumer's knees braced against the examiner's body. The second examiner provides support as needed and gently evaluates disturbed balance and response to corrective forces with the influence of gravity. In this position, the con-

Figure 4-1. **(A)** Evaluation of a consumer in the supine position. **(B)** The examiner measures the underthigh length and the distance from the popliteal fossa to the heel of a consumer in the supine position.

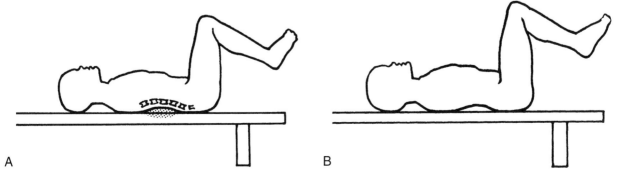

A   B

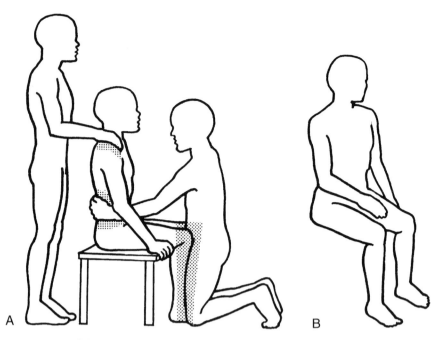

Figure 4-2. **(A)** Evaluation of a consumer in a seated position. **(B)** Seated dimensions are taken with the consumer in a totally supported position.

sumer should be asked to produce movements needed for function. The examiners should again use a hands-on approach similar to that used in the initial part of the evaluation to determine how support and position change affect functional movements.[1,9]

Seated dimensions should be taken at this time, with the consumer totally supported in the most optimal alignment (Fig. 4-2B). These measurements will be used to create a seated environment and will be available to the team for reference during design and creation of the system, should compromises be necessary. They will also be available for cross-checking at fittings and delivery.

STEP 3

GOAL SETTING

▶ The team should now have enough information to set goals and begin planning an intervention. The team should decide what goals they have that can be realistically influenced with seating intervention and additional enabling technology. Discussion must be honest and reality based, using all the information gathered to date. A well-planned seating system may

- Normalize tone
- Decrease pathologic reflex activity and abnormal movement patterns
- Achieve and maintain good pelvic alignment through facilitation and accommodation
- Improve postural symmetry
- Improve and/or supplement postural control
- Enhance range of movement

- Maintain and/or improve skin condition
- Increase comfort and sitting tolerance
- Decrease fatigue
- Improve function of the autonomic nervous system

The overriding goal is usually to provide a stable base of support and allow for good central control so that the consumer has a base for controlled distal movements. Good trunk position is necessary because all function, both central (control, alignment, internal organ function) and distal (gross and fine motor control in the head and arms), is based on position and control in the trunk and pelvic girdles.[1,10–12]

STEP 4

INTERVENTION PLANNING

▶ *System Properties* Once the team begins to plan the intervention, they will need to decide what properties are needed in the seating system and its components to achieve the stated goals.

- **Surface type:** describe the profile of the support surface
    Planar: flat
    Contoured: gentle to aggressive curves that are preformed, added with modular components, or carved to fit approximate body contours
    Molded: intimate curves provide contact to all body contours via a custom molding process
- **Dimensions:** size and shape of surfaces
- **Placement:** where the surface is attached to the seating system and where it makes contact with the person
- **Attachment**
    Removability
    Adjustability
    Strength/durability

Decisions will depend on the work needed from the system. When considering intervention, the team needs to follow an ordered progression. First, fixed "deficits" or body features must be accommodated. These can be limitation in joint range of motion, asymmetrical or prominent body contours (scoliosis, kyphosis, bony prominences, a stump), bracing, obesity, or other existing body features that cannot be changed. Once these accommodations are made, the team can use the information gathered during the physical assessment to determine how to inhibit or normalize the influence of tone or pathologic reflexes. Success with normalizing tone may free the consumer to allow facilitation of active responses through the strategic placement of supports and/or reorientation of the work site (e.g., moving a switch or joystick to a different position may facilitate better posture and, therefore, better distal function). Lastly, decisions must be made about offering additional postural support and/or control to assist the consumer in achieving the desired result.

Features such as the makeup of the support surfaces, their relationship to each other, and their orientation in space will affect the consumer. Again, using the information garnered in the physical evaluation, the team should decide what support surfaces are needed: primary (seat, back, head, feet, upper extremities) and secondary (lateral and anterior head; anterior shoulders; lateral and anterior trunk; lateral and anterior hips; medial, lateral, superior, and anterior knee; lateral, superior, and anterior foot). If the support is needed, what properties are necessary to provide the best result? Surface properties vary according to how much contact is needed between the consumer and the surface. More contact provides more support and distributes pressures over a broader area, resulting in more comfort and control.[13] Planar (flat) systems have minimal contact, contoured have more contact, and molded systems that are created from a body cast to fit the exact contours of a single user have the most contact. The dimensions refer to the height, length, depth, and width of the support. The placement of the support describes its relationship to the person and to the rest of the seating system (angulation, distance, pitch), as well as the relationship to the work. Angular relationships between the surfaces at the hip and knee joints (seat/back surfaces, seat/calf surfaces) must be determined by the range of motion results obtained in the physical assessment. Angles must respect and accommodate limitations in range of motion to allow for deformity and ensure proper alignment of body segments.[1] Changes of orientation in space affect the consumer's comfort level, pressure over skin surfaces, fatigue, and ability to work in gravity-eliminated and gravity-influenced positions.[5–7] The attachment describes whether the support swings away or is removable and how strong and durable it has to be.

Simulation The team will usually find it helpful to simulate its choices using a simulator chair or a series of commercially available components. At this stage, it is imperative to have the supplier (rehabilitation engineer or rehabilitation technology supplier) present to discuss options available to meet the team's goals. If the supplier was not present for the assessment and goal setting, he or she will want to be familiarized with the process to date. It is important that suppliers be included as an equal member of the team, with equal access to information so that they can recommend possible solutions to meet the goals determined by the team. The supplier will be able to explain the pros and cons and prices of various options to everyone involved and assist with informed decision making. Sometimes a seating solution will have to be custom fabricated, while others can be created using components from various commercial sources.

STEP 5

SUPPLY

▶ Once the components and sources have been determined, the process moves into the supply phase. It will be necessary to find funding and actually order and/or create the device as specified by the team. The supplier should keep all the team members appraised as the process moves along from submission through approval, ordering, and receiving. Once the system is complete, the supplier must deliver it as instructed by the prescriber (to the medical clinic, school, work site, or home of the user). At delivery, the prescriber should inspect the system and be sure that it meets the specifications, as well as observe and assist as the supplier makes the final adjustments. On final delivery, the supplier and prescriber should be sure that the consumer understands how to use and maintain the system and whom to call if there are problems.

STEP 6

SUPPORT

▶ Most interventions fail after the supply phase. Everything is adjusted and fitted well during supply. If modifications need to be made, they are made during that phase, and "supply" is considered complete once the system is working as it was intended. Once the system leaves the assessment/delivery arena, it needs continuous support. Some of the support is maintenance, which is the responsibility of the consumer and any caregiver. The seating system and wheeled mobility base should be treated like any other important item needed for daily functioning such as clothing, household appliances, or transportation vehicles. Normal maintenance includes using the device as it was intended, keeping it clean, maintaining connectors and batteries, and tightening loose parts.

Warranty repairs are the responsibility of the supplier. Each piece of equipment should come with manufacturer's warranty information that describes the warranty on each component. Labor is usually not covered under the warranty, and consumers should read the information carefully, and ask questions of the supplier and the team during the delivery of the equipment. Adjustments that are needed to accommodate changes should be handled in the environment in which the assessment was done, as they usually require some type of reassessment and decision making. Support of the system by the team and the supplier is imperative for the successful attainment of optimal seating in the different environments including school, home, or workplace.

REFERENCES

1. Bergen A, Presperin J, Tallman T: Positioning for Function: Wheelchairs and Other Assistive Technologies. Valhalla Rehabilitation Publications, Valhalla, NY, 1990

2. Cook A, Hussey S: Assistive Technologies: Principles and Practice. Mosby-Year Book, St. Louis, 1995

3. Zacharkow D: Posture Sitting, Standing, Chair Design and Exercise. Charles C Thomas, Springfield, IL, 1988

4. Bain BK: Steps in a problem solving evaluation for assistive technology. AJOT Technology Special Interest Section Newsletter. 5(2):1–3, 1995

5. Nwaobi O: Seating orientations and upper extremity function in children with cerebral palsy. Phys Ther 67(8):1209–1212, 1987

6. Nwaobi O: Seating orientations and upper extremity function in children with cerebral palsy. Dev Med Child Neurol 28:41–44, 1986

7. Nwaobi O, Hobson D, Trefler E: Hip angle and upper extremity movement time in children with cerebral palsy. pp. 39–41. In Proceedings of the 8th Annual Conference of the Rehabilitation Engineering Society of North America, Memphis, TN, June 24–28, 1985

8. York J: Mobility methods selected for use in home and community environments. Phys Ther 69(9):736–747, 1989

9. Zollars JA: Special Seating: An Illustrated Guide. Otto Bock Orthopedic Ind., Minneapolis, 1996

10. Curtis KA, Kindlin CM, Reich KM, White DE: Functional reach in wheelchair users: the effects of trunk and lower extremity stabilization. Arch Phys Med Rehabil 76(4):355–367, 1995

11. Trefler E, Hobson D, Taylor S et al: Seating and Mobility for Persons with Physical Disabilities. Therapy Skill Builders, Tucson, 1993

12. Zacharkow D: Proper backrest stabilization: the overlooked factor in wheelchair seating. Phys Ther Forum, April 21:4–6, 1995

13. Sprigle S, Chung K, Brubaker C: Reduction of sitting pressures with custom contoured cushions. J Rehabil Res Dev 27(2):135–140, 1990

SUGGESTED READINGS

Engstrom B: Ergonomics, Wheelchairs and Positioning. Posturalis, Hasselby, Sweden, 1993

Hedman G (guest ed): Rehabilitation technology. Phys Occup Ther Pediatr 10(2):1–173, 1990

Hill J, Presperin J: Orthotic management and positioning. In: Spinal Cord Injury: A Guide to Functional Outcomes in Occupational Therapy. Aspen, Rockville, MD, 1986

Miedaner J, Finuf L: Effect of adaptive positioning on psychological test scores for preschool children with cerebral palsy. Pediatr Phys Ther 177–182, 1993

Padula W: A Behavioral Vision Approach for Persons with Physical Disabilities. Optometric Extension Program, Santa Ana, CA, 1988

Presperin J: Seating systems: the therapist and rehabilitation engineering team. Phys Occup Ther Pediatr 10(2):11–45, 1990

Ward D: Prescriptive Seating for Wheeled Mobility. Vol. 1. Theory, Application, and Terminology. Health Wealth International, Kansas City, KS, 1994

Zacharkow D: The problem with lumbar support. Phys Ther Forum 9(35):1–5, 1990

Zacharkow D: Wheelchair Posture and Pressure Sores. Charles C Thomas, Springfield, IL, 1984

General Guidelines for Mobility Assessment

IDENTIFY

- Identify the task that the consumer wants to do but cannot because of the limitations of his or her positioning
- Be realistic, but use your imagination. Assume that a good assessment and match to proper technology will produce success
- List problems
- List expectations

ASSESS

- Gather information about consumer, environment(s), funding
- Observe consumer: present performance, posture, limitations to task performance
  Use your eyes and hands
- Do a thorough physical assessment:
  Supine: on a firm surface, determine potential for correction of alignment; determine limitations of range of motion that cannot be corrected; measure angles
  Sitting: on a firm surface with knees flexed to 90 degrees or more, determine response to corrective forces and ability to produce controlled movement with support; measure angles and dimensions

SET GOALS

- Determine what a seating system can do
- Provide a stable base of support and good central control as a base for controlled movement

INTERVENTION

- Determine what supports are needed
- Determine what properties they must have—surface type (planar, contoured, molded); dimensions; placement; attachment
- Accommodate fixed deficits; inhibit or normalize tone; offer postural support
- Use simulation to make decisions
- Be sure supplier is qualified to assist with assessment and decision making; supply what the consumer needs, and provide ongoing support
- Match features to products

SUPPLY

- Work with supplier to arrange for funding and ordering
- Check equipment at fittings and on delivery: be sure it is what you expected and that it works as intended
- Modify as needed

SUPPORT

- Instruct consumer in normal maintenance
- Provide warranty information
- Provide training in proper use
- Provide for repairs as needed

CHAPTER 5

JANE MILLER

Basic Electricity and Electronics

More than 200 years ago, Benjamin Franklin remarked that "electrical fluid … may … be of use to mankind."[1] This powerful and convenient form of energy has greatly affected our lives. Today, electricity and its many applications abound in our world. With the push of a button or the flick of a switch, we light our homes, listen to music, cook dinner, talk to friends on the telephone, and create documents on our computers. We tend to ignore its presence except when the alarm clock fails to go off in the morning, the television reception becomes fuzzy during a favorite movie, or a lightning storm interrupts a swim in the pool. Yet, most individuals have little or no understanding of what electricity is or of how it works.

This chapter is an overview of electricity and electronics, their applications, and general principles. It is intended only as a nontechnical survey and does not assume to usurp the expertise of qualified professionals. When the services of a licensed electrician or a rehabilitation engineer are required, these individuals must be contacted. Improper use of electrical devices can, and often does, have dangerous results.

Electricity is not a human invention. It is a naturally occurring phenomenon in such things as lightning, electric fish, and magnetic rocks. Even the neural signals in the human brain are electrical. The word *electricity* comes from the Greek word *elektron*, meaning amber. The ancient Greeks observed that rubbing a piece of amber (fossilized tree sap) with fur created what we now refer to as static electricity. Electricity is an invisible force that can produce heat, light, motion, and other physical effects. This force is due to an attraction or repulsion between electric charges. Sources of electricity are useful in many applications: conversion of chemical energy (batteries, electroplating), electromagnetism (generators, door chimes, magnetic lifting cranes, telephones), photoelectricity (incandescent and fluorescent lights, solar cells), and thermal emission (soldering irons, arc welders, flashers, circuit breakers).

Electronics is the science of controlling the movement of electrons and the creation of applications involving the control of electricity. Once involving only circuits with vacuum tubes, electronics now incorporates the transistor, integrated circuitry, and the microprocessor. A brief listing of electronic applications includes radar, AM/FM radio, microwave oven, television camera, photoelectric eye, x-ray machines, and computer technology. Environmental control units (ECUs) and augmentative and alternative communication (AAC) aids would not be possible without electronics.

BASIC CONCEPTS OF ELECTRICITY: TERMINOLOGY AND DEFINITIONS

Matter, having mass and occupying space, is composed of small particles or molecules that are made up of atoms. An atom consists of a nucleus (which is further broken down into protons having a positive charge and neutrons having no charge) surrounded by negatively charged electrons moving in orbit. Like charges (particles having the same polarity) will repel each other, whereas those with unlike or a different charge will attract one another. The push and pull of electric charges of these particles is the electrostatic force (which holds the electrons in orbit around the nucleus). Sufficient electron movement creates energy that when properly channeled and used will illuminate light bulbs, cause motors to turn, and enable radios to play. Electric energy is produced in huge generators powered by water, coal, oil, and nuclear fuel.

STATIC VERSUS CURRENT ELECTRICITY

Electrons are very light in weight and easily "rub off" while in motion. An atom attempts to lose or borrow free electrons to maintain a neutral or balanced situation. This hustling movement or friction creates electric activity. It is referred to as static electricity. When combing your hair or walking across a carpeted room, you may notice sparks or hear the crackling sound of electric current. Although it is a sudden and often uncontrollable energy form, static electricity can be used functionally in some devices such as capacitors and air cleaners. Note that static electricity can damage or cause malfunctions in sensitive electronic equipment such as a computer. Any electric charges should be "discharged" before handling a computer or magnetic storage media such as floppy disks. Installation of an antistatic floor or desktop mat can safely dissipate static.

Electric current, unlike static electricity, flows through a wire just like liquid in a pipe. Its current, or the electrons flowing through a cross section of wire, is measured in amperes (also referred to as amps, [A]). Each electrical device has an amperage rating. Circuits are also rated for the total number of amperes it can safely deliver. The strength or pressure of an electrical current is measured in volts (V). Household circuits are usually 120 V (for small appliances, lights, etc.), 240 V (for heavy-duty appliances such as ovens and clothes dryers), or low voltage. A low-voltage device might be a doorbell chime, thermostat, or household intercom system. These devices generally require less than the standard 120 V (typically 20 to 30 V). They require a transformer (an electrical device that changes the voltage of alternating current by raising or lowering the voltage) to "step down" or reduce the household power to the desired voltage. A transformer can be built into the appliance or is a separate unit plugged into the wall outlet. A watt (W) is the unit of power or the amount of electricity needed to operate a device. The formula for calculating wattage, volts × amps = watts, is helpful in figuring the load on an individual circuit. This information is generally listed on a sticker or plate on the appliance.

CONDUCTORS, INSULATORS, AND RESISTORS

Molecules within a wire vibrate in an irregular way, producing heat. When free electrons collide with these molecules, the molecules begin to turn and vibrate even faster, creating increased heat. A conductor, generally a solid or liquid metal such as silver, copper, or aluminum, allows electric current to move readily. These substances offer little resistance to the flow of current. Although not a metal, water and even your own body will conduct electricity due to the presence of ions (or charged particles).

Conversely, an insulator (e.g., rubber, wood, glass, cloth, paper, and porcelain) is a poor conductor. These materials prevent the flow of current in an electric circuit. Usually a nonmetal, an insulator keeps the electric current within the material (e.g., plastic casing or insulation over copper wire in an appliance cord).

A semiconductor is a material whose resistance is a combination of a conductor and an insulator. Materials such as silicon or germanium may be used as semiconductors. Their degree of conductivity can be controlled by the presence of impurities.

Resistance, the tendency of a conductor to inhibit the flow of current, is the degree of opposition to electron conduction of any wire or circuit measured in units called ohms. Resistance depends on the type of material, its length, and cross-sectional area. For example, a piece of copper wire has lower resistance than carbon of the same length and width. If two wires are made of the same material and have similar width, the longer wire is a better resistor; a thinner wire has higher resistance when comparing wires of identical material and length. A resistor is often added to a circuit to increase electrical resistance. Resistors are manufactured with a specific ohm value and are used to dissipate power without producing excessive heat.

ELECTRIC CIRCUITS

Electric current must flow in a complete path or circuit from its energy source (typically a battery or generator) through various fixtures and appliances and then back to the source. A circuit is the circular path of electric current. Any break or interruption in the circuit will stop the flow. Electron flow is actually from the negative terminal to the positive terminal (e.g., in a battery, from cathode to anode); however, conventional current is said to flow opposite: positive to negative.

Most circuits contain a switch that controls the flow of current. A switch is a component used to either open or close the path for electron flow in circuit. The switch is either completely on (closed) or off (open), such as a power switch or button on the television set or computer. A more detailed discussion of switches is provided in Chapter 6.

An electric circuit can be illustrated in pictorial form or as a schematic diagram. A schematic diagram is a "shorthand" method of indicating the components, the various electrical connections, and their functions using universally accepted symbols. Commonly, these diagrams are included with household appliances such as radios, stereos, and hair dryers. A building's electrical system is illustrated in the electrical or wiring plan that includes location of switches, lighting fixtures, receptacle outlets, and the wiring (Fig. 5-1).

A series circuit is an arrangement of components in which there is only one path (wired end to end from its negative to positive terminals). The current flows through all parts and back to its source. Therefore, if one bulb goes out (e.g., in a string of decorative lights), all will go out. All bulbs share the same amount of current. If there is a greater load (e.g., more lights added to the circuit), then the bulbs will be dimmer. Safety devices, such as fuses and circuit breakers, are usually in series circuits.

In a parallel circuit, there is more than one path for the current and two or more components are directly connected to the source of electricity. Parallel circuits are typical of household wiring and several appliances can be attached to the same circuit within the room. Each appliance, such as the refrigerator or lights, has a separate path or branch. An open circuit in one branch does not affect the others. However, an open circuit in the main line results in no current for all the branches. The total current in a parallel circuit is the sum of all currents in all the individual branches. The

Figure 5-1. A simple circuit containing a light bulb (load or "resistor") and a battery (energy source) connected with wires (the conductor) and a switch (control mechanism). The bulb will light when the switch is closed or in the "on" position.

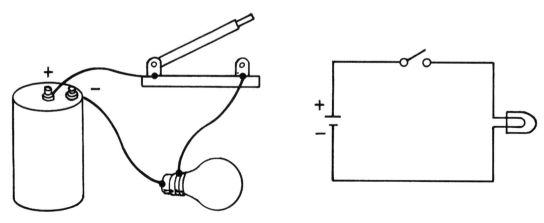

voltage across all appliances is the same. However, as the resistance is heightened, the current is decreased; and conversely, as the resistance is lowered, the current is increased.

Some appliances make use of combinations of both serial and parallel circuits. When integrating various technological devices (e.g., AAC aids and ECU), these may be connected to common or separate voltage sources. Depending on their specific use, voltage source, and circuitry, there may be a greater demand on the system. The manufacturer's listing of voltage and watts, which is usually marked on the back of appliances, must be checked for each appliance.

ELECTRIC CURRENT AND ELECTROMAGNETISM

Electric current is generally classified into two general categories: direct current (DC) and alternating current (AC). Direct current is usually identified with batteries. Alternating current is the form of electricity delivered to your home via overhead or underground power lines. The service wires provide power to operate 120-V and 240-V appliances.

DIRECT CURRENT

DC, such as a dry cell or car battery, has steady voltage and a unidirectional flow. It has to be a closed loop of conductors attached to voltage source. DC has fixed polarity, but the voltage may be steady or varying.

ALTERNATING CURRENT

In AC or typical household current, the voltage is "unsteady." First, the current flows in one direction, then in the opposite direction, with regular rhythm reversing 120 times per second. These reversals occur due to changes in polarity. Each back-and-forth motion is called a cycle. In the United States, this is referred to as 60-cycles per second AC or 60-cycle AC. AC is more readily produced, easier to lower or raise the voltage, and easier to transport via wires. Different countries have different electric voltage, and adapters must be used to transform the electric power to use appliances. Outside the United States, the voltage is usually 220/240, and adapters will reduce the voltage to 110/120. A travel agent or embassy should be consulted before traveling to ensure that the proper adapters are available to use and/or recharge any electric appliances.

ELECTROMAGNETISM AND THE ELECTROMAGNETIC SPECTRUM

Electricity and magnetism are closely related. Electric currents produce lines of force as in a magnetic field. When current flows through a straight wire, a magnetic field appears in the space surrounding the wire (the "field" or disturbance in radio reception when driving under high-tension power lines is an example of this). Electromagnets are used in many devices (e.g., doorbells, telephone receivers, electric motors, circuit breakers, relays, and alarms). A motor is an example of how current can react with a magnetic field to produce motion.

The advances in electronics (e.g., integrated circuits, remote controls, infrared technology) have expanded our use of the electromagnetic spectrum. Audio, radio, radar, infrared, visible light, ultraviolet, and x-ray frequency bands are included in this spectrum. Depending on its frequency, we may or may not be able to detect these electromagnetic forces. Many electronic sensors, such as thermostats, automatic door openers, or alarms, react to stimuli. Changes in light, heat, temperature, or position will affect the flow of electric current (e.g., sound an alarm, raise or lower the temperature, open a door).

PORTABLE SOURCES OF ELECTRICITY: THE BATTERY

An electrochemical power source or battery produces electricity by spontaneous chemical reactions. The battery converts chemical energy into electric energy (frequently in an electrolyte containing two metals with differing polarity). Commercial batteries have been manufactured for more than a century, providing relatively inexpensive, convenient, and portable energy sources. Batteries (offering direct current) are used where AC cannot be readily used (e.g., portable appliances, wristwatches, pacemakers, powered wheelchairs). A primary cell is a battery with a limited life span. The chemical reactants are consumed by the electron discharge. Secondary cells, by contrast, are able to be charged or recharged. A secondary battery is also considered a storage unit. The capacity of a storage battery is rated in ampere-hours. Batteries vary in size, total available energy, internal composition, and intended application. Batteries may also be classified as either wet or dry cells (although this does not apply to the entire range and latest battery technology). In the wet cell, the electrolyte is a liquid; however, in the dry cell, it is a moist paste.

A typical flashlight battery is a dry cell or a primary aqueous electrolyte cell. The electrical output is limited. The carbon rod is surrounded by a damp mixture in a tightly sealed zinc container. The rod and zinc can both react with the moist chemical filler, creating an electron pump: pushing electrons out of the cathode or negative (−) terminal and pulling electrons into the anode or positive (+) terminal. Attaching a wire to both battery terminals completes the circuit (Fig. 5-2). If a light bulb or some electrical device is also connected, the current will enter the device (e.g., lighting the bulb). With batteries in series, the total voltage is equal to the sum of individual values, and the current is the same throughout. In parallel, battery voltage is the same throughout, but the current is equal to the sum of the individual values.

Fitting the right battery to each device is not always easy. In addition to checking the manufacturer's recommendations, the correct equipment

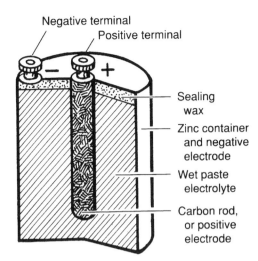

Negative terminal
Positive terminal

Sealing wax

Zinc container and negative electrode

Wet paste electrolyte

Carbon rod, or positive electrode

Figure 5-2. Dry cell.

must be matched to the intended use. Devices vary in availability, pricing, and amount of power offered.

Common carbon zinc batteries are sized D, C, A, AA, and AAA. These 1.5-V batteries, with varying current ratings, are sealed and cannot be spilled. They can be operated in any position at room temperature. Fresh batteries should be used. Shelf life can be extended by storage at 40° to 50°F.

In addition to the carbon zinc battery, there are many other primary batteries: zinc chloride (for heavy-duty use); mercury oxide (flat round button batteries having long life and constant voltage that perform well at temperatures greater than 130°F); and silver oxide (small button batteries found in communication equipment, hearing aids, pacemakers, cameras, and watches). Popular secondary batteries include lead-acid (e.g., 9-V and automotive batteries used when high current load and low voltage are necessary); nickel cadmium (nicads are common in cordless electrical devices such as toothbrushes, shavers, and power tools); and mercury, lithium ion, solar, plastic, and alkaline cells. Each has it own unique characteristics and properties. Many portable computers and some ECUs use long-lasting lithium batteries.

Alkaline batteries, either primary or secondary, are used when greater performance is required (e.g., heavy current drain for longer, continuous action in toys, radios, and electronic equipment). They function at lower temperatures and have a longer shelf life.

Powered wheelchairs and scooters tend to use deep-cycle, rechargeable 12-V batteries. These are not the same as an automotive battery. The deep-cycle battery provides a continuous source of power (whereas the car battery offers only a quick start until the alternator takes over). Three basic deep-cycle batteries are currently in use: wet lead acid, absorbed glass mat (AGM), and gel/sealed lead acid. The wet lead acid type is the least expensive, is not sealed, and requires maintenance (adding distilled water). These can spill during transport and are classified as hazardous materials. Use on commercial transportation, especially airlines, may be restricted to these batteries and their users. The other two types, AGM and gel/sealed lead acid, are easier and safer to transport. They are not classified as hazardous materials and generally do not have any transportation restrictions.

The life of a battery is dependent on its type and frequency of use. Typically, powered wheelchair manufacturers offer guidelines for minimum requirements under average operation. The Battery Council International (BCI) and the American National Standards Institute (ANSI) promote uniform standards for the industry.

The optimum method for recharging a storage battery depends on the type and characteristics of that specific secondary battery. Some batteries require deep discharge followed by recharge to maximum capacity. Others require only trickle charging or some form of taper charging. Some are more tolerant to overcharging (e.g., nickel-cadmium), whereas overcharging others can cause permanent damage (e.g., zinc-silver). The regimen suggested by the manufacturer should be followed.

SAFETY FACTORS AND DEVICES

The world of electricity and electronics is full of wonder and awe. However, electricity must be respected and handled carefully. Strict safety standards exist for electric and electronic procedures and equipment. Electric practices and procedures are governed by specific codes, such as the National Electric Code (NEC). The NEC establishes minimum safety standards for electric wiring and equipment. The Underwriter's Laboratory provides a safety label (UL label) that is applied to manufactured devices that have been tested for safety and approved by the UL. It is important to read the instruction manual before using any device. There are certain "rules" that must be obeyed!

- **Never** touch electrical devices with wet or damp hands. Always be sure that your hands are dry. This includes not handling switches or appliances while bathing or swimming. Be sure that you are standing in a dry place before using any electrical equipment.
- **Never** overload the electric outlet.
- **Never** put electric wires under rugs or carpets. Insulation can be worn away by traffic.
- **Never** touch a downed power line or electric cable.
- **Never** place anything except a plug into a wall socket. When receptacles are not in use, apply safety covers to avoid accidents.
- **Never** remain under or near a tree nor remain in a pool or lake during a thunderstorm.
- **Never** use worn or broken electric wiring or equipment. If the device can be safely repaired, do so immediately or replace it.

If AC is being used, the outlets must be properly grounded. Having properly grounded appliances and receptacles lessens the chance of accidental electric shock. Use only cables with a three-prong plug. The third prong must never be broken on a grounded plug to fit a two-slot outlet (grounded adapters must be used properly). A cable must be unplugged by grasping the plug, not the cord. Cords and plugs must be inspected regularly for damage or cracking. Extension cords should not substitute for permanent wiring. Cords should never be attached with tacks or pins.

When traveling with a computer, it must never be put through an airport metal detector. Loose batteries should not be carried in your pocket or handbag. Contact with a metal object, such as keys, can short-circuit the battery and may cause burns.

Cooling vents on electronic equipment must not be obstructed. Environmental "hazards" such as food, beverages, dust, temperature extremes, and overexposure to sunlight should be avoided. Surge suppressors must be installed to protect electronic units from voltage spikes. Lastly, smoke detectors and fire extinguishers must be installed in the home.

A short circuit occurs when two wires make contact (either bare or lacking insulation) or the circuit is overloaded (delivering too much current). When this occurs, the wire becomes very hot and may possibly burst into flames. To avoid the risk of fire, a fuse or circuit breaker are commonly used. The fuse is a piece of wire in the circuit that will melt, breaking the circuit if current level is too high. A circuit breaker is a control switch that opens if there is too much current. Each circuit is generally protected by a fuse or circuit breaker. These are located in the fuse box or service panel. The current will instantly cease if an overload occurs (e.g., drawing more amperage than the circuit can provide). A circuit breaker with an amperage rating higher than that specified for the circuit must never be installed.

This chapter has presented an overview of electricity and electronics, their application, and general principles. The prudent consumer, caregiver, and/or professional should follow these guidelines:

- Routinely check for exposed wires
- Use heavy duty extension cords and periodically check their condition
- Check fuse boxes and circuit breakers monthly
- Have a professional check all house and apartment wiring annually, especially in older buildings
- Watch battery indicators and replace or recharge as needed. Keep contact surfaces clean
- Do not combine different brands or old and new batteries. Store in cool, dry place
- Read all user manuals carefully; note voltage, watts, and UL markings; complete and submit warranty forms immediately
- Be aware of what can be maintained and/or repaired by the consumer, caregiver, or family and what will require the attention of a licensed electrician

Electricity, the throughput of many ATDs, is a wonderful source of power if used wisely. The next chapter in this section presents an overview of access methods for ATDs (switches).

REFERENCE

1. Vogt G: Electricity and Magnetism. Franklin Watts, New York, 1985

SUGGESTED READINGS

Groneman CH, Feirer JL: Getting Started in Electricity and Electronics. McGraw-Hill, New York, 1979

Gutnik MJ: Electricity: From Faraday to Solar Generators. Franklin Watts, New York, 1986

Institute of Rehabilitation Medicine: A Know-How Manual on Electricity for the Severely Disabled and Their Families. Monograph 65. New York University Medical Center, New York, 1979

Math I: More Wires and Watts: Understanding and Using Electricity. Charles Scribner's Sons, New York, 1988

Ryan CW: Basic Electricity. 2nd Ed. John Wiley & Sons, New York, 1986

Sinclair IR: The Harper Collins Dictionary of Electronics. Harper Collins, New York, 1991

Webster J, Cook A, Tompkins W, Vanderheiden G (eds): Electronic Devices for Rehabilitation. John Wiley & Sons, New York, 1985

Whyman K: Electricity and Magnetism. Gloucester Press, New York, 1986

Wolff TL: All charged up. Independent Living Provider 10:42–46, 1995

CHAPTER 6

BEVERLY K. BAIN

Switches, Control Interfaces, and Access Methods

A switch or control interface allows a person to access or activate a device. Switches are often referred to in the assistive technology (AT) literature as control interfaces because they allow the user to control or activate a device. Each AT system has four parts: (1) the switch, which is referred to as the input unit, which activates or sends a command to the device; (2) the throughput, which is the processing unit of the device; (3) the output, which is the result of a successful operation; and (4) the display, which is the visual, auditory, or tactile feedback that informs the user that the system is operational.

Switches enable people with impaired manipulative skills or sensory disabilities to interact with their environment, to increase their functional activities, and to extend their capabilities (Fig. 6-1). It has often been said that the most magnificent technological device is underused or useless if the person cannot effectively operate it; it can also be the most frustrating experience for the consumer and/or caregiver. With the ever-increasing advances in technology, people with any disability can activate a switch using virtually any body part: a finger, hand, arm, foot, head, tongue, eyes, breath, or voice (Fig. 6-2). The body part that is used to activate the switch is known as the control site.

ASSESSMENT FOR SWITCH OR CONTROL INTERFACE

Before the selection of any assistive technology device (ATD), an assessment of the consumer, the tasks, and all the environments is necessary, as delineated in Chapter 3. The Bain Assistive Technology System (BATS) is a

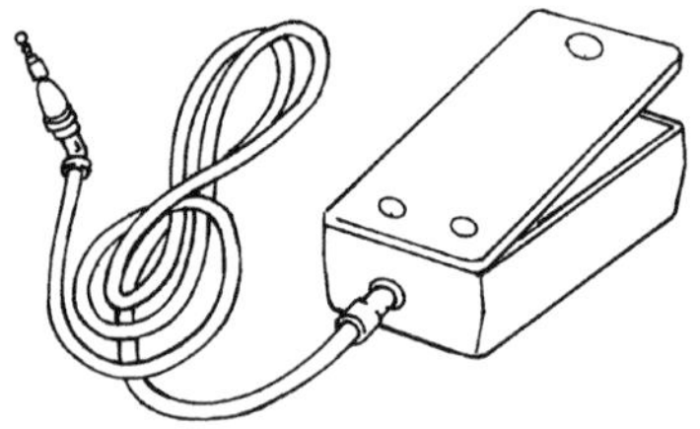

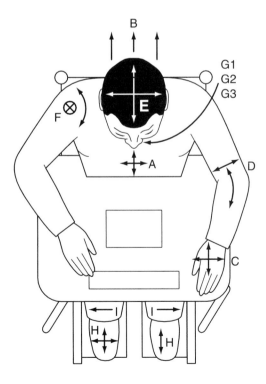

Figure 6-1. Simple switch plate for computer.

synergistic evaluation that includes four components: the task, the consumer, the device, and the environment. One of the first and often the most important activities of the technologist and consumer is to determine the most accurate, reliable, and efficient movement that the person with a disability can use to activate the switch.[1] If done correctly, this will require numerous trials with a variety of switches; therefore, it is strongly recommended that the rehabilitation technology team carefully review the initial evaluation of the consumer, consider all ATDs that the consumer may need to activate, all the environments in which the devices will be used, and all the activities of daily living (ADL) tasks that the consumer and the caregiver must perform and, most important, ensure that the consumer feels comfortable with the switch and the mounting system (see Table 6-1 for assessment guidelines and Appendix 6-1 for sample assessment forms).[2]

Figure 6-2. Examples of switch activation using various body parts as the control site. Common control points are identified by letter: A, chin control; B, headrest control; C, hand control; D, arm/elbow control; E, head control; F, shoulder control; G, face control; H, foot control; I, knee control.

Table 6-1. Guidelines for Switch or Control Interface Assessment

1. Establish the optimal position for the consumer, noting all other functions, especially ADL.

2. Determine which ATDs the consumer needs the switches to interface (toy, wheelchair, ECU, AAC, computer, or other).

3. Evaluate the consumer's abilities, considering the sensorimotor, cognitive, and psychosocial components (voluntary control, active range of motion, endurance, speed of response, vision, etc.).

4. Note all precautions (seizures, respiration, fatigue, etc.).

5. Discuss with the consumer and caregiver their thoughts, opinions, and desires.

6. Test the consumer for two or three possible control sites by observation, formal testing, interviewing, and reviewing the initial assessment (if the consumer cannot communicate, be sure to observe all voluntary motions that are accurate, reliable, and efficient, and interview the caregiver). Make a written list or notes.

7. Evaluate the operational features of the switch: activation, force requirements, distance switch must travel, size of the control surface, durability, feedback, connector type, and momentary or latching mode.

8. Analyze the selection technique required by the ATD (direct selection, scanning, or encoding).

9. Determine where the switch will be used (in bed, on wheelchair; at desk, work station, or other site).

10. Mount the switch temporarily. DO NOT hold the switch.

11. Try the switch with a temporary mounting. If this is not successful, try another switch or change the mounting. If it is successful, mount the switch permanently and make notes (picture and words) to aid caregivers in the proper placement and use of the switch.

12. Reevaluate periodically.

Copyright 1993 BK Bain.

CLASSIFICATION

Switches can be classified as mechanical, electromagnetic, biopotential, or sonic.[3] Mechanical switches that require pressure to close the circuit are the most frequently used for powered wheelchairs, environment control units (ECUs), and computers. Examples include joystick, pillow or cushion, treadle, rocking lever, tongue, chin, and pneumatic or sip and puff (Fig. 6-3). Electromagnetic switches, often referred to as lightbeam or optical pointer or light-emitting diode, are usually mounted on the person and activate photosensitive sensors in augmentative and alternative communication (AAC) aids. Another example of an electromagnetic switch is the electromyographic switch that is used in myoelectric prostheses, where an electrode is placed over the desired muscle site and a slight muscle contraction activates the switch. Infrared or biopotential switches are used to activate televisions, video cassette recorders, and ECUs. In performing an evaluation of the environment, the technology team should be aware of the different signals of each type of activation device.

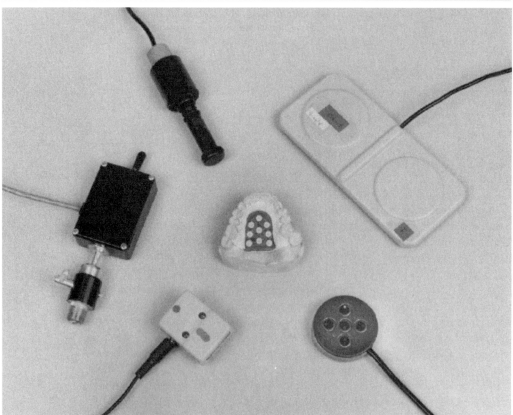

Figure 6-3. Some mechanical switches used to activate devices. (Photographs copyright 1997 Tony Velez.)

Infrared beams send signals that must be in direct line with the infrared receiver, whereas mechanical switches can send signals through walls and at greater distances. Sonic switches are ultrasound or voice-activated switches that convert sound levels to a switch closure and must be used in close proximity to the device because sonic waves do not pass through walls and are extremely sensitive. Ultrasonic switches are used with some ECUs. Currently, there is an increase in the use of voice-activated computers and ECUs that must be carefully programmed to recognize the consumer's voice in a noise-free environment.

Switches are often referred to as single, dual, or multiple switches. For a simple on/off toy, a single cushion switch may be used; for an ECU that requires scanning and selection, a dual pneumatic switch may be required. For a powered wheelchair that moves in many directions, a multiple joystick is needed. See Table 6-2 for more information.

OPERATIONAL FEATURES

To select the most effective switch for a person with any disability, there are several important operational features to consider, including

- How much pressure is required to activate the switch?
- Can the force required to activate the switch be graded from light to hard pressure? (some catalogs list the sensitivity in ounces of pressure)
- How much time and how much motion is needed to move off the switch to deactivate it?
- What is the feedback mode: tactile, auditory, visual, or proprioceptive?
- What is the size of the contact surface? (3 inches or the size of a straw)
- What connector type is needed, a ⅛th-in. mini plug, a 9 pin, a 25 pin, or a circular 6 pin? (*note:* there are available connector interfaces that can alter the connector type)
- What selection method is required? (direct or indirect)

OPERATIONAL MODES

The operational mode of a switch must also be considered to ensure the most appropriate switch selection. The major modes are momentary, latching, and proportional. A momentary switch is activated and remains on/off until the circuit is closed/open (pressure is released) (e.g., a car horn or an electric bed). A latching switch requires a single motion to turn on/off a device that remains on/off until the switch is activated a second time (e.g., a light switch or the on/off control of a computer). A proportional switch mode is most important in starting the slow smooth acceleration of a powered wheelchair, allowing for a gradual buildup of

Table 6-2. Switch or Control Interface Comparison Chart

Number of Switches or Control Interfaces Name	Single Treadle	Dual Pneumatic	Multiple Joystick
Operational Features			
Activation	Light-to-heavy pressure	Blowing and puffing	Touch
Force required	Can be graded	Breath minimal	Can be graded
Feedback: T, tactile; A, auditory; V, visual	T/A		T/A
Momentary	✓		✓
Latching		✓	
Size of contact surface	¼ to 3 in.	Straw	1 to 2 ½ in.
Connecter type	⅛-in. mini phone	Stereo mini phone	9-pin DIN
Selection Technique			
Direct selection	✓		✓
Scanning		✓	✓
Encoding		✓	✓
Mounting			
Flexible (gooseneck)	✓	✓	
On body	✓		✓
Universal	✓		✓
Other	Head band	Caterpillar	Chin
Interface with			
Augmentative communication	✓	✓	✓
Computer	✓	✓	✓
ECU/telephone	✓	✓	✓
Powered wheelchair	✓	✓	✓
Cars and vans			✓
Other (e.g., toy)	✓		✓

Copyright 1992 BK Bain. Revised 1994.

speed instead of an abrupt lurching forward motion. Currently, there are interconnectors available that can change switches from momentary to latching, or vice versa, and many powered wheelchairs have damping switches that allow for persons with irregular or spastic motions to control a powered wheelchair smoothly.

SWITCH INPUT METHODS

Switches can activate, deactivate, or control a device by direct and indirect selection and certain encoding techniques or input methods. Direct selection is a straightforward time- and energy-efficient approach to sending commands to devices. It can be accomplished with a single motion such as a finger or a mouthstick, a light pointer, or a wand inserted in a universal cuff and used for row, column, or linear scanning; however, it does require some degree of motor control. Indirect selection requires "intermediate steps between indicating the choice and actually sending the command" to the device.[4] These intermediate steps increase both the time and effort and require a higher level of cognitive ability. They can also be accomplished with a finger or any of the input methods listed above and are applicable in the various scanning methods (linear and row-column). Encoding is another method of switch selection, applicable with computers and AAC aids in which a letter, word, picture, or icon can symbolically represent a complete sentence or phrase frequently used. Encoding—also known as "macros" when used with computers—conserves time and energy; however, it requires a higher level of cognitive ability than direct or indirect selection.

MOUNTING

Another crucial factor when selecting the best switch or control interface is how and where the switch will be mounted. There are numerous places to mount a switch, including on the body of the consumer, on a bed frame, on a wheelchair, or on a desk (Fig. 6-4). Wherever the switch is mounted, it must be comfortable for the consumer and should not interfere with other daily activities or caregiving. Whenever possible, one switch is selected to activate several devices; for example, a powered wheelchair that can be programmed to control an AAC aid, an ECU, and a computer. Note that some powered wheelchairs manufactured before 1993 are compatible with only specific ECU systems; therefore, the technology team must consider this factor in their final selection of an integrated AT system. In addition, the mounting system must be placed so that it is readily accessible to the consumer, and, when possible, transferable to accommodate the consumer when in bed or in a wheelchair and at school, home, or work. This is especially important for the emergency or assistance call switches. Refer to Table 6-1 for guidelines on switch or control interface assessment.[2]

Switches can be mounted on or worn by a person, including

- Those mounted on the head, such as the infrared head pointer that is attached to a head band, or a mouse that is used to access a computer, or an eyebrow switch

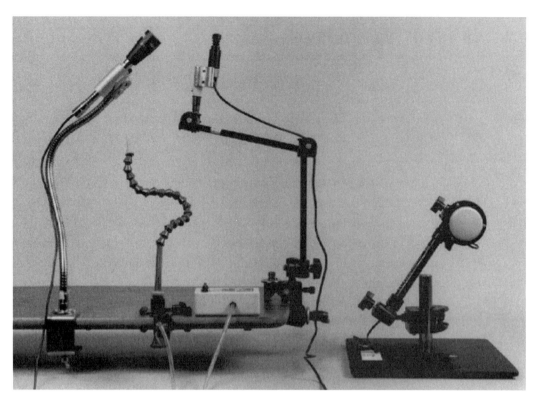

Figure 6-4. Various ways to mount a switch. (Photograph copyright 1997 Tony Velez.)

- A tongue switch that is inserted in the roof of the mouth and activated with tongue
- Those worn on the chest, such as the chin joystick
- Those worn on the wrist, such as a wrist extension mercury switch attached to a static hand splint
- A knee- or foot-mounted pressure switch can be attached to the body part with a strap or Velcro

Switch mounting systems that are most frequently used are (1) the flexible gooseneck; (2) the universal, which is clamped to a stationary surface and has add-on rods that can be adjusted to various configurations by turning knobs at one to five or six joints (similar to a camera stand); (3) a caterpillar flexible mounting system with a clamp that can readily be transferred from a bed frame to a wheelchair (used mainly with pneumatic or sip and puff switches, in which the tubing is threaded through the center of the interlocking pieces); (4) interlocking mounting rods that can be adjusted for height, length, angles, and pressure (they usually have a clamp for desk or tray mounting, and some can be fitted into a wheelchair clamp); and (5) Velcro strips that can be attached to bed frames or wheelchair trays or desks and newly developed adhesives that prevent slippage on flat surfaces.

The technology team should review the many switch catalogs that usually include various mounting systems and/or versatile mounting kits before carefully selecting the most practical, accessible, safe, and adjustable system from the consumer and caregiver's perspective. Furthermore, it is highly recommended that the mounting system be checked frequently to ensure that all clamps and adjustments are secure.

SWITCHES FOR BATTERY-OPERATED DEVICES

Severely involved children are first introduced to AT when they use switches to control battery-operated toys. The use of switches and ATDs gives children the opportunity to interact with their environment by controlling appliances such as the television, thereby teaching cause and effect and increasing their independence. Children can interact with others by learning these skills and controlling aspects of their environment. Switch control is the first and essential component of introducing a child to ATDs, because they must be able to activate, control, and deactivate the device. To counter the possibility of learned helplessness, a child should be encouraged to perform many tasks independently and at a very early age. The introduction and use of simple access devices will promote the sense of accomplishment that is developmentally important, particularly for a child with any type of disability. Switches can also be used to help a severely involved child to learn head-righting control (Fig. 6-5).

Simple custom switches can be fabricated by therapists or rehabilitation engineers. The cost of materials can be less than $5.00, but the labor time may negate the savings and an off-the-shelf switch may be more economical if an appropriate one can be located for the particular needs of the consumer. The technology team should have a supply of different commercially available switches and mounting systems to use for evaluation purposes. (See Appendix 6-2 for additional information.)

Any commercially available battery-operated toy can be switch activated by using a battery adapter. A typical battery adapter has a copper disk at one end that is placed between the battery and the battery contact; the other end has a phone jack that is plugged into a switch (Fig. 6-6).

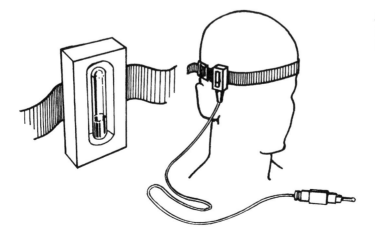

Figure 6-5. Mercury switches used to help a severely involved child to learn head-righting control.

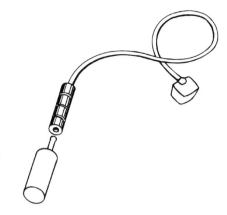

Figure 6-6. A typical battery adapter with a copper disk that is placed between the battery and the battery contact.

Jack adapters are also available in the event that the plugs are not the same size, and most of these adapters can be obtained at electronic stores. Additionally, series adapters are available that enable the consumer to activate two switches simultaneously, and many other configurations are possible with the flexible adapters and switches currently on the market.

Recently, a cordless switch became available that sends radio signals to either a battery-powered receiver (toy) or a small appliance receiver. The cordless switch can also be used with a "control unit" that has four modes of control; direct, timed seconds, timed minutes, and latch. The control unit connects electrical appliances to a switch for easy activation by plugging the control unit into a standard electrical outlet, plugging any switch into the control unit, or plugging any battery-operated toy or electrical appliance into the control unit (Fig. 6-7).

Figure 6-7. A cordless switch sends radio signals to either a battery-powered receiver (e.g., in a toy) or a small appliance receiver.

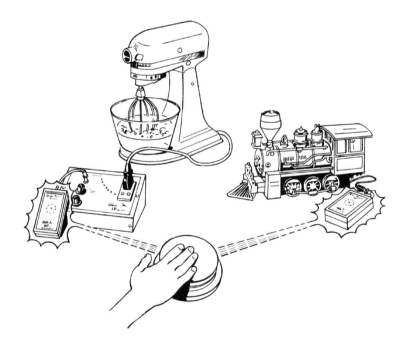

These are only a few switch and mounting suggestions. The possibilities are limited only by the creativity of the rehabilitation technology team, which includes the consumer and the caregiver. It is highly recommended that a member of the team contact AbleData for a list of switches.

REFERENCES

1. Wright C, Nomura M: From Toys to Computers: Access for the Physically Disabled Child. 2nd Ed. San Jose, CA, 1991

2. Bain BK: Technology. pp. 333–337. In Hopkins H, Smith H (eds): Willard and Spackman's Occupational Therapy. 8th Ed. Lippincott-Raven, Philadelphia, 1993

3. Webster JG, Cook AM, Tompkins WJ, Vanderheiden GC (eds): Electronic Devices for Rehabilitation. John Wiley & Sons, New York, 1985

4. Church G, Glennen S: The Handbook of Assistive Technology. Singular Publishing, San Diego, 1992

SUGGESTED READINGS

Angelo J: Assistive Technology for Rehabilitation Therapists. FA Davis, Philadelphia, 1997

Burkhart L: Homemade Battery Powered Toys and Educational Devices for Severely Handicapped Children. Special Needs Project, Santa Barbara, CA, 1989

Cook A, Hussey S: Assistive Technologies: Principles and Practice. Mosby, St. Louis, 1995

Goossens' C, Crain SS: Utilizing Switch Interfaces with Children Who Are Severely Physically Challenged. Zygo Industries, Portland, OR, 1992

Lee K, Thomas D: Control of Computer-Based Technology for People with Physical Disabilities. University of Toronto Press, Toronto, 1990

McGregor G, Arango GA, Fraser B, Kangas K: Physical Characteristics Assessment: Computer Access for Individuals with Cerebral Palsy. Don Johnston Inc., Wauconda, IL, 1994

*Switch or Control Interface Evaluation**

Consumer Name _____ Name of Switch_____

Age _____   Disability_____

1.   Why does the (consumer/user) need or want this switch?

_____

_____

_____

2.   (a)   What is the <u>major</u> functional goal for using the switch?

_____

_____

_____

(b)   What are 2 secondary goals?

(1)   _____

_____

(2)   _____

_____

3.   Where will the user use the switch? (all environments)

_____

_____

4.   What type of feedback is <u>best</u> for the user? Why? _____

_____

_____

*Copyright 1994 BK Bain.

5. List 2 or 3 possible control sites/body parts the consumer/user <u>can</u> use to activate the

    switch (Be as specific as possible).

    (1) _____

    (2) _____

    (3) _____

6. How much force does the user have to activate the switch?
    minimum _____   moderate _____   maximum _____

7. How much contact surface does the switch require?
    under an inch _____   more than 1 inch _____   2 to 3 inches _____

8. Can the consumer hold the switch:
    3 to 5 seconds _____   6 to 8 seconds _____   10+ seconds _____

9. Can the consumer release the switch upon command?

10. Does the user need momentary or latching switch control?
    Explain.

    _____

    _____

    _____

11. Describe the <u>best</u> mounting system for the switch.

    (a) where _____

    _____

    (b) how _____

    _____

    (c) type _____

    _____

12.   List 3 activities that the user <u>can</u> perform with this switch.

(a)   _____

(b)   _____

(c)   _____

13.   How will using the switch as described above influence the consumer's function with respect to the following areas:

(a)   physical/motor   _____

       _____

(b)   psychosocial   _____

       _____

(c)   cognitive _____

       _____

(d)   social   _____

       _____

(e)   sensory-integrative _____

       _____

(f)   other areas (i.e. ADL, work, leisure, school)

       _____

       _____

       _____

       _____

Names of Evaluator(s)_____   Date _____

_____

Resources

MAJOR SWITCH MANUFACTURING COMPANIES

AbleNet Inc.
Minneapolis, MN
(800) 322-0956

APT Technology Inc.
(formerly Du-It)
Shreve, OH
(216) 567-2001

Crestwood Company
Milwaukee, WI
(414) 352-5678

Don Johnston, Inc.
Wauconda, IL
(800) 999-4660

Prentke Romich Co.
Wooster, OH
(800) 642-8255

Tash
Ajax, Ontario
(800) 463-5685

Toys for Special Children
Hastings-on-Hudson, NY
(914) 478-0960

Words+, Inc.
Palmdale, CA
(800) 869-8521

Zygo Industries, Inc.
Portland, OR
(800) 234-6006

JULIE S. DeMICCO
LINDA STERN

CHAPTER 7

Communication in the Workplace

Anne walked into the office at 9:00 am and started perusing her mail. At 9:05, her telephone rang. While talking on the phone to a customer, she glanced at her calendar and saw that she had a 9:30 meeting. At 9:15, her boss stopped by and they discussed a strategy for dealing with a difficult customer. Anne jotted down her boss's suggestions before joining the staff meeting.

Communication is considered the "lifeblood of every organization."[1] Can you imagine a day spent without talking to someone in person or on the telephone, writing a memo, reading a letter, writing important reminder notes, or entering data into a computer? The above segment of Anne's workday is not atypical.

In a recent analysis of the help wanted advertisements in the *National Business Employment Weekly*, a publication of *The Wall Street Journal*, 71 percent of the job listings included specific communication skills that were essential for the job described.[2] Vital communication is omnipresent in the workplace. What happens when there are individuals who have impairments that may interfere with their ability to communicate effectively? What happens to Sam, who recently had a laryngectomy (removal of the larynx) and has almost inaudible speech production? Or Sally, who has cerebral palsy and cannot use a standard computer keyboard? How is Bob, who is visually impaired, going to read that important memo the boss just sent? And what about Joseph, who cannot hear over a standard telephone? The purpose of this chapter is to explore the assistive technology devices (ATDs) that may be used by people with visual, hearing, speech, and/or motoric impairments to enable them to communicate effectively in the workplace, at home, and at school. This section focuses primarily on workplace adaptations.

Technology has provided many persons with disabilities the opportunity to enter or return to the workplace. For example, Ted lost his vision when he was in his mid 40s. Without technology, Ted would be unable to have his present successful career as a travel agent. He uses a talking calculator to quote prices of trips, a tape recorder with raised symbols to record client information, and a talking computer to retrieve and store information on trips, clients, and expenditures. These three devices, along with a telephone, have allowed Ted to remain a viable and productive member of the workforce. Assistive technology (AT) has contributed dramatically to increasing the quality of his life.

LEGISLATION

With the passage of the Americans with Disabilities Act (ADA) of 1990, employers, employees, and potential employees must be cognizant of the available options for people with impairments that interfere with their ability to communicate. As discussed by Witt,[3] a recent Harris poll indicated that 23 percent of individuals with disabilities who are *not* working or who are working part-time stated that they lack equipment that would assist them in communicating with others.

Both Title I and Title IV of the ADA are related to communication. Title IV requires that telephone companies provide telecommunications relay services 24 hours a day, 365 days a year to individuals who have impairments with hearing and/or speech production.[3] Title I of the ADA strives to protect individuals with physical or mental impairments from discrimination in the workplace. Individuals who have difficulty performing communication tasks essential in the workplace may require reasonable accommodations when applying for a job, being trained for a position, and/or performing a job. The ADA defines reasonable accommodations as "a modification or adjustment to a job, the work environment, or the way things usually are done that enables a qualified individual with a disability to enjoy an equal employment opportunity."[4]

REASONABLE ACCOMMODATIONS

The following reasonable accommodations related to communication in the workplace are examples outlined by the Equal Employment Opportunity Commission.[5]

- Telephone amplifiers for people with hearing impairments
- Special software on computers to enlarge print or convert print to spoken words for people with visual limitations
- Speakerphones for individuals whose mobility may be limited
- Training materials on tape or in large print for the visually impaired
- Tape recorders if a written examination is required during the job application process, so that a person with visual impairments or decreased motoric capabilities may record test answers

TYPES OF COMMUNICATION

The ADA highlights the need to be aware of existing technology. Before discussing the specific ATDs to facilitate communication, it is important to consider the two general types of communication in the workplace.[1] The first is internal communication to other employees in the same organization.

Internal communication is critical in relaying information within the company, informing people of meetings and other important events, building morale, providing training information, and relaying recommendations. The second type of communication is external messages to people outside the company. Good communication is essential to attract and retain customers, do business with other companies, and manage the inventory and financial control of any organization.[1]

Internal and external communication can be either verbal and/or nonverbal. Nonverbal communication includes appearance, body language, facial expressions, gestures, postures, smell, voice quality, use of silence, timing, and sounds such as laughter and clearing the throat.[1] Both verbal and nonverbal communication can be affected by the impairments discussed above. For example, a person with multiple sclerosis may be able to handwrite a note to a customer, but due to decreased fine motor coordination, there are frequent crossouts and the paper gets somewhat crumpled. Is there a nonverbal message that may inadvertently be communicated here (e.g., the person is careless)? Use of a computer may enhance the impression given by this otherwise well-qualified worker in her relations with customers and coworkers.

ELEMENTS OF COMMUNICATION

In addition to understanding the components of communication, it is also critical to review the elements of communication. According to Murphy and Hildebrandt,[1] the five elements are

- **Sender-encoder**—This refers to the person who initiates the communication (e.g., the writer or the speaker).
- **Message**—As discussed above, the message can be verbal (written or spoken) or nonverbal.
- **Channel and medium**—This refers to how the message is sent. For example, information within an organization to coworkers could be conveyed in a memo, through electronic mail, through company newsletters, through a group conference, and/or through a personal telephone call to each employee.
- **Receiver-decoder**—This is the person who receives the message (the reader or listener).
- **Feedback**—The receiver of the message will generally react in one way or another. When considering ATDs for persons with disabilities, it is necessary to consider all the above aspects of communication. For example, a person with dysarthria (poor speech production resulting from impairments in the tongue or other muscles related to speech) may feel comfortable communicating verbally and the family may understand him or her well. Yet, the less familiar listener (receiver-decoder) in the workplace must ask the speaker to repeat her- or himself frequently and must strain to understand the speaker. This is far from effective communication in the workplace and may place the speaker at a competitive disadvantage.

CATEGORIES

Before researching ATDs, it is first essential to conceptualize and organize the types of communication in the workplace. Table 7-1 categorizes communication into seven major areas: face-to-face, telephone, printed, handwritten, computer-generated, paged communication, and miscellaneous (videos, slides, charts, etc.). Within each overall communications category,

Table 7-1. Types of Communication in the Workplace

Communication Category	Types of Communication within Category	Tasks That May Present a Problem for Individuals with Visual, Hearing, Speech, and/or Motoric Impairments
Face-to-face communications	One-to-one	Listening
	Group	Speaking
	Videoconferencing	
Telephone communications	One-to-one	Listening
	Conference call	Speaking
	Speakerphone	Picking up/ putting down receiver
	Voice mail	Holding receiver
	Answering machine	Dialing
		Reading/seeing numbers
		Reading message light, numbers on display
Printed communications	Business cards	Reading
	Rolodex cards	Typing
	Mail	Turning pages
	Newsletters	For photocopier/fax:
	Magazines	Operating buttons
	Books	Installing paper
	Memos/letters	Feeding document
	Newspapers	Removing document
	Catalogs	
	File cabinet labels	
	Tabs on hanging folders	
	Labels on manila folders	
	Computer printouts	
	Photocopied documents	
	Faxed documents	

(Table continues.)

Table 7-1. *(Continued)*

Communication Category	Types of Communication within Category	Tasks That May Present a Problem for Individuals with Visual, Hearing, Speech, and/or Motoric Impairments
Handwritten communications	Phone messages	Writing with pen/pencil
	Notes	Reading
	Memos/letters	Stabilizing paper
	Photocopied documents	Detaching paper from pad
	Faxed documents	For photocopier/fax:
		Operating buttons
		Installing paper
		Feeding document
		Removing document
Computer-generated communications (on screen and/or paper)	Electronic mail	Reading screen
	Telecommunications	Reading printed document
	Memos	Reading keyboard
	Letters	Inputting/accessing via keyboard/mouse
	Reports	Listening (auditory feedback)
	Data entry	Inserting disk
		Turning computer on/off
Paged communications	Beepers	Listening (receiver)
	Office intercom	Speaking (sender-intercom)
		Dialing/operating
		Reading (display on beeper)
Miscellaneous	Videos	Reading
	Slides/overheads	Seeing
	Charts/easels	Listening

types (channels) are itemized. For example, under telephone communications, the following types are listed: one-to-one, conference call, speakerphone, voice mail, and answering machine. It is important to remember that no one list can be all-inclusive of the vast array of communication channels available in a business environment.

The last column in Table 7-1 is the most critical. It provides a brief activity analysis, a tool commonly used by interdisciplinary team members, for each communication category. In an activity analysis, each activity is closely examined and divided into distinct components. For example, the components of telephone communication include picking up the

Table 7-2. Assistive Devices for Individuals with Visual Impairments

Devices	Tasks Addressed						Communication Category				
	Seeing	Dialing	Reading	Typing	Writing	Inputting	Face-to-Face	Telephone	Printed	Handwritten	Computer Generated
TeleTalker Enhanced Telephone Amplifier (with large buttons)	✓	✓						✓			
Basic Clarity Phone	✓	✓						✓			
3M Braille Labeler	✓		✓						✓		
Perkins Brailler	✓	✓	✓	✓					✓	✓	
Handi-cassette Recorder/Player			✓	✓					✓	✓	
Optelec 20/20 Optelec 20/20+	✓		✓		✓				✓	✓	
The Reading Edge	✓		✓					✓			
Braille 'n Speak			✓		✓						
MAGIC			✓						✓		
Zoom Caps										✓	
Speaqualizer Speech Synthesizer			✓								✓
Intelli Keys	✓			✓		✓					✓
Max-Eye Portable Handheld Electronic Magnifier	✓		✓					✓	✓	✓	
Page Magnifier	✓		✓					✓	✓	✓	
Big Button Plus Phone		✓					✓				
Voice Dialer		✓					✓				

Manufacturer/ Dealer Phone	1996 Price Range
Williams Sound Corp. 800-328-6190	$$
HELLO Direct 800-444-3556	$
The Lighthouse Inc. 800-829-0500	$
Howe Press 617-924-3434	$$$
American Printing House for the Blind 800-223-1839	$$
C-Tech 800-228-7798	$$$$
C-Tech 800-228-7798	$$$$
American Printing House for the Blind 800-223-1839	$$$
Microsystems Software, Inc. 800-828-0500	$$
American Foundation for the Blind Product Center 800-829-2600	$
American Printing House for the Blind 800-223-1839	$$$
Intelli Tools, Inc. 800-899-6687	$$
C-Tech 800-228-7798	$$$
S + S Adapt Ability 800-266-8856	$
HELLO Direct 800-444-3556	$
HELLO Direct 800-444-3556	$$

Key: $, Less than $100; $$, $100–500; $$$, $501–1500; $$$$, $1501+.

Table 7-3. Assistive Devices for Individuals with Hearing Impairments

Devices	Tasks Addressed		Communication Category	
	Listening	Speaking	Telephone	Computer
43-178 Fone Flasher	✓		✓	
Basic Clarity Phone	✓		✓	
Telebraille III	✓	✓	✓	
Teletalker Telephone Amplifier System Large Buttons	✓		✓	
XB-1 Transmission Booster (voice amplifier)	✓	✓	✓	
43-237 Compact Handset Amplifier	✓		✓	
Call Alert	✓		✓	
Deluxe Vari Tone Ringers (Telephone Signal)	✓		✓	
In-Line Handset Amplifier	✓		✓	
Telephone Hearing Amplifier	✓		✓	
Amplifier Handset	✓		✓	
Dialogue VCO	✓		✓	
Pocketalker Pro System	✓		✓	
AT&T Advanced TTY	✓	✓	✓	
WIO In-Line Amplifier series	✓		✓	
Speech Adjuster Tone	✓		✓	
SeeBeep Software	✓			✓
Big Button Plus Phone	✓		✓	
Call Signaling Device	✓		✓	
Sure Sound Tone/Volume Amplifier	✓		✓	

Manufacturer/ Dealer Phone	1996 Price Range
Radio Shack Division of Tandy Corp. 800-843-7422 or local Radio Shack	$
HELLO Direct 800-444-3556	$
Telesensory Corp. 800-227-8418	$$$$
Williams Sound Corp. 800-328-6190	$399.00 (headset option $90.00)
RDM Sales 213-851-2786	$
Radio Shack Division of Tandy Corp. 800-843-7422 or local Radio Shack	$
Ameriphone 714-897-0808	$
Communications Products and Equipment Company 800-833-4273	$
Ameriphone 714-897-0808	$
S+S Adapt Ability 800-266- 8856	$
Ameriphone 714-897-0808	$
Ameriphone 714-897-0808	$$
Williams Sound Corp. 800- 843-3544	$$
HELLO Direct 800-444-3556	$$
Walker Equipment Corp. 800-426-3738	$
HARC Mercantile, LTD 800-445-9968	$$
Microsystems Software, Inc. 800-828-2600	$
HELLO Direct 800-444-3556	$
HELLO Direct 800-444- 3556	$
HELLO Direct 800- 444-3556	$

Key: $, Less than $100; $$, $100–500; $$$, $501–1500; $$$$, $1501+.

Table 7-4. Assistive Devices for Individuals with Visual and Hearing Impairments

Devices	Tasks Addressed		Communication Category	Manufacturer/ Dealer Phone	1996 Price Range
	Listening	Speaking	Face-to-Face		
Telebraille III	✓	✓	✓	Telesensory Corp. 800-227-8418	$$$$

Key: $$$$, $1501+.

receiver, reading/seeing numbers, dialing, listening, speaking, holding the receiver, putting down the receiver, and reading message lights/phone numbers on display.

Once the components of a task such as telephone communication are identified, it is then important to examine the skills needed to perform the activity.[6] For example, a person with quadriplegia (paralysis of all four extremities and the trunk) will have difficulty picking up/putting down a telephone receiver, dialing, and holding the receiver on a conventional telephone. Therefore, this individual would need ATDs to accomplish these components of the task.

Tables 7-2 to 7-6 focus on ATDs that may be used by persons with visual, hearing, visual and hearing, speech, and motoric deficits, respectively, to increase their ability to communicate in the workplace. These tables explain the specific ATDs, vendors, 1996 price range, and the various tasks around the office they address. We have included both devices that

Table 7-5. Assistive Devices for Individuals with Speech Impairments

Devices	Tasks Addressed	Communication Category		Manufacturer/ Dealer Phone	1996 Price Range
	Speaking	Face-to-Face	Telephone		
HandiCHAT Software	✓	✓		Microsystems Software, Inc. 800-828-2600	$$$
Intelli Talk with Speech	✓	✓		Intelli Tools, Inc. 800-899-6687	$
Speechmaker Personal Speech Amplifier	✓	✓		HARC 800-445-9968	$$
XB-1 Transmission Booster	✓		✓	RDM Sales 213-851-2786	

Key: $, Less than $100; $$, $100–500; $$$, $501–1500.

are "low" technology (e.g., a plastic pencil grip) and "high" technology (e.g., a sophisticated communication device). The ATDs in the charts are organized by overall communication category as outlined in Table 7-1. Also highlighted are the relevant types of communication within each category.

APPLICATION

The practical use of these tables is shown in the following example. An employer of a person with a visual impairment may refer to Table 7-2 and identify the communication category of concern: telephone communications. The employer may perform a market search and conclude that a "big button" telephone would be ideal to assist the employee in the task of "seeing" the telephone keypad.

Because there is a plethora of ATDs in the marketplace, these tables only provide an overview for the person with a disability, the allied health professional, and/or the employer. Manufacturers or vendors may be contacted for a more complete listing of products available. In addition, resources for more information are provided at the end of Chapter 8.

Arnold discussed the perceived disadvantages faced by any prospective worker (with or without a disability) who lacks training on the latest technology that a company uses. She recommends that both employers and workers remember that "success in business will depend, as it always has, upon words, not technology."[2] In this way, one can say that it is the disabled person's words (the message) that count, not the technology or method used to produce those words. The technology is the enabler to express the words and thoughts already present within the individual.

Let us take another look at Anne, the worker discussed in the introduction to this chapter. If Anne were a person with sensory, speech, and/or motoric impairments, she could still accomplish her job functions with the use of an ATD such as that described in the tables. For example, if Anne were visually impaired, she could use a telephone with large numbers and a braille dot on the number five for easy orientation. She may also use a *Perkins Brailler* for jotting down her boss's suggestions and writing down her appointments. Anne may also have a magnifier to enlarge the written copy on her mail. If Anne were hearing impaired, she may use a teletypewriter for her telephone communications. If Anne were speech impaired, she might use a speech amplifier for face-to-face communications and a transmission booster for telephone communications to increase the volume of her voice. If Anne were motorically impaired, a specially equipped computer work station would enable her to pick up/put down the telephone receiver, dial, type notes, and access written information via the use of a special input device such as a chin control.

All the above devices could be effectively used in the office environment for a reasonable cost to the employer. Home-based employment is another option for consumers of AT. "Recent advances in assistive and computer technology have spurred a renewed interest in home-based computer work for persons with disabilities."[7]

Communication is an essential element of every organization, and without ATDs it would be impossible for millions of people with visual, hearing, speech, and/or motoric impairments.

Table 7-6. Assistive Devices for Individuals with Motoric Impairments

Devices	Tasks Addressed							Communication Category		
	Picking Up/Putting Down Receiver	Dialing	Holding Receiver	Writing	Stabilizing Paper	Inputting via Keyboard or Mouse	Turning Pages/Cards	Telephone	Printed	Computer Generated
Quad Quip	✓							✓		
Remote Control Speakerphone Model RC 3000	✓	✓						✓		
Slip-On Keyboard Aid		✓						✓		
T-140 Series Puff & Sip Speakerphones	✓	✓						✓		
LIAISON Computer Workstation	✓	✓	✓		✓	✓		✓		✓
E.A.S.I. DIALER #2110	✓	✓						✓		
Handiphone System Windows	✓	✓						✓		
Fone Holder			✓					✓		
Contour Rheumatics Pen				✓				✓		
One-Handed Writing Board					✓			✓		
Triangular Pen/Pencil Grip				✓				✓		
HandiKey						✓			✓	
Headmaster Plus						✓			✓	
Handishift Software						✓			✓	
Keyguard						✓				✓
Ergorest Articulating Arm Support						✓				✓
Macintosh Touch Window						✓				✓
The Eyegaze Computer System						✓				✓

Manufacturer/ Dealer Phone	1996 Price Range
Sammons Preston 800-323-5547	$
Ameriphone, Inc. 714-897-0808	$$
Sammons Preston 800-323-5547	$
Environmental Control, Inc.	$295.00 to $475.00
APT Technology Inc. 216-567-2001	$$$$
TASH, Inc. 905-686-2600	$$$
Microsystems Software, Inc. 800-828-2600	$$
Sammons Preston 800-323-5547	$
Sammons Preston 800-323-5547	$
Sammons Preston 800-323-5547	$
Sammons Preston 800-323-5547	$
Microsystems Software, Inc. 800-828-2600	$$
Prentke Romich 800-262-1984	$$$
Microsystems Software, Inc. 800-828-2600	$
TASH, Inc. 800-463-5685	$
Sammons Preston 800-323-5547	$$
Don Johnston Development Equip. 800-999-4660	$$
LC Technologies, Inc. 800-733-5284	$$$$

(Table continues.)

Table 7-6. *(Continued)*

Devices	Picking Up/Putting Down Receiver	Dialing	Holding Receiver	Writing	Stabilizing Paper	Inputting via Keyboard or Mouse	Turning Pages/Cards	Telephone	Printed	Computer Generated
Co-Writer Software for the Macintosh						✓				✓
Select-Ease Keyboard						✓				✓
Dragon Dictate for Windows						✓				✓
Slip-On Typing Keyboard Aid						✓				✓
Ke:nx 2.0						✓				✓
Intelli Keys						✓				✓
Mini-Keyboard						✓				✓
Next Page Turner #4600							✓		✓	
Vacuum Wand							✓		✓	
Electronic Rolodex File/Organizer							✓		✓	
Desktop Rolodex Database							✓		✓	

Tasks Addressed spans columns "Picking Up/Putting Down Receiver" through "Turning Pages/Cards"; *Communication Category* spans "Telephone," "Printed," and "Computer Generated."

REFERENCES

1. Murphy HA, Hildebrandt HW: Effective Business Communications. 5th Ed. McGraw-Hill, New York, 1988

2. Arnold VD: The communication competencies listed in job descriptions. Bull Assoc Business Communication LV(2):15–18, 1992

3. Witt MA: Job Strategies for People with Disabilities. Peterson's Guides, Princeton, NJ, 1992

4. Americans with Disabilities Act (ADA) of 1990. PL 101-336, Title 42 U.S.C. 12101 et seq: U.S. Statutes at Large, 104, 327–378, July 26, 1990

Manufacturer/ Dealer Phone	1996 Price Range
Don Johnston Developmental Equip. 800-999-4660	$$
Sammons Preston 800-323-5547	$$
Dragon Dictate 800-TALK-TYP	Personal Edition $$ Classic Edition $$$ Power Edition $$$$
Sammons Preston 800-323-5547	$
Don Johnston Developmental Equip. 800-999-4660	$$$
Intelli Tools, Inc. 800-899-6687	$$
Don Johnston Developmental Equip. 800-999-4660	$$
TASH, Inc. 905-686-4129	$$$$
Sammons Preston 800-323-5547	$
Reliable Home Office 800-869-6000	$$
Reliable Home Office 800-869-6000	$$

Key: $, Less than $100; $$, $100–500; $$$, $501–1500; $$$$, $1501+.

5. Equal Employment Opportunity Commission: A Technical Assistance Manual on the Employment Provisions (Title I) of the Americans with Disabilities Act. EEOC, Washington, DC, 1992

6. Trombly CA: Activity selection and analysis. pp. 303–310. In Trombly CA (ed): Occupational Therapy for Physical Dysfunction. Williams & Wilkins, Baltimore, 1989

7. Vagnoni J, Horvath L: Home-based employment for persons needing assistive technology. Technol Disability 1(4):77–84, 1992

CHAPTER 8

LINDA STERN

Telephone Communications in the Home

A VITAL LINK TO THE OUTSIDE WORLD

89

Telephone
Communications
in the Home:
A Vital Link to the
Outside World

Within a few seconds, the telephone can provide us with a communication link to the outside world and linkages to other people, connecting homes to schools, workplaces, and the community. The word *telephone* is derived from two Greek words meaning *far* and *sound*.[1] The telephone helps bring people who are a physical distance from one another closer together, thereby lessening isolation and enhancing communication. The telephone provides a means for socialization, allows us to conduct our personal business, and provides access to emergency resources when needed. The use of the telephone is critical to everyone but is particularly crucial for persons with disabilities who may be more physically and socially isolated. Since Alexander Graham Bell patented the telephone in 1876, phone usage has exhibited steady growth, skyrocketing from 700 telephones in the United States in 1877 to more than 110 million telephones in the United States by 1990.[2]

The home telephone is critical for convenience, socialization, and conducting personal business. It is also crucial for safety and security.[3] For example, individuals may need to summon help due to illness, falls, burglary, assault, etc.; in fact the first telephone exchange in 1877 started as an adjunct to a burglar alarm system.[2] Both the psychosocial and safety needs for a telephone are particularly crucial for individuals with physical, sensory, and/or cognitive disabilities. Different categories of communication and the problems faced by persons with disabilities are presented in Table 7-1.

A study by Mann et al[4] examined the role the home telephone plays in the life of frail elders. Almost 10 percent of the sample of 354 frail elders were having some difficulty with the usage of the telephone. The problems these elders experienced were visual, mobile (not being able to answer the telephone in time), fine motor, cognitive, hearing, safety (e.g., wiring across floor), and miscellaneous issues such as interfering background noise. During intervention, all the phone-related problems were solvable with existing commercially available products, at an average equipment cost of $70.45 (exclusive of personnel time).

This chapter reviews five disability categories: hearing, visual, speech, motor, and cognitive impairments. Each of these categories is reviewed with respect to potential problems individuals within the disability category may have accessing the telephone, and possible product/service solutions are discussed. The tables in Chapter 7 are also referred to throughout this chapter. A resource list with company names and telephone numbers is included in Appendix 8-1 for reference purposes.

Many products are readily available through local stores or through consumer catalogs. In addition, local telephone companies are an excellent resource for products/services that assist people with disabilities with telephone access. For example, in New York City there is a Communication Center for People with Disabilities, where a plethora of information on products is available at cost (with shipping and handling costs waived) to people with disabilities. At the center, various smaller products (e.g., a magnifying glass for the visually impaired) are also given for free. In addition, specific telephone company services are available at no charge to persons with disabilities and are usually delineated in the front pages of most telephone directories.

The products and services offered through the local telephone company are generally available to persons with a "certified" disability. To qualify, a consumer would need to have their disability certified by a licensed physician, specialist (e.g., a speech pathologist), or an authorized agency. In addition, there is often an application form to complete.

The products mentioned below are included for instructive purposes only and are not intended to be inclusive of all products available or as product endorsements. In addition, similar products are often provided by more than one company.

HEARING IMPAIRMENTS

Individuals with hearing impairments may experience difficulty hearing the ringer on the telephone or hearing the person on the other end of the telephone. The type of technological solution to this difficulty depends on the degree of hearing loss (see Table 7-2). Additionally, Table 7-3 provides information for persons with both visual and hearing impairments.

Many consumer products are commercially available to aid persons with hearing impairments. Many companies sell or lease telephones that have a hearing aid–compatible handset. There may be technical difficulties that prevent persons with hearing aids from using plain handsets, because they may cause feedback. Some hearing aid–compatible handsets are equipped with a voice coil that generates a magnetic signal that will eliminate the clarity problem common with most handsets.

Increasing the volume of the incoming voice on a telephone does not necessarily address the issue of clarity of the incoming voice. Some products are available that give the consumer the flexibility of adjusting the frequency for maximum clarity. One such telephone has several critical features that address the needs of a person with impaired hearing. It amplifies a caller's voice up to 10 times as loud as a standard phone while suppressing background noises. The user can adjust ringer loudness as well as tone control. There is also a red indicator light that flashes with each ring, providing a visual signal that a call is incoming. This type of indicator light or amplified ringer is commonly available from many telephone companies.

Teletypewriters (TTYs) are critically important for many persons with hearing impairments. This equipment (also called telecommunication devices for the deaf [TDD]) sends typewritten words over telephone lines to another TTY. A TTY consists of "a small computer with a screen, keyboard, and modem. To communicate, there must be a TDD at each end of the telephone line. ... At one end, the sender types a message into the telephone system. At the other end, the message is visible as a line of text on a special telephone equipped with an LCD readout display."[5]

Relay services enable a person with a TTY to speak with a person without a TTY and vice versa through the use of a hearing operator (called a communications assistant) who uses a TTY. This relay service vastly increases the telephone communication capabilities of persons with hearing impairments.[5] Many TTYs are available commercially, including a 24-character mini-printer, a portable TTY, and a pocket-sized TDD. Another sophisticated TTY is available that offers a combination TTY text telephone/TTY answering machine that can also be used as a regular telephone.

In addition to providing many products at cost, local phone companies may also reduce phone usage charges for consumers who are hearing impaired and use a TTY. Telephone directory listings may also indicate the presence of a TTY.

91

Telephone
Communications
in the Home:
A Vital Link to the
Outside World

VISUAL IMPAIRMENTS

Individuals with visual impairments may have difficulty seeing and reading the telephone dial (and thus dialing correctly), seeing and reading telephone numbers from the telephone book, and reading telephone bills.

Most telephone companies offer the following aids free of charge: enlarged number rings for rotary phones; enlarged stick-on numbers for push-button phone keypads; a magnifying glass; and a dial "0" overlay that fits over the standard push-button keypad, allowing the user to access the operator when any key is pressed.

Persons with visual impairments may also be exempt from specific telephone service charges. For example, some phone companies may provide a special phone credit card that allows operator-assisted calls from pay phones at the lower direct-dial rate. There may be exemptions from directory assistance charges, and dial operator privileges may be provided free of charge. Braille and large-print bills may also be available. The consumer, caregiver, and/or technology team should contact the local telephone company to determine the services available and their cost if any.

Products for consumers with visual impairments—particularly large button keypads—are frequently available in department stores that sell telephones (see Table 7-2). For example, some stores have telephones with extra-large buttons that may also feature three color-coded emergency buttons. The braille "flashing" telephone has oversized buttons and braille characters. Another telephone has a large-number keypad and provides a color choice of white with black numbers, ash with gray numbers, and white numbers with a black background. Some telephone companies also provide large-print telephone books on request.

SPEECH IMPAIRMENTS

Persons with speech impairments may have difficulty expressing themselves clearly to the person on the receiving end of the telephone. Understanding a person with a speech impairment when he or she uses the telephone is generally more difficult than in person due to the lack of visual cues (e.g., observing lip movements or environmental context). One type of product that is available is a headset/amplifier that increases the volume of the speaker's voice for consumers with a soft or weak voice.

Another product of unique value to a person who has had a laryngectomy is a hand-held lightweight device that can be used to reproduce the sound of the voice when held to the speaker's throat. This equipment, which has a wide frequency range, can be used to communicate both in person and on the telephone.

TTYs and fax machines can also be invaluable for a person with a speech impairment (see Table 7-5). In addition, local telephone companies may have reduced telephone usage charges for customers who have a speech disability and use a TTY. The telephone company may also provide listings for TTY users.

MOTOR IMPAIRMENTS

The difficulties that a person with motor impairments may encounter when using a telephone are multifold and may even preclude use of this important communication device. The problem areas include picking up and putting down the receiver, holding the receiver, and dialing. In addition, the consumer may have difficulty getting to the telephone before it stops ringing.

A raised push-button grid and a dial "0" overlay (fits over push-button keypad and dials the operator when any key is pressed) may be available free of charge from local telephone companies to persons with certified motion disabilities. In addition, consumers with disabilities may be exempt from charges for making operator-assisted calls from a pay telephone, for directory assistance, and for operator assistance from home telephones.

The level of technology involved in assisting a person with a motoric impairment varies according to the severity of the disability (see Table 7-6). The following are some "off-the-shelf" solutions to milder problems. A giant push-button telephone adapter with larger push-buttons that have more space between each number is useful for some persons with disabilities, as are large-button telephones that can be accessed with a mouthstick or pointer. Telephone shoulder rests help to ease shoulder stiffness and pain. Many companies also sell headsets that can reduce telephone fatigue and provide for freedom of the hands. Headsets are available in both corded and cordless versions.

Many products and services are also available for individuals who may have difficulty getting to the telephone in time. For example, leather holders are available that allow an individual to hook a cordless phone to his or her pants or belt. Some companies sell cordless phones that can be equipped with a headset (Fig. 8-1), and the handset can hook onto the user's belt or clothing. Telephone companies also provide a service that allows an individual to access the last number that called—in the event that the person is unable to answer the phone before it stops ringing. An answering machine is another useful device for persons who cannot respond quickly to a ringing telephone.

Specialty companies produce telephones that address the needs of consumers who are more physically involved. One product allows for sip'n'puff calling (Fig. 8-2). A person sips into the mouthpiece to initiate an outgoing call. Then he or she would puff gently to connect to the operator (who would dial the number). The conversation would be ended by sipping into the device. Phones can also be equipped to respond to a verbal command: the consumer says "Hello" from anywhere in the home any time after the second ring to answer the phone. Conversely, phones can be instructed to make outgoing phone calls using verbal commands.

Remote-control speakerphones are available for persons with disabilities. These are hands-free speakerphones designed specifically for individuals who are disabled and/or elderly. A remote-control telephone has one-touch remote control for dialing and answering and provides hands-free conversations from up to 15 ft away. Assistive technology devices (ATDs) such as a sip-and-puff switch, pressure foot switch, and lapel microphone can be used to control this type of telephone.

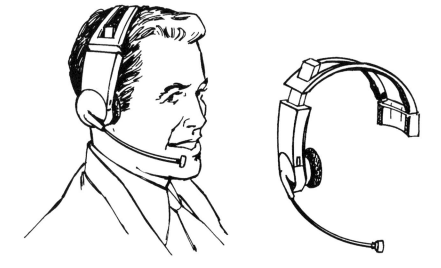

93

Telephone
Communications
in the Home:
A Vital Link to the
Outside World

Figure 8-1. Cordless telephone equipped with a headset.

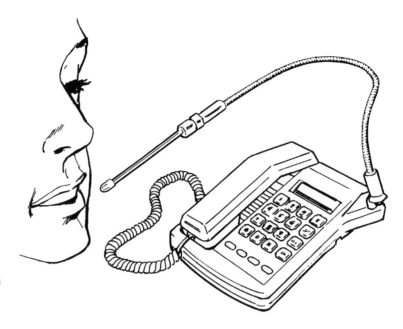

Figure 8-2. Telephone equipped with a sip'n'puff device.

An expanded use of the telephone is through an environmental control unit (ECU). ECUs are "a means to purposefully manipulate and interact with the environment by alternatively accessing one or more electrical devices via switches, voice activation, remote control, computer interface, and other technological adaptations … in order to maximize functional ability and independence in the home, school, work, and leisure environment."[3] One of these appliances is the telephone. Access to the ECU can be through switches, computer interface, voice activation, chin controllers, tongue/lip controllers, etc. (see the Resources list at the end of this chapter for a listing of major ECUs that have telephone capabilities).

COGNITIVE IMPAIRMENTS

The most significant problems faced by a person with cognitive impairments when using a telephone are remembering telephone numbers, locating the telephone, and having difficulty understanding the functions on more complex telephones. One feature of most commercially available telephones is memory dialing. Only a single button needs to be pushed to access a particular number, eliminating the need to remember the entire phone number. The amount of memory for easy speed-dialing varies between telephone models. A speed-calling service may also be available from the local phone company. This allows the consumer to dial frequently called numbers by using either a one- or two-digit code. In addition to memory dialing, telephones may also have one-button access for emergency numbers. For example, some telephones have colored emergency symbols on keys 1–2–3 for one-button access to the fire department, police, and medical alert. If an individual cannot remember where he or she has placed a cordless telephone handset, a paging feature can be used that sends an audio signal from the telephone base to the handset and prompts a beeping or alarm.

CONCLUSION

In the home, telephones are a link to communication with others. Rehabilitation professionals can profoundly affect the life of consumers with limited access to the telephone by enabling them to use this important communication medium through readily available products and services. It is recommended that rehabilitation professionals and/or consumers check with local telephone companies to discern which products and services are available and whether the consumer is eligible for discounted or free services.

REFERENCES

1. The World Book Encyclopedia. Vol. 19. World Book Inc., Chicago, 1995

2. Encyclopedia Americana. Vol. 26. Grolier, Danbury, CT, 1991

3. Bain BK: Technology. pp. 333–337. In Hopkins H, Smith H (eds): Willard and Spackman's Occupational Therapy. 8th Ed. Lippincott-Raven, Philadelphia, 1993

4. Mann WC, Hurren D, Charvat B, Tomita M: The use of phones by elders with disabilities: problems, interventions, costs. Assis Technol 8(1):23–33, 1996

5. Mann WC, Lane JP: Assistive Technology for Persons with Disabilities: The Role of Occupational Therapy. American Occupational Therapy Association, Rockville, MD, 1991

95

Telephone
Communications
in the Home:
A Vital Link to the
Outside World

Resources

TRACE Resource Book, 1996-97 Edition
(608) 263-2309

New York Telephone Communication Center
  for People with Disabilities
(800) 482-9020

Lucent Technologies Accessible Communication
(800) 233-1222

Formerly AT&T Special Needs Center
National center for communications products

TELEPHONES & RELATED PRODUCTS

Communication Products & Equipment Company, Inc.
(800) 033-4273

Tel-Ease

Hear You Are, Inc.
(201) 347-7662

Catalog of products for hearing-impaired
adults and children

HELLO Direct
(800) 444-3556

Catalog of telephone productivity tools

HITEC Group International
(708) 654-9200

Call Alert; Miniprint 425;
Big Button Plus Telephone;
The Remote Control Speakerphone
(Model RC 3000)

IBM Phone Communicator
(800) 426-4832

Dials, prints, and saves telephone conversation on
IBM-compatible computer screen (for individuals
with hearing & speech impairments)

The Lighthouse Inc.
(800) 829-0500

The Big Button Braille Flashing Telephone;
Big Print Address/Telephone Book

RDM Sales
(210) 051-2706

XBI Transmission Booster

Reliable Office Solutions
(800) 735-4000

Telephone shoulder rests

Sammons Preston
(800) 323-5547

Telephone adapter with larger push buttons

The Sharper Image
(800) 344-4444

Receiver hook, cordless phone with headset

Siemens Hearing Instruments, Inc.
(800) 333-9083

Servox

Temasek Telephone, Inc.
(415) 075-6666

Sip'n' puff calling; Tell It To Answer phone;
Tell It To Call phone

Walker Equipment Corporation
(800) 426-3738

High-frequency Clarity Telephones;
W7 Series Transmit Amplifier

ENVIRONMENTAL CONTROL UNITS (ECU) WITH TELEPHONE CAPABILITIES

APT Technology Inc.
(216) 567-2001

Liaison, Deuce

Madenta
(403) 450-8926

Proxi

Prentke Romich
(800) 262-1984

Control I and HECS-I, EZ Phone Director
& Scanning Director

97

Telephone
Communications
in the Home:
A Vital Link to the
Outside World

Quartet Technology, Inc.
(508) 692-9313
Simplicity 5,6,7 Series

Salko
(602) 731-9805
SenSei

TASH
(800) 463-5685
Unidialer, Kincontrol, Relax

Teledyne Brown
(800) 944-8002
Imperium 200H

Words +
(800) 869-8521
U-Control

CHAPTER 9

HILDY S. LIPNER

Augmentative and Alternative Communication

Tom is an 18-year-old with athetoid cerebral palsy and poor speech intelligibility who has just been accepted as a member of the incoming freshman class at his local university. In preparation for his entry into college, Tom requested an interdisciplinary assessment at an assistive technology (AT) resource center. The speech-language pathologist recommended a change from a dedicated to a computer-based augmentative communication system with additional word processing capability and capacity for environmental control. The physical therapist recommended necessary modifications to his powered wheelchair to accommodate the mounting of a new laptop computer and to assist his access to a large plate switch selected by the occupational therapist as the most efficient method for computer access given Tom's physical limitations. Tom will operate his computer via row-column scanning.

Effective verbal communication requires coordination within and among the respiratory, phonatory, and articulatory subsystems of the speech-producing mechanism. The respiratory system, consisting of the diaphragm, lungs, and thoracic musculature, provides the breath support and muscle control required to produce the prolonged controlled exhalation (airstream) on which we speak. The phonatory system, consisting of the vocal folds and cartilages of the larynx, is responsible for the production of voice and pitch control. The articulatory system, consisting of the lips, tongue, teeth, jaw, and velum (soft palate), is responsible for changing the shape of the oral/nasal resonance chamber. It provides a series of varied constrictions of differing durations, which impede the outgoing airstream. In combination, this system produces the vowel and consonant sounds that we organize into sequences and recognize as spoken words. A variety of congenital (e.g., cerebral palsy, Duchenne muscular dystrophy, spinal muscular atrophy, developmental apraxia of speech) and acquired (e.g., amyotrophic lateral sclerosis, Parkinson's disease, multiple sclerosis, stroke, traumatic brain injury, spinal cord injury) impairments can affect this delicate balance of timing and coordination to varying degrees of severity throughout the speech-producing mechanism. When the intelligibility of spoken language is so severe that it is inadequate for self-expression and significantly limits participation in activities of daily living or success in school or in the workplace, it becomes essential to explore appropriate augmentative and alternative communication (AAC) strategies.

The American Speech-Language-Hearing Association has estimated that approximately 2 million Americans have severe temporary or permanent communication disorders.[1] Augmentative communication systems can be used as an alternative or as support for existing verbal communication skills. Augmentative communication additionally incorporates the technology developed to assist with written as well as verbal communication when physical disability precludes legible handwriting.

LOW VERSUS HIGH TECHNOLOGY

AAC systems span a continuum from "low" (nonelectronic) to "high" (electronic) technology. Low technology may include, but not be limited to, the use of gestures and manual signs, picture or alphabet boards, communication notebooks, and picture wallets. High technology can range from the simple to the sophisticated, requiring time-intensive structured training programs for both the consumer and caregiver. Simple electronic systems range from single-button switches producing one 20-second prerecorded message (e.g., "Please come, I need help") to more complex multileveled voice output communication aids and computer-based synthesized speech output systems.

Prerecorded natural speech is digitized and stored on a microchip. Devices that rely on digitized speech technology have a predetermined recording capacity measured in seconds to minutes. Lengthening recording time may be possible by purchasing extended memory (additional microchip storage), but in many devices, use of extended "talking time" results in some compromise in the clarity of speech output.

"Synthesized" speech is artificially generated by a voice synthesizer. The clarity and quality of synthesized speech have improved significantly over the past 10 years, making the synthesized voice more acceptable and comprehensible to both the listener and augmentative communication user. Technology has introduced multiple voices including male and female adult, young child, and whispered speech. Synthesized speech is also becoming available in a variety of foreign language versions. The ability to switch back and forth from a native to a second language would make this the ideal option for a bilingual speaker; it allows flexible use of the same device across a variety of communication settings. However, synthesized speech still remains artificial sounding and may require a greater degree of attention and some additional processing time on the part of the listener to ensure comprehension. The more natural sounding digitized speech output has been found to be more acceptable to the younger language learner or the AAC candidate with less-than-average cognitive functioning (intelligence) and is a better choice for encouraging peer interaction within those groups.

DEDICATED VERSUS NONDEDICATED SYSTEMS

AAC devices can be either dedicated or nondedicated. A dedicated communication device was designed for the single purpose of substituting for verbal speech production. Dedicated communication devices can range from simple, which provides just a few choices with limited vocabulary, to complex programmable devices with liquid crystal displays and multiple connecting levels with access to a vast stored dictionary of vocabulary. Varied models of dedicated augmentative communication devices are available with either digitized or synthesized speech output.

Computer-based augmentative communication systems, or non-dedicated systems, are software programs that can be loaded into fixed or portable laptop computers. Computer-based programs provide the user with the flexibility to use the same system for multiple applications, including communication, word processing/desktop publishing, environmental control, and information gathering on the internet. The use of a computer-based augmentative system permits both augmented verbal and written communication. "An augmentative writing system for the physically disabled (user) has the following components: a microcomputer, word processing software and adaptive input modifications. The computer and the word processor are used to complete writing assignments by allowing the (user) to enter text and edit using the keyboard or an alternative entry method in place of handwritten script."[2] The computer user who is visually impaired and physically disabled is also able to use augmented writing systems in either of two modalities, dependent on the extent of the visual impairment. An enlarged-print system uses a large-print monitor or print enlargement software. A second system uses auditory rather than visual prompts to facilitate computer operation.[2] For the blind computer user, keyboards with raised braille symbols and software programs that reformat electronic documents for printing in braille are also available.

Computer-based systems are typically limited to synthetic voice output, although this is changing in the dynamic world of computer technology. In addition, manufacturers of many dedicated communication devices have recognized the need to extend beyond their primary purpose and have designed more recent models to accept interfaces with both computers and environmental control units (ECUs).

DIRECT SELECTION VERSUS SCANNING MODALITIES

Both dedicated and nondedicated augmentative communication systems can be accessed via direct selection or scanning modalities. Direct selection requires the ability to apply pressure to activate a single space or individual key on either a membrane or computer keyboard. Direct selection can also be accomplished by touching a defined area on the surface of a liquid crystal display or on a touch-sensitive window mounted directly over a computer screen. Direct selection typically requires isolated finger mobility and dexterity with the ability to apply a specific level of direct pressure for a brief duration followed by removal from the target. The target may often be as small as a ½-in.-square defined area. For users unable to perform isolated finger movement, direct selection may be accomplished by striking a key or defined area with a hand-held dowel, headpointer, or mouthstick. Some devices permit adjustment in the amount of pressure required to activate a key or can be adapted to activate only on release of pressure. A keyguard, typically a lightweight plastic cutout overlay, fits over a computer or membrane keyboard, isolating each individual key. This can help to increase the precision of direct selection and eliminate accidental keystrokes to neighboring keys adjacent to the target. For some computer systems, software that disables the automatic repeat feature of individual keys is available. Computer-based augmentative system users may also take advantage of alternative keyboards. These include enlarged keyboard designs, miniature keyboards for users with adequate pointing skills within a decreased range of mobility, numeric keyboards, and modified keyboard arrangements in an alphabetical or frequency of occurrence organization instead of a standard QWERTY pattern. Alternate keyboards usually require the use of a separate hardware unit to interface between the keyboard and the serial port, but newer models are capable of direct attachment to the keyboard port.[3]

For the more physically challenged AAC user, direct selection access may be precluded by the severity of the physical disability. For these users, the scanning modality is the optimal mode for access to either a dedicated or nondedicated augmentative system. A single switch activated by a reliable body movement (e.g., head, hand, foot, elbow, knee, eye gaze, eyebrow, or facial movement) is connected to the appropriate port of a dedicated device or via interface to a computer-based system. Switches are mounted appropriately for easy access. Decisions related to switch selection and placement should be part of the assessment process when a scanning modality is determined to be the best choice for user access. See Chapter 6 for additional information about switches.

Commonly used switches for AAC include the following: button, plate, leaf, pillow, rocker, infrared, sound, touch, sip-and-puff, and arm slot control.

Scanning may be manual or automatic. In automatic scanning, a light (dedicated device) or cursor (computer-based system) typically moves in a row-column display. Switch activation stops the scanner and identifies the selection. Scanning speed and patterns can often be modified to fit the needs of an individual user. Manual scanning involves user control of the scanning light or cursor. Each switch activation moves the scanner toward the intended target. Manual scanning extends response time even more significantly than automatic scanning but is often optimal for younger consumers with cognitive impairments and/or multiple disabilities.

Many dedicated AAC systems are programmed to accommodate both direct selection and scanning. Computer-based AAC systems may require special software with built-in scanning arrays.

ICONIC VERSUS GRAPHIC REPRESENTATIONS

Augmentative communication programs fall within one of two classes: iconic or picture based, fulfilling the needs of the preliterate user; and graphic programs, requiring some level of functional reading and spelling skills. Iconic systems impose picture representations on both picture-producing (e.g., apple, bed, sun) and non-picture-producing vocabulary (e.g., happy, gentle). The ability to recognize a picture symbol and assign meaning to it requires life and social experience within a culture, familiarity with signs and symbols, cognitive skill including the ability to make within-class associations, a learning process, and the absence of any significant visual impairment.[4] As vocabulary increases, assigning meaning to picture symbols requires increasing cognitive skill because individual picture symbols can be combined into various sequences and used to represent more than one idea.

Some examples of commonly used picture symbol systems include

- Mayer-Johnson PicSyms
- Minspeak (Prentke Romich Co.)
- Blissymbols
- Rebus
- Imaginart Symbol Set
- Intellitools Picture Library
- DynaSyms (Sentient Systems)

Many picture symbols are also identified by the written word that fosters emergent literacy in the AAC user with the cognitive potential for learning to read.

To be able to produce spontaneous productions unlimited by device capacity and programming, spelling ability is essential. Graphic-based augmentative communication programs offer unlimited communicative potential to the user. A general all-purpose graphic program allows a direct selection user to type text and have it synthetically voiced. Many programs also contain a menu of preprogrammed words and phrases that can be "quick voiced" with a single keystroke even as additional text is being typed. Additional "quick voice" phrases can be customized to suit the needs of an individual user.[2] Graphic-based programs are also accessible via scanning. Word prediction software programs are especially beneficial to the user dependent on the scanning modality. "As the user types the first letters of a word, the word prediction program compares it to a dictionary of words beginning with those same letters. A window appears on-screen with the list of words; if the user finds his or her intended word in the list, he or she enters one key stroke and the word is inserted into the document. If not, the user continues typing until the program presents him or her with a match."[3] The word prediction software dictionary can be customized over time to be the most responsive to an individual user. Abbreviation/expansion programs allow a user to type in a standardized or customized abbreviation for frequently used vocabulary. The computer recognizes the abbreviation and types in the complete word. Software that assists in the reduction of key-strokes decreases response time in conversation and increases the productivity of augmentative writing programs.

Iconic-based programs are available for use with both dedicated and nondedicated systems. Graphic programs can be run on only the most sophisticated high-technology dedicated devices and most computer-based augmentative systems.

ASSESSMENT

The Bain Assistive Technology System (BATS) should be part of the evaluation process for AAC, as with any assistive technology device (ATD) (see Ch. 3). This holistic BATS approach includes an evaluation of the consumer, the device, and all the environments in which the desired task will be performed. In addition, evaluating consumers for an AAC system requires decisions about

1. Appropriate communication modality to suit the user's needs and cognitive ability
   Low versus high technology
2. System selection and access
   Dedicated versus computer-based augmentative system
   Direct selection versus scanning with switch access
3. Programming options
   Iconic versus graphic representation
4. Integration of the system into daily routines
   Flexibility of systems(s)
   Portability of systems(s)
   Education and training of user and communication partner
5. Who will pay for the system
   Identification of funding sources

A multimodal approach to AAC combines an assortment of augmentative communication modes, often high and low technology, into a communication network designed to address a broad range of communicative functions.[5,6] Evaluation is best accomplished at an AT resource center or augmentative communication laboratory where a variety of equipment is available for diagnostic trial.

Assessment for AAC should be coordinated by a speech-language pathologist with training and experience in the holistic review of communication needs and design of an augmentative communication network that will successfully address all identified needs.[7] The speech-language pathologist should be part of an interdisciplinary team of professionals including an occupational therapist, physical therapist, and rehabilitation engineer. Each team member has specific responsibilities and contributes to the evaluation process within their area of expertise. (The following information is adapted from the New York State Medicaid Guidelines for Augmentative Communication Systems Evaluation.[8])

SPEECH-LANGUAGE PATHOLOGIST

1. Assessment of language skills (comprehension, expression, and interactional abilities)
2. Communication needs assessment
   Typical communication partners
   Message needs
   Communication environments (home, school, workplace, community)
3. Exploration of various communication devices/modalities to determine individual suitability
4. Determination of appropriateness for iconic versus graphic representation
   Identification of specific symbol system
   Identification of specific software program options
5. Knowledge of funding sources and assistance in obtaining funding for purchase of equipment by providing written documentation/justification
6. Interval consultation/training sessions for both consumer and caregiver(s) to optimize use of selected system(s) and provide assistance and support for successful integration of the augmentative communication network into the home, school, workplace, and broader community

OCCUPATIONAL THERAPIST

1. Assessment of fine motor skills, visual-motor coordination, and sensory-motor integration as applicable to the user's ability to fully access the selected AAC
2. Identification of optimal access technique(s)
3. Identification of appropriate supports to ensure successful use of selected AAC
   Keyboard modifications and/or additional supports for direct access
   Switch selection
   Interfaces required
   Scanning speed
   Modifications for visual field reductions
   Large-print screens and/or large-print software

PHYSICAL THERAPIST

1. Assessment of mobility status
2. Determination of optimal positioning as related to pelvis, trunk, head position, and control site (switch), if applicable
3. Recommendations for seating modifications
4. Integration of mobility with AAC and other AT

REHABILITATION ENGINEER

1. Provides physical adaptations (hardware) necessary for positioning of AAC and system control(s) to achieve best view and access
2. Implements seating modifications as directed by the team

In the area of AAC assessment, any evaluation team is only as strong as the sum of its members. This becomes especially true when assessing the consumer with severe physical disabilities who will require input from all team members to address his or her multiple programming, access, and positioning needs. The field of rehabilitation technology is rapidly changing and evolving. Hardware and software applications that exist today did not 10 and even 5 years ago and will be replaced by new and more responsive technology within the next 5 to 10 years. It is incumbent on all interdisciplinary professionals providing AAC and AT evaluation and treatment services to keep current of technological development to best serve the consumer.

EARLY TRAINING IN THE USE OF "LOW-TECH" AAC

Children who are early candidates for AAC evaluation and training demonstrate acquisition of the following prerequisite skills:

- Age-appropriate eye contact, attending behavior and nonverbal social interaction skills (e.g., reciprocal smiling, joint attention)
- Development of prelinguistic cognitive skills (object permanence, operational causality, means-end relationships)
- Receptive language comprehension at a minimum of an 18-month to 2-year level when formally evaluated, including emerging object-to-picture matching and beginning symbolic representation skills
- Indicating "requests" and expressing "choices" via eye gaze, pointing, or gesturing, demonstrating development of communicative intent

The successful implementation of even the most basic AAC system requires that the user understand that each initiation (e.g., pointing to an object or picture on a communication board) will elicit a response from a communication partner and/or bring about a change in the immediate environment. The user must ultimately understand that the AAC system acts as an interface to facilitate communication. Many children and older cognitively impaired individuals will require preparatory therapeutic intervention with a focus on establishing these prerequisites to communication before achieving readiness for AAC training.

Before the development of picture identification skills, object recognition and association of objects with actions and/or primary function are established. Introduction of AAC is possible at this level through the use of direct selection or scanning object boxes (Fig. 9-1). Depending on the

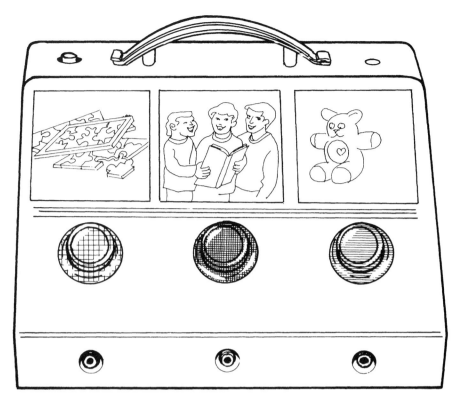

Figure 9-1. Low-tech AAC: nine-box compartment.

capability of the user, objects can be used to elicit simple choice making (juice box versus cookie) or to represent a particular activity ("cup": thirsty/want a drink; "refrigerator": hungry/want something to eat; "toy car": want to go for a ride). Choices available range from 2 to 10. Direct selection is made by triggering the appropriate buzzer or light corresponding to the selected object. Scanning practice at this level is typically manual, with the user activating a switch to bring a light to the appropriate box corresponding to his or her choice. These battery-operated systems are generally inexpensive and simple to operate.

As a child progresses from identification of objects and photographs to early symbolic recognition, an iconic-based picture symbol system must be chosen to expand augmentative communication potential. This symbol system should be able to "grow" with the child and later be integrated with higher-level technology when the introduction of a dedicated or computer-based AAC system is deemed appropriate. As the child is simultaneously learning to assign meaning to the labels (words) and concepts of his or her native language, learning to assign meaning to specific symbols and symbol sequences has been hypothesized to be "analogous to second language learning."[9] Aided Language Stimulation is one technique for teaching picture symbol comprehension and stimulating symbol use as a means for self-expression. Aided Language Stimulation requires the speaker (mother, father, teacher, therapist, etc.) to point out the symbols on a communication display simultaneous with his or her verbal utterances (Fig. 9-2), just

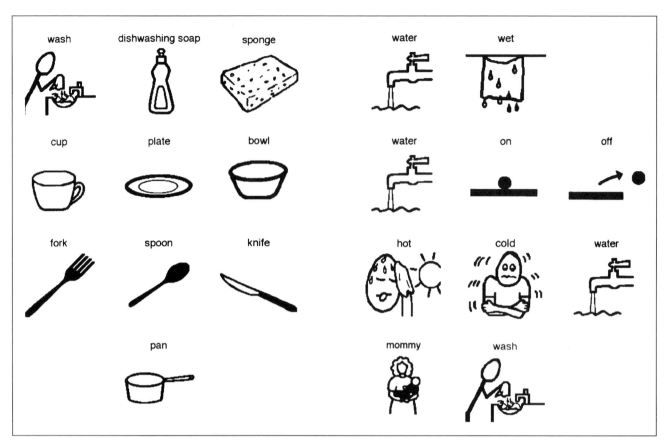

Figure 9-2. Picture symbol vocabulary.

as a speaker would sign simultaneously while speaking when communicating with the deaf. In this way, a child receives consistent modeling of the use of the communication system.[9,10] Goossens' et al[9] further postulated that Aided Language Stimulation was most effective when presented via an "immersion approach" requiring accessible display of picture symbol vocabulary (objects, actions, modifiers) strategically placed throughout the environment to reflect associated tasks (e.g., picture symbol vocabulary placed adjacent to the kitchen sink of a 3-year-old augmented communicator: wash, plate, bowl, cup, pan, fork, spoon, knife, wet, water, on/off, hot/cold, soap, sponge). Goossens' et al[9] called this approach to teaching "engineering the environment," and it has been recommended for the preschool classroom in which the augmented communicator is included, as well as the home. As for the 3-year-old, picture symbol vocabulary accessible to the mother above the sink may not be accessible to the child due to physical disability. Therefore, duplicate picture symbol vocabulary could be placed on the tray table attached to the prone stander (covered with clear contact paper to prevent getting wet or torn) and accessed via a headpointer, so that the child and his or her mother could "converse" while doing the dishes.

The described technique is one very effective method of integrating augmentative communication training and "low-tech" AAC into daily routines that can be taught to parents, teachers, family members, babysitters, and any other significant caregivers. There are many other techniques and low-tech AAC solutions that may be individualized for a particular user. Interval follow-up with parents is essential to success to expand vocabulary across communication environments. School consultations with teachers will coordinate vocabulary selection with preacademic and academic curriculum.

There is no preset age at which an augmented communicator automatically becomes eligible for introduction of electronic communication devices or systems. This decision is made based on evaluation of current communication needs and the adequacy of the present system(s) to meet these needs. Training requirements for the use of a selected electronic system (e.g., coordinating switch access, learning scanning routines) may delay the integration of that system into all communication environments at once, and the user may continue to rely on low-tech AAC as appropriate. Low-tech AAC modalities may also become a permanent part of that user's communication network as they may remain most effective in some settings (e.g., water-resistant communication folder poolside for swimming lessons). Low-tech does not automatically preclude use of graphic representation. Older adults may choose not to progress from low-tech AAC (e.g., alphabet, word, and phrase boards) to electronic systems. The severely cognitively impaired user may function best with low-tech AAC but not always! The reality of financial concerns may also limit the capacity of some users to consider transition to costly electronic systems.

TRAINING AND INTEGRATION

As previously discussed in this chapter, electronic or "high" technology AAC systems can range from the simple to the sophisticated. An alphabet board user with the ability to achieve precise keystrokes to hit closely spaced ¼- to ⅛-square-in. targets with accuracy may easily make the transition to a portable, calculator-size, dedicated communication device that produces typed hard copy or a liquid crystal display of words. A lightweight 8- or 16-key direct selection access keyboard with voice output small enough to fit in a pocket or pouch may be just the solution for the ambulatory AAC user for whom portability of his or her computer-based system is a problem and who is ready for an upgrade from the picture communication wallets he or she uses to facilitate communication when participating in community-based recreational and social activities. Transition from a low-tech picture communication board to a simple 32-key dedicated voice output communication aid (Fig. 9-3) may be the next step for the consumer in a wheelchair who has a small core vocabulary and is ready for a "voice" of his or her own that will command the attention he or she does not seem to get as quickly when quietly pointing to pictures. However, electronic dedicated communication devices with symbol sequencing capability and various software applications can extend the capacity of 32 keys into a vocabulary of many words, phrases, and simple sentences, making a "simple" device no longer seem so simple.

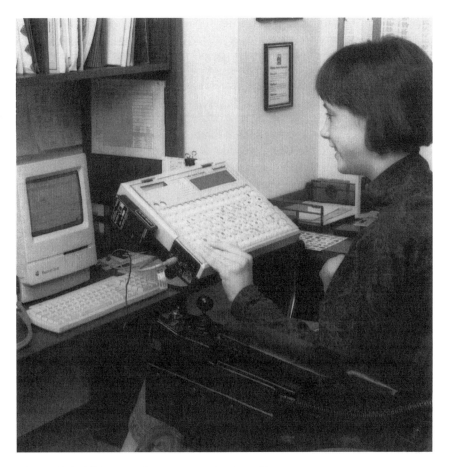

Figure 9-3. Thirty-two-key communication aid.

As the capacity of any device or system increases, a higher level of cognitive ability is required to fully realize device potential. Programming demands for digitized as well as synthesized voice output communication systems also increase in complexity and can become an overwhelming task for the caregiver responsible for the input of this programming if appropriate education, training, and support are unavailable. Securing a sophisticated dedicated or computer-based system for a prospective user without honest discussion of the training component, technician to provide the training, frequency of instruction, and duration of training that will be provided can lead to underuse, poor usage, and ultimate dissatisfaction with even a very appropriately chosen system.

The decision to upgrade to a sophisticated high-tech augmentative communication system is an important one. The prospective user must be motivated to accept the challenge of learning and integrating a complex system, be willing to devote a significant amount of time to that learning, and have access to an adequate level of support from a competent educator to provide the necessary training and technical assistance. Prospective users who travel long distances to evaluation centers may find few avenues for obtaining this assistance from a knowledgeable provider when they receive their augmentative systems back in their home community. It is unfortunate that many funding sources will pay for the actual communication device or system but not the follow-up training and support necessary for learning to use the device to its full potential. The need for learning of sophisticated access modalities as well as software applications may extend typical training time for use of a system significantly.

Dedicated AAC devices that use iconic-based programs can be as complex to learn as computer-based graphic systems. Device selection must meet communication needs and be matched with the consumer's cognitive ability to facilitate successful learning. The design of a system includes decisions relative to system access and related hardware needs, as well as programming and software needs. At this juncture, the interdisciplinary assessment team may require additional consulting members. An educational consultant or learning disabilities specialist may be of assistance when making decisions related to augmented writing programs for document generation, note taking (e.g., spell checking/proofing software, editing programs including audible text editing), and other educational software applications when the goal of the AAC user is readiness to participate in a secondary or postsecondary educational setting.[2] Prior discussion with a vocational counselor who has expertise in employment counseling for consumers with physical and/or developmental disabilities may be beneficial when making system choices for the augmentative communicator whose goal is employment.

For the adult user, verbal and written augmentative communication systems and other related ATs provide the opportunity for greater independence through the achievement of personal choice and the control and enhancement of both educational and employment skills.[11] Once the parameters of an AAC system have been defined, the training component must be developed. If, as already discussed, learning to effectively use an AAC system requires "immersion" in natural environments, the question remains as to how we can adapt this concept to developing training programs for the adult user. Augmentative Communication and Empowerment Supports (ACES), an education and advocacy group at Temple University in Philadelphia, provides the adult equivalent of an immersion program by offering 2-week intensive residential institutes in which participants receive 60 hours of intensive instruction in the use of their new or upgraded AAC and AT system. Participants live together in university housing and learn to depend on their AAC system to accomplish activities of daily living (e.g., telephone calls, eliciting information), educational/prevocational (e.g., note taking, word processing), and social/recreational (e.g., shopping, eating at a restaurant) activities. Each participant attends the immersion program with a one-to-one "tutor" from his or her home community who is trained at the institute to provide follow-up support on return to home at the end of the 2-week intensive instruction period. Opportunities to interact with program graduate mentors and coursework that focuses on independent living skills, money management, vocational training, and personal empowerment are also an integral part of this model program for persons with disabilities.[11]

Bryen et al[11] conducted a study of 17 adults ranging from 17 to 50 years of age with assorted diagnoses and AAC system needs who had completed the ACES institute program and responded to a follow-up questionnaire a minimum of 1 year after completing the course. These researchers found that participants thought that acquisition of their augmentative communication system had made the greatest positive impact on their ability to "communicate, maintain an income, and learn."[11] They report that the ACES institute experience suggests that most individuals require between 100 to 200 hours of additional instruction (following initial 60 hours training) to master the "language" of the device's software and its full operation, to learn how to customize it for current and future educational or vocational needs, to integrate its use into daily life, and to learn how to maintain the equipment—in other words, to become a fluent, competent communicator.[11]

AAC, AT, AND ENVIRONMENTAL CONTROL

The ability to communicate extends beyond the spoken word. It implies mastery of old and new forms of electronic communication: the telephone, the fax machine, electronic mail (e-mail), and travel on the information superhighway, the internet. Using telephone equipment features such as a large-button dialing pad (accessible via headpointer, mouthstick, or handheld dowel), preprogrammable memory for single-button access to frequently dialed or emergency numbers, or voice-activated dialing features and "hands-free" speakerphone technology, the dedicated voice output communication aid user can now achieve independent telephone communication. A computer-based AAC system can easily be designed to provide access via modem to all forms of electronic communication. Electronic communication has and will continue to create new and exciting employment opportunities for individuals with severe disabilities within the growing arena of telecommuting (working from home with computer hook-up to the office). Information gathering and interactional opportunities available on the internet provide persons with disabilities with up-to-date information related to computer technology and have supported the creation of national and international advocacy groups.

Independence for persons with physical disabilities is achieved not only by establishing communicative competence but is further enhanced by the ability to take charge of or "control" the immediate environment. Physical disability often implies reliance on others to assist with performance of many activities of daily living (e.g., getting out of bed, bathing, turning on a light, changing a television channel). The purpose of ECUs is to create additional opportunities for independence (ECUs are discussed in greater detail in Ch. 10). Although many persons with physical disabilities may still require the assistance of another person to perform grooming and transfer activities, the development of ECUs has permitted independent access to lights, appliances, televisions, VCRs, stereos, and in some cases, the programming features of sophisticated dedicated communication devices. ECUs use various remote technology to send signals from a transmitter to a receiver in the same manner as a hand-held remote control unit sends signals to a television. The transmitter can be mounted independently at the bedside, connected to an auxiliary port of a powered wheelchair, mounted directly to some dedicated communication devices, and connected through an interface to a computer-based system. Receivers interface directly with lamps and appliances or replace standard wall switches. Some ECUs can be accessed via direct selection or scanning with switch access. ECUs interfaced with computer-based systems require specialty software and are controlled through manipulation of on-screen computer display. Some remote ECUs can enable the user to send commands from one room to another throughout the house to turn on a light in the bedroom before entering or turn off a radio or television in the next room. Currently, the integration of sophisticated AAC systems, ECUs, and even the introduction of trained animal assistants are enhancing independent living opportunities for persons with disabilities and reducing the amount of time needed for support from outside caregivers.

FUNDING OF AUGMENTATIVE COMMUNICATION SYSTEMS

An important part of the evaluation process, in addition to the selection of an appropriate AAC system and associated AT, is the identification of a funding source to facilitate purchase of the equipment. Augmentative communication equipment can range in cost from a few hundred dollars for the simplest devices with minimal access requirements to more than $10,000 for sophisticated electronic systems with multiple hard- and software adaptations, as well as associated interface with ECUs. There is nothing more frustrating to a potential consumer and/or evaluator than to design an appropriate communication network for an augmentative communication candidate and later find that this equipment will be unavailable to that person due to its prohibitive cost. It is the responsibility of the evaluator and/or evaluation team to make realistic equipment recommendations based not on cost, but on the consumer's communication needs. However, it is very important that the evaluator select the most fiscally reasonable system that meets the prospective user's current communication needs with approximately a 5-year allowance for growth potential in skills but that does not excessively exceed current needs or attempt to address the potential needs of a lifetime, especially when evaluating a young child. Most funding sources will consider a new request for AAC within 5 to 7 years after the initial purchase and may be willing to provide payment for less costly system upgrades in 2 to 3 years. With continuing improvements in technology, it is reasonable to assume that a new and better system will be available when it is time to reevaluate a consumer's needs.

Traditional sources for funding of AAC systems include private medical insurance, government-supported health care programs (Medicare, Medicaid), state departments of vocational rehabilitation, school districts, and on a very individualized basis, private service organizations (e.g., Lion's Clubs, Knights of Columbus). Many vendors of dedicated communication devices have funding departments with personnel who will assist an evaluator or, in some cases, a caregiver in preparing the appropriate written documentation or justification for submitting payment requests to private insurance companies, government funding sources, or school districts. When making a written request for funding, it is essential to address not only the cost of the device itself, but also the total cost of all the components necessary to make the system viable, including switches and other hardware adaptations, interfaces, mounting materials, labor costs, and software programs needed. Private and government insurers additionally require a physician's prescription including a "statement of medical necessity" explaining the medical diagnosis related to the inability to speak, prognosis for "recovery," and the medical needs this equipment will address (e.g., permitting communication with health care professionals for safety and self-report of physical state).

Electronic communication systems may be considered as a "prosthetic device" or be characterized as "durable medical equipment" and become eligible for payment by insurers whose contracts provide such coverage. Given new managed care guidelines, many private insurers have implemented strict prior approval and preauthorization criteria that must be closely adhered to in order to qualify for the mere consideration of payment for the augmentative communication evaluation and/or funding of the actual equipment. In New York, a panel of speech-language pathologists under the auspices of the state's professional association created standardized guidelines relative to eligibility requirements for receiving augmentative communication equipment, evaluation protocols for appropriate equipment selection, and protocols for funding of system upgrades, modifications, replacement, and repairs. These were accepted by the state government department responsible for overseeing Medicaid fund disbursement in this area. Compliance with these protocols is essential to obtain Medicaid funding for AAC in New York State but is not a guarantee of approval.[8]

Augmentative communication devices or systems have also been funded by local school districts under the Individuals with Disabilities Education Act (IDEA), consistent with achievement of its primary tenet of ensuring a "free and appropriate public education" to all children regardless of disability. In this case, the equipment must be deemed as necessary for the child to fully participate in a specialized educational setting (e.g., special education or related services) or be educated in the "least restrictive environment." The child's individualized education plan (IEP) must include specification of the device and how and when it will be used to achieve performance of specific academic skills. When the parent and school personnel responsible for creating the IEP cannot agree to the inclusion of AAC or other AT, the parent may seek independent evaluation as a second opinion and follow his or her local school district's appeals process. When a school district does purchase an AAC, questions of ownership arise. Although the AAC device is the actual property of the school district, it has been determined that if the technology is required at home to accomplish school assignments (e.g., homework, projects, reading books), it must be made available for that child. This is a vastly simpler and less costly task when discussing portable (dedicated or nondedicated) versus fixed computer-based systems and should be taken into consideration when designing systems or selecting devices for children when the school district is regarded as the most likely prospective funding source, if possible. Given that the AAC is school property, many school districts have required that it be returned to the school on graduation for use by other students. However, many school districts have also permitted purchase of the AAC by the consumer or the family and have accepted payment in an amount that reflects both the age and depreciation of the device.

Provisions under the American with Disabilities Act implemented as an amendment in 1994 focus on supporting efforts to increase access to AT and services by improving funding through consumer-friendly financial loan programs. The Tech-Related Assistance Act of 1994 provides for availability of federal government grants to states to encourage but not mandate the creation of specialty loan programs for funding of AT. Specialty loan programs may feature assistance with the application process, relaxation of credit history requirements, low or no-interest, extended or variable repayment terms, creation of revolving funds into which repayment money is recycled into future loans for the same purpose, approvals for loan cosigners, and specific loan appeal procedures.[12]

Lawsuits have been initiated in many states by consumers and/or their families against private insurers, Medicaid, and school districts for failing to fund AAC. Lawsuits can become more costly than the technology itself, making them less than an ideal option for most prospective users. However, precedent-setting lawsuits have paved the way for increased access to funding for AT across funding sources. Self-advocacy groups for the disabled have been active in supporting landmark cases. These groups are also involved in advocating for consumer protection against faulty AAC and AT. Legislation, commonly known as lemon laws, has been enacted in several states, but at this time, it predominately covers defective powered wheelchairs and not communication equipment. An essential task of self-advocacy groups as well as the professionals who serve and assist persons with disabilities is to convince society of the fiscal reality that AAC equipment and AT increases independence, facilitates education, and leads to employment; therefore, it more than pays for itself over time when compared with the cost of dependence and full-time residential care. In addition, failure to meet the mandate of providing access to AT for all who can benefit from it robs everyone of the contributions of an important segment of our society.

REFERENCES

1. American Speech-Language-Hearing Association: Augmentative and alternative communication. ASHA, suppl. 5, 33:9–12, 1991

2. Horn C, Shell D, Benkofske M: Technology usage in post-secondary education. Closing the Gap Newsletter Aug./Sept. 1989

3. Wilson L, Kotlas C, Martin M: Assistive technology for the disabled computer user. Institute Academic Technol Nov. 1994

4. Gangkofer MH: Is it easy or hard to "read" a picture? ASHA Special Interest Div (Augmentative Alternative Communication) Newslett 5(2):4–5, 1996

5. Zarella S: Toward communicative competence: matching nonverbal clients with appropriate AAC. Adv Speech-Language Pathol Audiol 5:6, 1995

6. Blischak DM, Lloyd LL: Multimodal augmentative and alternative communication: case study. Augmentative Alternative Communication 12:37–45, 1996

7. American Speech-Language-Hearing Association: Competencies for speech-language pathologists providing services in augmentative communication. ASHA 31:107–110, 1989

8. Guidelines for Augmentative Communication Systems. Bureau of Standards Development, New York State Department of Health, Albany, NY, 1992

9. Goossens' C, Crain SS, Elder PS: Engineering the Preschool Environment for Interactive Symbolic Communication. 2nd Ed. Southeast Augmentative Communication Conference Publications Clinician Series, Alabama, 1994

10. Goossens' C: Aided communication intervention before assessment: a case study of a child with cerebral palsy. Augmentative Alternative Communication 5:14–26, 1989

11. Bryen DN, Slesaransky G, Baker DB: Augmentative communication and empowerment supports: a look at outcomes. Augmentative Alternative Communication 11:79–88, 1995

12. RESNA Technical Assistance Project: Financial loan programs. TAP Bull Nov./Dec. 1994

SUGGESTED READINGS

Fishman I: Electronic Communication Aids: Selection on Use. College Hill Publications, Boston, 1987

Lazzaro JJ: Adapting PCs for Disabilities. Addison-Wesley, Reading, MA, 1996

Lazzaro JJ: Adaptive Technologies for Learning and Work Environments. American Library Association, 1993

Lewis RB: Special Education Technology: Classroom Applications. Brooks/Cole, 1993

Assistive
Technology:
An
Interdisciplinary
Approach

Resources

ORGANIZATIONS

American Speech-Language-Hearing
  Association (ASHA)
10801 Rockville Pike
Rockville, MD 20852

Baruch College Computer Center for
  the Visually Impaired
The City University of New York
17 Lexington Avenue, Box 515
New York, NY 10010

Blissymbolics Communication
  International
250 Ferrand Drive, Suite 200
Don Mills, Ontario M3C 3P2, Canada

EASI: Equal Access to Software
  and Information
c/o American Association for
  Higher Education
One Dupont Circle, Suite 360
Washington, DC 20036

International Society for Augmentative
  and Alternative Communication
  (ISAAC)
P.O. Box 1762, Station R
Toronto, Ontario Canada L8N 3K7

RESNA Technical Assistance Project
1700 North Moore Street, Suite 1540
Arlington, VA 22209

Trace Research and Development Center
  on Communication Control
  and Computer Access
University of Wisconsin—Madison
S151 Waisman Center
1500 Highland Avenue
Madison, WI 53705

United States Society for Augmentative and
    Alternative Communication (USSAAC) Newsletter
1850 Sand Hill Road, Apartment 10
Palo Alto, CA 94304

PUBLICATIONS

Closing the Gap (newsletter)
P.O. Box 68
Henderson, MN 56044

Computer Resources for People with Disabilities
The Alliance for Technology Access
Hunter House Publishing, 1994

The Guide to Augmentative and Alternative
    Communication Devices (1996 edition)
Rehabilitation Engineering Research Center on
    AAC Applied Science and Engineering Labs
University of Delaware/duPont Institute
P.O. Box 269, 1600 Rockland Road
Wilmington, DE 19899

MANUFACTURERS

Don Johnston Developmental Equipment, Inc.
P.O. Box 639
Wauconda, IL 60084

Mayer-Johnson Co.
P.O. Box 1579
Solana Beach, CA 92075

Prentke Romich Co.
1022 Heyl Road
Wooster, OH 44691

Sentient Systems Technology, Inc.
2100 Wharton Street
Pittsburgh, PA 15203

Technical Aids and Systems for the
    Handicapped, Inc. (TASH)
Unit 1, 91 Station Street
Ajax, Ontario L1S 3H2, Canada

Words +, Inc.
P.O. Box 1229
Lancaster, CA 93535

Zygo Industries, Inc.
P.O. Box 1008
Portland, OR 97207

CHAPTER 10

Environmental Control Systems

Harry has a 10:00 AM presentation to give to his advertising group. In order to review and finalize his audio-visual material, he arrives at work before the office is open. By pressing a switch placed at wheelchair level near the door, Harry is able to activate the heavy office door that automatically opens and closes after he enters. By changing his powered wheelchair control from the "drive" mode to the "ECU" mode, he can turn on the lights, lock the door behind him, turn on the air conditioner, listen to his telephone messages, and activate the slide and overhead projectors to view his presentation.

Harry's independence and increased productivity are possible by controlling his workplace remotely through environmental control units (ECUs). He physically lacks fine hand manipulative skills, but he can push buttons and switches to access devices in his office as well as in his home and in limited community places. ECUs are "a means to purposefully manipulate and interact with the environment by alternately accessing one or more electrical devices via switches, voice activation, remote control, computer interface, and other technological adaptations."[1]

ECUs can be used by even small children who need assistance in accessing electronic equipment in the home or at school. Sam, an elementary school student with nonfunctional manipulative hand skills, participates in a cooking class with his peers by using an ECU that he controls with his head. By using his head to push a switch that is connected to a control unit, Sam can activate an electric mixer that the teacher has connected to the control unit, which is also plugged into an electrical outlet. While Sam presses on the switch, the mixer operates, and he makes a positive contribution to the class project. When he is at home, Sam can help in the kitchen as well, where he activates an electric corn popper and microwave oven. ECUs enable Sam to turn on the lights and television, and with other assistive technology devices (ATDs), Sam can change the channels.

Margaret is a widow who wants to continue living independently in her own home after recovering from a stroke that impaired her right arm, right leg, and vision. Margaret wears an emergency call pendant that she can press to summon help in the event of a medical or other emergency. In this way, she feels more secure and independent, and she can use other ECUs to control the lights, television, and small kitchen appliances. Margaret has also been able to "teach" her infrared (IR) remote ECU to change the channels and volume of her television.

This chapter presents some background information on ECUs, including why people with disabilities need them, where they can be used, how they operate, and how they are integrated with other ATDs to maximize the functional ability and independence of persons with physical and sensory disabilities. An ECU assessment is discussed that was developed by five therapists working in different rehabilitation settings with a variety of populations.[1] Examples are provided of different types of ECUs and the many ways in which they can be used at home, in school, and in the workplace. A resource list of major manufacturers is also included.

Environmental control systems in this chapter include remotely operated systems for electrical appliances, telephones, and monitoring systems (Fig. 10-1). Both "high" (complex) and "low" (simple) systems are mentioned, but the final selection of which system is most appropriate can only be determined after an assessment of the user, the tasks that need to be accomplished, the operative ability of the system, and the environment(s) in which it will be used.

Figure 10-1. ECU (voice, switch, remote) access methods and appliances.

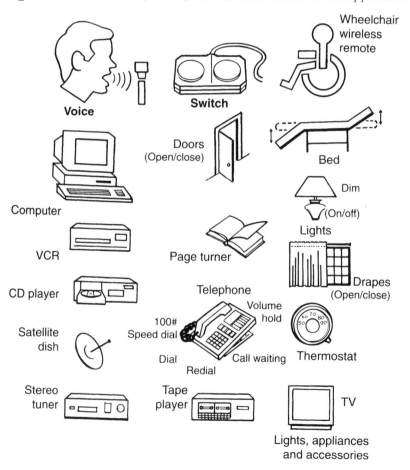

APPLICATIONS OF ECU

There has been an explosion in the variety of commercially available technology devices designed to increase the comfort, safety, convenience, energy, and time of consumers. Today, rehabilitation professionals and persons with both physical and sensory disabilities are using these devices to increase their ability to live alone and feel secure, to conserve their energy and time, to reduce the expenses of attendant care, and to become functionally independent. Here are a few examples of how ECUs can benefit persons of all ages. They can be used to

- Safely call for an assistant by pressing a pillow switch or using a monitor system
- Turn on house or room lights via remote control before entering
- Change the channels and volume of a television, radio, or VCR by using a sip-and-puff switch instead of the small buttons on most remote control units
- Turn on a fan or change the room temperature by regulating a thermostat
- Turn on the coffee pot in the kitchen from a bedside ECU with large manageable buttons
- Participate in group games or activities
- Remind a person to take medicine or make an important telephone call by programming an ECU to turn on a light at a designated time. (For people with hearing impairments, this can be an added advantage for doorbells, telephones, or fire alarms; for people with visual impairments, alarms can be programmed to detect dangerous situations such as a pan boiling over or a buzzer to note approaching footsteps)

Most ECUs are used by persons with severe disabilities when they are in bed or in a wheelchair, and they are also effective throughout the home, at school, and in the workplace.

METHODS OF CONTROLLING ECUs

The major means of controlling ECUs for the past 15 years has been through AC house wiring, IR, radio frequency (RF), and ultrasound. In recent years, there have been an increasing number of systems that can be voice activated or computer driven. For details, see Table 10-1.

Most ECUs consist of the four standard ATD components:

- **Input or access,** which includes mechanical switches, sonic (both ultrasound and voice activation), IR, RF, light beams, voice activation, and computer commands. This is the means by which the user activates the device.

Table 10-1. Comparison of Environmental Control Methods

Control Method	Components	Advantages	Disadvantages	Examples (Manufacturers)
AC Power Line (House Wiring)	Command Control Center	Very flexible	Requires programming of units and house codes	X-10 (X-10 USA)
AC Power plus modules	Basic receiver	No extra wiring needed	May receive nonprogrammed signals	DEUCE (APT Technology)
	Appliance modules	Single control center		Control 1 (Prentke Romich) Can be used with "Light" and "Touch" Talkers
		Add-on units (expandability)		Home Control Interface
		Travels through walls and ceiling		Mini and Maxi Command Center (Heath Co.)
		Can control inside and outside		EZRA (KY Enterprises)
		Controlled from bed and wheelchair		Plug 'n Power System (Radio Shack)
		Programmable with computer		Home Control System (SEARS)
		Varies in price from $100–$500 (base unit)		HECS (Prentke Romich)
		Can be programmed for time		
		Has battery back up		
Ultrasound	Ultrasound control command transmitter receiver	Does not require "line of sight"	Operates only 2 or 4 appliances in same room as transmitter	Ultra 4S, 4L, 4J, 2P, 2T (TASH)
	4 color-coded modules	Wireless setup and operation	Ultra 4S has very small buttons	Commercial "Clap Hands"
		Small and portable		
		Can send 2 (Ultra 2P or Ultra 2T) or 4 signals (Ultra 4S, 4L, 4J)		
		No extra wiring or cable		
		Has large keypad for access		
		Can be mounted to wheelchair or table top		
Voice activated	Command center	No switch or motor control necessary	Must be programmed	Master voice

(Table continues.)

Table 10-1. (*Continued*)

Control Method	Components	Advantages	Disadvantages	Examples (Manufacturers)
	Mic	Hands are free to do other activities	Voice can change due to cold	Simplicity (Quartet Tech)
	X-10 modules	Can interface with X-10	Mic must be close	Voice navigator (Madenta)
			Noise in room can change command	PROXI (Madenta)
Computer driven	Computer software	Transparent	Must have computer interface	TEAM (Microsystems)
	Controller	Can interface with X-10	Expensive	Sensei (Safko)
	Receiver	Use most switches	Can be accessed only with a computer	X-10 Power House (X-10 USA)
	Computer interface			
	X-10 modules			
Infrared (IR)	Transmitter	Flexible method for coding control commands	Needs a "line of sight" for transmission	Relax (TASH)
	Receiver	Light in weight, also very portable	Incompatibility of different remote systems	Kincontrol (TASH)
	Can also use X-10 IR receiver	Some can interface with X-10 system	Needs trainable transmitters	Scanning Director (Prentke Romich)
			Signal cannot travel through walls	Imperium (Teledyne)
Radio frequency (RF)	Transmitter (through the air)	Travels through walls and ceilings	Limited distance control signal can travel (50–200 ft)	Scanning X-10 Powerhouse (Prentke Romich)
	Receiver	Transmits and controls wide ranging of appliance	Subject to interference causing false devices to operate	Radio Shack's Wireless Remote Control System
		Does not require wiring or cabling		Powermid (Prentke Romich)
		Can convert IR signals to radio signals to control IR appliances		

- **Through-put or transmission,** which includes AC house/building current plus a module, batteries, sonic, radio waves, and IR. This is how the ECU receives the input, processes it, and then sends a signal to the appliance.
- **Output,** or the action of the appliances, which includes lights, electrical appliances, security devices, thermostats, door openers, and intercoms. The output is the manner in which the appliance is activated or deactivated when the signal has been received and processed correctly.
- **Feedback,** which is usually a visual, auditory, or tactile display relaying to the person that the system is operating. It can involve flashing lights or beeping to signal that the device has been activated, especially for consumers with visual or hearing impairments.

To remotely control a lamp from the bed, the consumer would press both a "number" button and the "on" button of a command center, which sends a signal to a coded module plugged into a standard wall outlet (input). The lamp has been plugged into the module and turned to the "on" position. The house wiring receives the message from the command center and activates the lamp (throughput), which remotely turns on the lamp (output) and the consumer receives the visual feedback (Fig. 10-2). This can be diagrammed as

Input		Throughput		Output		Feedback
Command center buttons	→	House wiring plus module	→	Lamp on	→	Visual light

For a comparison of various control methods and examples, see Table 10-1.[2] For various throughput methods, carefully read the manufacturer's

Figure 10-2. ECU control sequence. (Illustration courtesy of CM Burwell.)

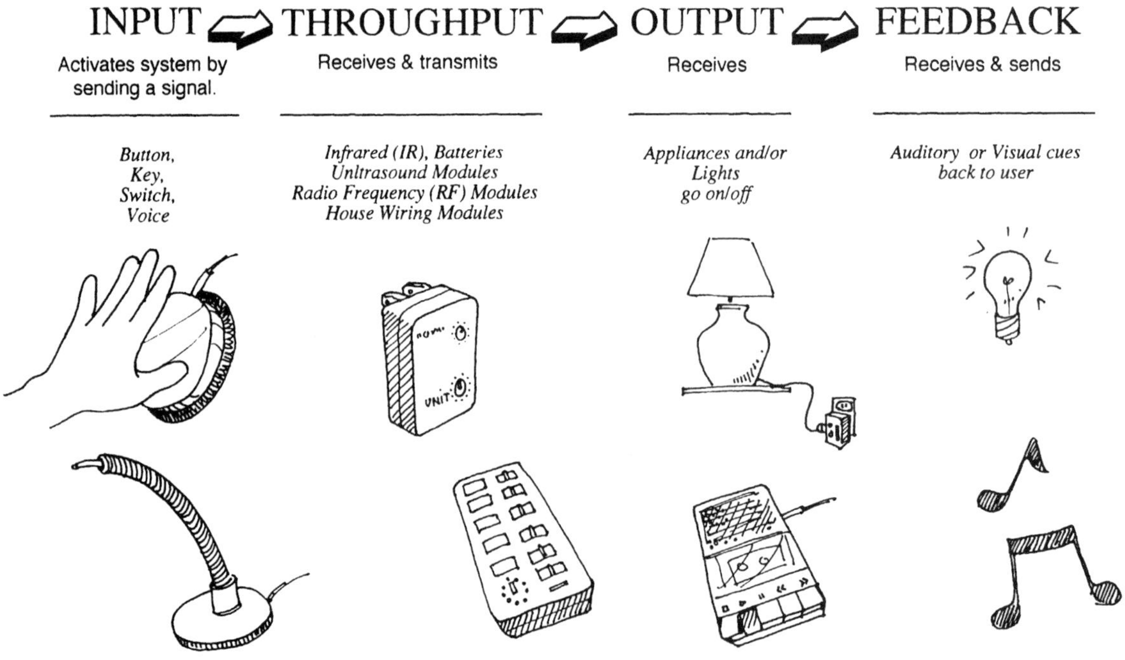

INPUT ⇨	THROUGHPUT ⇨	OUTPUT ⇨	FEEDBACK
Activates system by sending a signal.	Receives & transmits	Receives	Receives & sends
Button, Key, Switch, Voice	Infrared (IR), Batteries Ultrasound Modules Radio Frequency (RF) Modules House Wiring Modules	Appliances and/or Lights go on/off	Auditory or Visual cues back to user

literature to determine the portability of an ECU. The number and receiving method of appliances or peripherals that the consumer needs to operate presently and in the projected future must be analyzed. For instance, the television remote control receives a different IR signal than that transmitted by the ECU command center; however, IR signals can be taught to each other by first changing the transmitter to the "learn" or "teach" mode and then placing the television receiver close to the IR command transmitter until the receiver learns the new signal (see the operator's manual for specific details). In several other IR ECU systems, IR signals are sent from the IR transmitter to an IR receiver that converts the signal to control modules that operate on house current. In addition, the distance that an IR signal can be sent can be extended to cover larger areas, using devices such as Powermid or Leap Frog (Prentke Romich Co.).

In the final selection of an effective and efficient ECU system, the team must review the manufacturer's literature, speak to users of the system, and consider the number of appliances that the consumer needs to control. Computers are becoming the preferred tool for home, school, and work use, due to the development of sophisticated computer-driven ECUs. Voice-activated ECUs are particularly useful for consumers who need to work hands-free, but there must be consistent voice quality for the system to operate effectively. In some cases, voice-activated ECUs can be used in conjunction with augmentative and alternative communication (AAC) aids, and additional features are being developed as computer technology continues to improve.

The ECU compatibility with other ATDs (powered wheelchairs, computers, and telephones) is critical because some ECUs are compatible with only one specific wheelchair and some AAC aids can be controlled by only one specific ECU. Another major factor in the selection of an ECU is cost, because they are rarely covered by insurance plans. One solution might be for the rehabilitation team to consider an inexpensive ($50 to $200) system that controls only the on/off operations of appliances and a portable telephone less than $100 rather than an expensive ($2,000 to $5,000) system that can scan, control appliances, and perform various telephone operations (Fig. 10-3). As stated previously, the technology team must be cognizant of commercially available devices that are generally less expensive, making certain that the needs of the consumer and caregivers are not compromised. Tables 10-1 and 10-2 can be helpful when comparing different systems. The team also needs to calculate the hours and cost of attendant care that can be saved when the consumer gains independence because of using an ECU.

Currently, most ECUs do not require hardwiring installation to operate, but a few, such as some hospital call buttons, two-way wall switch modules, electric door openers, and some alarm systems, require the services of a licensed electrician. When planning to operate ECUs in various environments, especially in older homes, schools, and work sites, the technology team must take the wiring of old and new buildings into consideration, for it has a direct effect on the safety and expense of ECU installation. In the future, "smart homes" and schools will be wired for ECUs. An increasing number of public places are becoming more accessible, including shopping malls, stores, theaters, bus depots, train stations, airports, and sporting arenas with easily accessible door openers, water fountains, and lights that are controlled by "magic eyes," voice amplification telephones

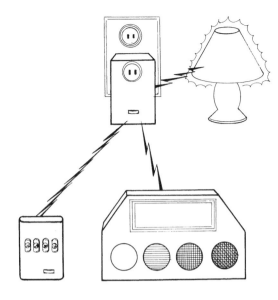

Figure 10-3. Remote control devices.

for people with hearing impairments, and large, clearly printed or braille signs for visually-impaired people.

A key to selecting the best operating system is to recall that IR can be transmitted only in "line of sight"; sonic waves transmit only in one room; RF and building currents can be transmitted throughout the structure and in the proximity of the building.

ASSESSMENT

Before undertaking an ECU assessment, the seating and positioning of the consumer must be evaluated, and care must be taken to ensure that an ECU does not interfere with any other ATDs or routine activities of daily living. The assessment of a consumer for an ECU requires an exact evaluation of the four parts of the Bain Assistive Technology System (BATS): the consumer's abilities, all the tasks for which the ECU is needed, all the environments in which the tasks will be performed, and the various ECU systems available. A review of Chapter 3 is recommended for details on the assessment protocol for ATDs.

The ECU Needs Assessment provided in Appendix 10-2 can be used to determine the consumer's needs, possible access methods, feedback, integration with other equipment, and funding concerns. Important considerations include

- What devices need to be controlled?
- What access methods are possible for this consumer?
- What feedback does the consumer require?
- Can the ECU be integrated with other ATDs? Is the ECU compatible with other ATDs?
- Can the ECU be expanded in the future, as the consumer's needs change?
- What funding is available, and are there creative ways to overcome financial constraints?

Table 10-2. Classifications of ECUs

Level I

Devices are available off the shelf

Devices do not require an adaptive switch

Devices use direct selection and may be used with adaptations such as mouthstick, typing pegs, hand splints, and so forth

Devices offer primarily latching control but very limited momentary control

Devices allow control of on/off functions of appliances and lights (which can also be brightened and dimmed); includes telephones, multiple stand-alone devices, or small units that will control more than one appliance

Devices may use infrared and radio frequency remote controls

Level II

Devices are available through specialty equipment manufacturers

Devices are controlled by an adaptive switch

Devices use direct selection or scanning

Devices offer primarily latching control

Devices allow control of on/off functions of appliances, lights (including brightening and dimming), television, VCR, and adapted access to telephone functions

Devices may use remote control through infrared, radio frequency, and ultrasound transmissions

Level III

Devices are available through specialty equipment manufacturers

Devices are controlled by an adaptive switch

Devices use scanning, with the exception of voice activation

Devices offer both latching and momentary control

One system allows control of all functions of multiple devices, including full telephone and bed control

Devices may use remote control through infrared, radio frequency, and ultrasound

Level IV

Devices are available through specialty equipment manufacturers

Devices are controlled by adaptive switch

Devices use scanning

Devices offer both latching and momentary control

One system allows control of all functions of multiple devices, including full telephone and bed control

Devices incorporate integration with other electrical devices such as augmented or alternative communication aids, power wheelchair electronics, and computers using the same switch to access all functions

Level V

Future developments integrating technology into the community

(Adapted from Bain et al,[8] with permission.)

The most valuable portion of the assessment is the evaluation of the sensory, motor, perceptual, and cognitive abilities of the consumer plus his or her motivation to use the ATD and psychological acceptance of assistive devices (see Table 3-1 and Table 10-2). The assessment should include the physical/motor abilities of the consumer, including positioning (lying, sitting, standing), and the placement of the control site (head, eye, tongue, and lower extremity, as well as hand/arm activation). Cognitive abilities are also a concern in the assessment of a consumer for an ECU. It is important to establish that the consumer can attend, read, and follow instructions; has sequencing skills; and has long- and short-term memory. Many ECUs can be used with simple commands, whereas others require complex sequencing skills.

Psychosocial issues must also be considered, taking into account the consumer's attitudes toward technology and the caregiver and/or family's feelings and expectations. Some ECUs can enhance the consumer's independence and ability to attend school, obtain employment, and engage in community activities.[3] Attitudes of peers and coworkers should also be considered, and the appearance of any ATD should be unobtrusive, if not attractive, to the consumer and others. Some system for maintenance and repair of equipment should be in effect to prevent injury, malfunction, and abandonment.

The evaluation should consider all the present and possible future physical environments where the system will be used. The technology team should not forget the social environment or the availability of assistance from the caregiver or others when required. Finally, the team must integrate all the various systems that the consumer will use with the ECU. Appendix 10-2 can be used as a guide when comparing the operational features, functional capabilities, and flexibility of the ECU. The goals and preferences of the consumer are paramount. In addition, the following should be noted:

- Safety of the consumer with regard to the electronic and electrical components
- Dependability of the manufacturer to loan equipment on a trial basis, to deliver the system in a reasonable time, and to promptly service the system
- Ease in purchasing or adapting a well-constructed product
- Maintenance and replacement provision of the warranty
- Expandability for future educational, vocational, and avocational needs
- Ability to interface with various switches or access methods
- Programmability by the consumer and/or caregiver
- Ease of access by the caregiver
- Flexibility, including the adjustable rate and method of scanning
- Portability of the ECU and/or remote control unit
- Noninterference with the daily care or other medical equipment needed by the consumer
- Training requirements, including the cognitive and physical abilities of the consumer, the fee for services of the trainer, and the places where the training will be conducted

Two additional guides to selection of the most appropriate ECU are provided in Fig. 10-4, a flowchart based on the consumer's abilities, and

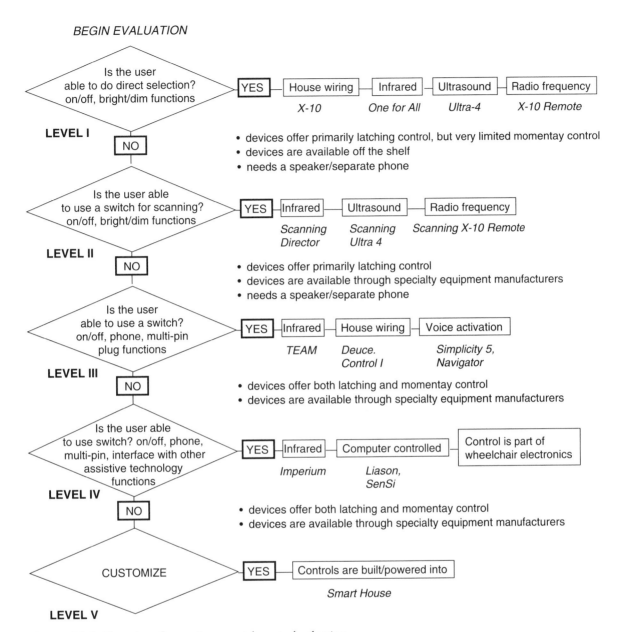

Figure 10-4. Flowchart for environmental control selection.

Table 10-2, a classification system for ECU based on availability, switch control, and transmission methods.

EVALUATING THE OPERATIONAL FEATURES OF ECUs

The following steps should be taken when evaluating an ECU:

- Determine the activation or input to the ECU: if a switch is required, how it will be accessed (selection, scanning, encoding, voice), and the nature of the feedback (auditory or visual)
- Evaluate the functional capabilities of the ECU: what kind of control is required (momentary or latching), how many appliances can be

controlled, and whether the telephone is integrated or separate from the system
- Assess the flexibility of the ECU to make sure that it is the most efficient for the tasks desired. This should also take into account the integration of the ECU with other ATDs and the mode of transmission that will be used in various settings
- Determine if the assistance of a licensed professional electrician is required for installation of the ECU
- Ensure that the ECU meets the goals of the consumer
- Consider the consumer's opinion of the ECU, its functionality, and mounting
- Compare the cost of the ECU and other options that may perform the same task in a different—possibly "low-tech"—manner, and choose the ECU that best fits the needs, desires, and financial requirements of the consumer
- Consult with the technology team and use clinical reasoning to assess other options

Implementation of this evaluation may require consultation with specialists in assistive technology (AT), either occupational therapists or rehabilitation engineers who are trained and/or certified in AT. This is particularly important for evaluating the functional abilities of the ECU and the flexibility of the system to meet the needs of the consumer and interact with other ATDs.

The ECU can send signals to the appliance in four different ways: IR, ultrasound, RF, and AC electrical wires. The first three send remote control signals, usually to a control module that is connected to various appliances (Fig. 10-5). The control module processes the signal and determines the function desired (e.g., turn on/off, dim or brighten lights).

Figure 10-5. ECU control module receives a remote signal that prompts it to activate various appliances.

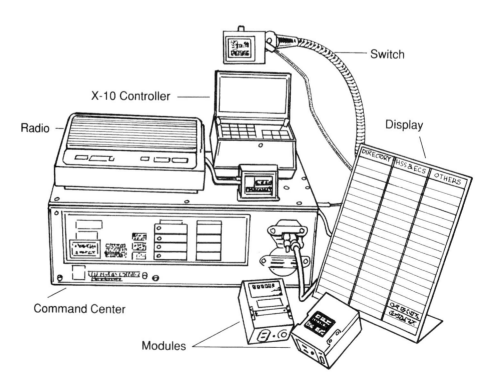

IR transmission works in direct line of sight to an IR receiver. An IR ECU signal can be recognized by other appliances, such as televisions, if they are programmed properly and the IR signal can be transmitted to other rooms by using technology such as Leap Frog or Powermid (Prentke Romich Co.). Radio signals are needed for room-to-room transmission. This can have the unwanted effect of triggering other appliances, sometimes in other apartments, that respond to the RF.

The environments in which the ECU will be used must be evaluated before selecting the control and transmission methods. The technology team should determine if the appliances will be able to receive the signal from a remote ECU and then if an IR or ultrasound signal can be used. If the appliance is in the same room or direct line of sight, an IR signal can be used. If four different appliances are to be used in one room, then ultrasound signals are used. And if a large number of appliances are to be controlled both inside and outside the building, house wiring may be used along with programmed modules (Fig. 10-6).

In summary, the assessment process requires time and diligence of both the consumer and members of a knowledgeable rehabilitation technology team, but the time and effort is well spent if the future independence and enhanced function of the consumer is accomplished. ATDs can be underused or abandoned once the consumer has been discharged unless proper training and routine reevaluations are carried out.

Because there are numerous different ECUs with various means of operation, other points to remember are the "newest" is not always the "best," the system with the most controls requires the most training and maintenance, the consumer must be properly trained in the use and full capabilities of the system, and routine reevaluations must be carried out. A key to the final selection of an ECU is to "keep it simple and usable." The result of these extensive evaluations should be a reduced rate of equipment abandonment.[4]

INTEGRATION OF ECUs AT HOME, SCHOOL, AND WORK

ECUs can be used in almost any environment, in one form or another. Many ECUs can also be integrated with powered wheelchairs and AAC by installing an ECU controller. An AAC aid and ECU may each require from 4 to 6 hours of power each day and therefore should use an independent power source when possible, so that the wheelchair batteries are not drained by the other ATDs. As always, consultation with technology specialists and licensed electricians is recommended when integrating electronic devices in any setting.

In the home, at school, and in the workplace, many lights and various appliances can be controlled by ECUs. For the person with a physical or sensory impairment, ECUs are available that can remotely control lights, kitchen appliances, security systems, thermostats, and door openers in a variety of environments. For persons with limited coordination and manipulative skills, off-the-shelf appliances are available at most stationery or office supply stores that can be controlled by ECUs, including electric pencil

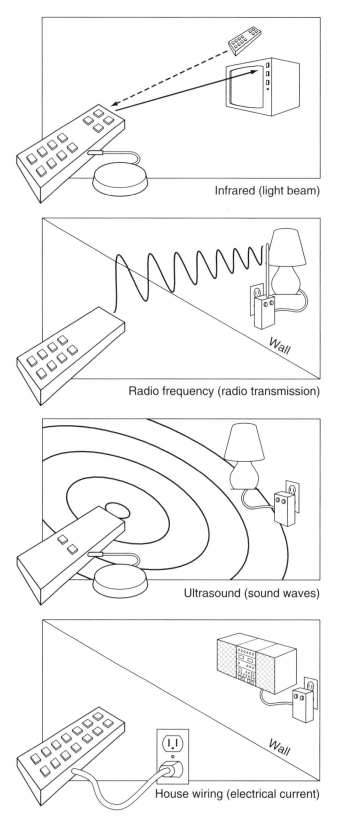

Figure 10-6. ECU transmitters (infrared, radio, ultrasound, AC).
(Copyright 1995 BK Bain. Graphics by CM Burwell.)

sharpeners, letter openers, electric staplers, and automatic paper folders. For persons with limited reaching ability, there are electric revolving trays commonly known as "Lazy Susans" or carousels that provide easy access to canned goods, paper files, or frequently used supplies. There are also electric page turners, roll-o-dex, fax machines, and paper shredders that can be managed by ECUs. Computer-driven ECU systems are transparent (e.g., they are programmed to operate without interfering with word processing, computer-aided design, or information retrieval programs). Some computer-driven and voice-activated systems can also control telephone operations.

Another important aspect of ECUs is telephone control. Telephones are discussed in greater detail in Chapters 7 and 8, but it is important to consider the integration of ECUs and telephones. New telephones are widely available with features that are especially useful to persons with disabilities. These include headsets, voice activation dialing and speaker-phones, cordless portables, and memory features that include automatic dialing and redialing, answering machine and fax features, and sophisticated print capacity telephone devices for the deaf (TDD). Any and all of these features can be adapted for "big-button" or mouthstick access but must be integrated with other ECUs to be most effective. As with any ATD, a careful assessment of all the tasks involved in telephone use will determine the optimal choice for the individual consumer (e.g., voice activation may be appropriate for a consumer with low functioning hands but not for someone with a speech disorder).

CONCLUSION

The ultimate ECU is a robot that can greatly enhance the independence of persons with disabilities. Robots are "stand-alone" aids that increase the functional abilities of humans (not only persons with disabilities).[5] Although some believe that in the future, robots will displace human labor in the workplace and reduce housekeeping chores, their best present use is to lend a hand to a person with a disability. The components of a robot are a manipulator or arm with a specific range of motion; a gripper or pincer "hand," a "brain" that responds to signals by performing specific actions, such as lifting or grasping; and a mode of transport or "legs" that move the robot according to instructions.[6] An example of a device created for use by consumers with disabilities is a robotic arm.[7] The robotic arm is a light-weight hydraulic lever that attaches to a wheelchair and can be operated using a sip-and-puff or joystick control (Fig. 10-7). Robotic arms are being developed that are very lightweight and flexible, with extremely fine motor control. As they become more affordable, many persons with disabilities can benefit from the seemingly limitless capabilities of these devices.

Larger free-standing robots are being used in assembly lines to manufacture everything from automobiles to vitamins, to serve food to hospital and extended-care patients, and to deliver mail in office buildings. Regardless of these technological advances, robots cannot replace human workers; rather, they act as an extension or augmentation of human capability. In the same way, ECUs are a technological means to enhance the mental and physical abilities of persons with disabilities, to increase their independence through participation in school, work, and community activities.

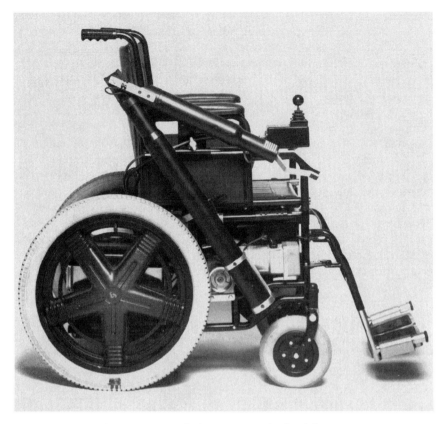

Figure 10-7. Robotic arm installed on powered wheelchair.

Any device that enhances the independence of an individual should be considered by the technology team when considering ECU options for a consumer with a disability.

REFERENCES

1. Bain BK: Technology. p. 333–337. In Hopkins H, Smith H (eds): Willard and Spackman's Occupational Therapy. 8th Ed. Lippincott-Raven, Philadelphia, 1993

2. Bain BK: Environmental control and robotics. In Hammel J (ed): Technology and Occupational Therapy: A Link to Function. American Occupational Therapy Association, Bethesda, MD, 1996

3. Efthimiou MA, Gordon WA, Sell GH, Stratford C: Electronic assistive devices: their impact on the quality of life of high level quadriplegic persons. Arch Phys Med Rehabil 62:131–134, 1981

4. Phillips B: Technology abandonment from the consumer point of view. NARIC 3:2–3, 1992

5. Webster J, Cook A, Tompkins W, Vanderheiden G: Electronic Devices for Rehabilitation. pp 289–296. John Wiley & Sons, New York, 1985

6. Mann WC, Lane JP: Assistive Technology for Persons with Disabilities. (2nd Ed) pp 44–52. American Occupational Therapy Association, Bethesda, MD, 1995

7. Seredos S, Taylor B, Cobb C, Dann E: The helping hand electromechanical arm. In: Proceedings of the RESNA 1995 Annual Conference. RESNA Press, Arlington, VA, 1995

8. Bain BK, DiSalvi M, Gold J et al: Environmental Control Systems: Assessment, Selection, and Training. Paper presented at AOTA Annual Conference, Cincinnati, OH, 1991

SUGGESTED READINGS

Bach JR, Zeelenberg AP, Winter C: Wheelchair-mounted robot manipulators: long-term use by patients with Duchenne muscular dystrophy. Am J Phys Med Rehabil 69:55–59, 1990

Batavia A, Hammer G: Toward the development of consumer-based criteria for the evaluation of assistive devices. J Rehabil Res Dev 27:425–435, 1990

Church G, Glennen S: The Handbook of Assistive Technology. Singular Publishing, San Diego, CA, 1992

Cook A, Hussey S: Assistive Technologies: Principles and Practice. Mosby, New York, 1995

Dickey R, Loeser A, Specht E: Environmental control units for persons with disabilities. pp. 257–286. In: Orthotics: Clinical Practice and Rehabilitation Technology. Churchill Livingstone, New York, 1995

Dickey R, Shealey SH: Using technology to control the environment. Am J Occup Ther 41:717–721, 1987

Lange M: Selecting an ECU. Team Rehabil 11:43–45, 1995

Minsky M: Will robots inherit the earth? Sci Am 4:108–111, 1994

Sell G, Stratford C, Zimmerman M et al: Environmental control and typewriter control systems for high-level quadriplegic patients: evaluation and prescription. Arch Phys Med Rehabil 60:246–252, 1979

Van der Loos H: VA/Stanford rehabilitation robotics research and development program: lessons learned in the applications of robotics technology to the field of rehabilitation. IEEE Trans Rehabil Eng 3:46–55, 1995

Resources

MAJOR ECU MANUFACTURING COMPANIES

APT Technology Inc., (formerly Du-It)
Shreve, OH
(216) 567-2001

Crestwood Company
Milwaukee, WI
(414) 352-5678

Don Johnston, Inc.
Wauconda, IL
(800) 999-4660

Prentke Romich Co.
Wooster, OH
(800) 642-8255

Quartet Technology, Inc.
Tyngsboro, MA
(508) 692-9313

Radio Shack (Tandy)
Fort Worth, TX
(817) 390-3011

TASH, Inc., Ajax
Ontario, Canada
(800) 463-5685

Teledyne Brown Engineering
Huntsville, Alabama
(800) 944-8002

X-10 (USA), Inc.
Closter, NJ
(201) 784-9700

X-10 LTD
Hong Kong
(852) 344-6848

Environmental Control Systems Needs Assessment

CLIENT NAME: _____ AGE: _____ SEX: _____

DIAGNOSIS/DATE OF ONSET: _____

REASON FOR REFERRAL: _____

DEVICES TO BE CONTROLLED

Devices	Quantity	Location/comments
Call bell		
Emergency call system		
Telephone		
Intercom		
Bed		
Television		
VCR		
Stereo		
Radio		
Tape recorder		
Light		
Fan		
Temperature		
Computer		
Page turner		
Door opener		
Door lock		

Comments _____

ENVIRONMENTS AND LOCATIONS WHERE ECU WILL BE USED

	Wheelchair	Bed	Work Station	Other
Home				
Institution				
School				
Work				
Other				

Comments: _____

_____

ACCESS METHOD

	Client Positioning		Comments
Access Method	Supine	Sitting	
Direction selection			
Scanning			
Encoding			

DOES THE CLIENT REQUIRE FEEDBACK?   [ ] Yes   [ ] No

Type of Feedback	Switch	ECU System	Comments
Auditory			
Visual			
Tactile		N/A	

DOES THE SYSTEM NEED TO BE INTEGRATED WITH OTHER EQUIPMENT?
[ ] Yes   [ ] No   If yes, with what other devices?

Equipment	Manufacturer/Model
Wheelchair	
Computer	
Communications aid	
Other	

Comments: _____

_____

Assistive
Technology:
An
Interdisciplinary
Approach

EXPANDABILITY FOR FUTURE USE

What are the client's goals?

Vocationally

Avocationally

Educationally

Medical status: (prognosis/potential for improvement)

FUNDING

Additional Comments: _____

(From Bain et al,[8] with permission.)

139

Environmental
Control Systems

CHAPTER 11

KENNETH F. DOOLEY

Introduction to Computers

Joan was a typist who developed carpal tunnel syndrome. Her employer assigned her to other duties for 2 months; however, she had to return to her normal duties by the end of that time or she would lose her job. A vocational rehabilitation counselor suggested that assistive technology (AT) could help Joan return to work.

One possible solution for Joan could be computer technology. For example, there are computers that are voice controlled through speech recognition technology, which allows virtually hands-free operation. If Joan could use such a system, her work problem might be ameliorated. A major advance in AT has been the application of computer technology to accomplish tasks and the development of technology to enable or facilitate the use of computers by people with disabilities.

Why does a person with a disability use a computer? For the same reasons anybody else does—word processing has replaced the typewriter in many offices, schools, and homes. People use computers for accounting, finance, weather forecasting, architectural design, engineering, and graphics design. They use them for audio-visual presentations. They use them to store and retrieve enormous amounts of information. They use them to control various devices such as tools, equipment, and the environment. They use them for inventory control, sending and receiving electronic mail and faxes, ordering products from a catalog, managing bank accounts, doing library searches, and many other things. A computer is essential for access to the "information superhighway."

Unfortunately, computers still intimidate many people, who are often afraid of looking or feeling stupid. The jargon associated with computers may also seem bewildering—words such as *RAM, ROM, kilobytes-megabytes-gigabytes, CPU, peripherals, hard drives* and *floppy disks,* and *hardware* and *software*. Moreover, wildlife and vermin appear to inhabit them—things such as bugs, mice, and viruses.

One should be clear on an important point at the outset: a computer has no more intelligence than a tack. But, like a tack, a computer is a tool that has many uses. For example, it can give people the power to make things happen through voice control alone.

The development of computers in some ways parallels the development of automobile and other technologies, each of which also has its

141

Introduction to
Computers

own jargon. When automobiles were new, it was wise to know a lot about how they worked before owning one; today, one does not need to know much more about the technology than what kind of gasoline to put in and to remember to have it serviced regularly. Similarly, great technical expertise is no longer necessary to be an intelligent computer user.

In this chapter, the term *computer* is used to refer specifically to microcomputers, as distinct from larger computers such as "minicomputers" and "mainframes." Microcomputers are often called personal computers and include desktop, notebook, and laptop computers. Their ability to run programs installed by the user distinguishes them from other devices that also use microprocessor technology, such as pocket calculators, electronic notepads, and calendars.

DEFINITIONS

COMPUTER

A computer is an electronic device that manipulates information (data) according to a set of instructions (programs). A computer system is composed of physical pieces (called hardware because it has physical substance you can touch and feel) and programs and data (called software because, unlike hardware, it has no tangible physical substance). The software must be in the computer's memory for the computer to work with it.

HARDWARE

Computer hardware, like the human nervous system, is divided into central and peripheral parts. The central part is called the central processing unit (CPU), which is the actual microprocessor. The peripheral parts include everything that is outside of the CPU—such as a monitor, printer, keyboard, disk drives—and these are called peripherals.

A computer has electronic doorways or gates, known as ports, that enable its CPU to communicate with the peripheral devices and, through them, with the outside world (which may include another computer). These ports allow input (the "putting-in" of information, such as commands or data; this may be from a keyboard, a mouse, a disk file, a microphone via a speech recognition system, etc.) and output (the "putting-out" of information such as data or control codes; this may be text on a screen, a printout, a message on the phone lines, a file to a disk drive, etc.). A typical system would use a keyboard and/or mouse for user input and a monitor and printer for output.

It is important to remember that the computer deals with electronic code. This is what passes through the ports. The computer has no interest in where the code comes from or where its code goes to. It is only necessary to get correct code to and from the operating system. The code is in binary digits (e.g., a numbering system in which there are only two digits—a 0 and a 1). These digits are called bits for *b*inary dig*it* and are grouped in 8-bit units called bytes. This allows 256 possible combinations in one byte.

Because the CPU deals only with code, alternatives to the standard devices can be devised (e.g., any device that gets the correct code to the CPU will cause it to execute the instructions; any device that can translate the output code correctly can be controlled by the computer). For example, anything that can transmit the code 01000001 can transmit the letter "A"—press a key and hold it for a brief time, then press it again for a little longer and you have done Morse code for the letter "A" and anything that can convert this to 01000001 can communicate this to the computer. Similarly, anything that can interpret the code 01000001 as the letter "A" can receive the output, even if it then converts the 01000001 to a short tone and a long tone (similar to Morse code). There are special programs called drivers that translate the code for specific devices.

SOFTWARE

Computer software can be looked at globally as being either system software, which is the software that controls the system and makes it work (the operating system), or applications software, which tells the system software what to do. The operating system handles everything that happens in the computer, and programs send their instructions through the operating system to make them happen. Without the software, a computer can still be used as a very expensive paperweight, but it would not be good for much else (if it has a monitor, it could be a nightlight.). For example, an application may want to send text to a speech synthesizer, so it sends the necessary code to the operating system to make this happen. The operating system then takes this code—which contains its instructions, including the location of the text—and sends it to the speech synthesizer. Each type of software may have associated data files. Application programs are written to work with specific operating systems, and code written for one system may not work on another.

MEMORY

Within the computer are small silicon chips that are outside the CPU and are used for holding information for use by the CPU; these are collectively called the computer's memory. This memory is ordinarily of a type known as RAM (random access memory), because the CPU can access any location directly by knowing its address. RAM is generally quite volatile (e.g., when you turn the power off, its contents are erased). Consequently, anything the user wants to keep must be saved to a long-term storage area such as to a disk. However, RAM is also quite fast—access time is measured in nanoseconds. The amount of RAM a computer has is critical to its being able to perform tasks, because some programs, including some AT software, are so large they cannot operate with small amounts of RAM.

There is also a permanent type of memory inside the computer, known as ROM (read only memory). This contains software needed for the system to perform. Although there is variation in how much system software is stored in ROM, at a minimum it contains the bootstrap program (from the expression "pull yourself up by your bootstraps"), which directs the computer to look for, load into memory, and run the system software every time the computer is turned on, a process known as "booting up." Before loading the system software, it usually does some checking of the hardware to make sure there is no problem (e.g., faulty memory) that would prevent the computer from operating properly.

In most computers, the system software is on the hard disk. The bootstrap program tells the computer exactly where to look for it on the disk. Sometimes the system software and some application software are also contained in ROM—this is most often found on portable computers.

Although there are other types of devices in use, every modern computer has at least one floppy (or flexible) disk drive and at least one hard (or fixed) disk drive for long-term or permanent storage. A disk is an electronic file cabinet; the drive is the electromechanical device that makes it work under control of the computer. The software is stored as a file on the disk. A "floppy disk" is also known as a "flexible diskette" because the disk is flexible, even if stored in a rigid plastic case; a "hard disk" is also called a "fixed disk" because it is made of metal and is rigid. In either case, the disk is coated with the magnetic medium to store the files. (No magnetic storage medium should be brought near a magnetic field or the contents may be altered or erased. Magnetic fields exist around electric motors, electric bells and telephones, speakers, etc. Instructions come with disks on how to protect them from other hazards and should be followed.)

PCs AND MACs

Although computers have been around for a long time, microcomputers did not come into existence until the 1970s. Initially, they were difficult to use and primarily for hobbyists. However, they developed rapidly, and they are now in common use. The two most common types are those based on the IBM personal computer (PC) and those based on the Macintosh by Apple. *PC* is a term used to refer to IBM computers or compatible machines. The Macintosh is often called simply a MAC.

PCs and MACs are based on microprocessors made by different manufacturers and having different instruction codes and operating systems; they are not usually compatible with one another. Consequently, software written for a PC will not run on a MAC, and vice versa, unless some special interface device is used to translate the code. Many new MAC computers have the interface built in so that they can read both types of diskettes.

Since its introduction, computer technology has made spectacular advances, and advances continue at a very rapid pace. Fortunately, there have also been spectacular reductions in their prices. One can get a fifth-generation PC today for less than the cost of the first-generation PC—and the dollar is not worth as much now as it was in 1981!

Not only has the technology become more powerful and less expensive, it has also become increasingly easy to use—for the general population and for persons with disabilities. This is the result not only of design improvements aimed at the general user but also of deliberate commitments made by the major producers of computer hardware and software to make computers accessible to persons with disabilities. A small but significant change involved moving the power switch from the rear to the front of the machine. This makes it possible for some people with disabilities to control the on-off switch and easier for nearly everyone else. Special features are developed for special needs; for example, there is software that permits pressing two keys in sequence rather than simultaneously, for people who may be unable to press two keys together. Other software changes can modify the speed with which a pressed key will repeat. There is also word prediction software that monitors text as it is being entered and tries to predict what the next word will be to reduce the task of entry. Additional features, adaptations, and special software are discussed below and in Chapter 12.

USE OF COMPUTERS BY PERSONS WITH DISABILITIES

If the user has a disability, then AT might be needed to use the computer. Such AT is generally either or both of two types: technology to facilitate input, and technology to facilitate use of output.

Assistive input devices are simple devices that enable use of the standard keyboard, such as a keyguard; software modifications in the way the system performs, such as altering the repeat rate on the keyboard; or alternative input devices, such as speech recognition or alternative code devices, our Morse code device from before, or perhaps various kinds of switches coupled to sensors (e.g., sensors that detect eye movements, motion, pressure, light).

Assistive output devices, which enable the user to get information back from the computer, may include software to enlarge the text on the screen, optical magnifying devices, speech synthesizers to read the screen to the person, braille devices, etc.

The computer, with or without special adaptations, might also be the AT needed for a person with a disability to perform various functions. Many of the uses listed at the start of this chapter and others might be specifically assistive for a person with a disability. Additional examples include devices that can read printed text and convert what is read to synthesized speech to assist persons with visual or motor impairments or a telephone directory on the computer that can dial the telephone automatically. Often, technology that is assistive for people with disabilities is also quite useful for people who do not have disabilities.

CHOOSING ASSISTIVE TECHNOLOGY

It should be apparent from this overview that selecting assistive computer technology (AT to use a computer, and use of a computer as AT) can be complicated. Many decisions have to be made, and making them sensibly requires information and expertise. It is important to use the Bain Assistive Technology System (BATS), described in Chapters 2 and 3 when undertaking an evaluation of a person with a disability. The BATS is a synergistic system that takes into consideration the consumer, the task, the environment, and the device. All these elements must be in balance for the AT to be useful in assisting the consumer to accomplish the task and achieve his or her objective.

Technology is a tool or a way of doing things, and choosing the right technology for the job is important. To choose, you have to know what the task is. It is worthwhile to remember that many jobs that might otherwise be dismissed as too difficult or impossible may seem reasonable once you know what the potential of the technology is. For example, tearing down a house and clearing out the lot can be daunting if you have to do it by hand, but it is not so difficult if you have a good bulldozer. Consequently, the expertise of various persons may need to be called on, such as the vocational rehabilitation counselor, the occupational therapist, the rehabilitation engineer, the AT center, the product manufacturer or vendors, and others to form a team of consultants. Jobs must be analyzed to discover the essential tasks, and the tasks must be analyzed to discover alternative ways of accomplishing them; various technologies need to be considered to identify those that accomplish the tasks adequately, and which of the alternatives is the best choice for the consumer.

The consumer must explore and evaluate his or her interests and goals, abilities, areas of functioning difficulties, and technological assistance to achieve the goals. Often, this will require the help of the team. It is not likely that any single individual will have all the knowledge and expertise needed to make the best AT decision.

The focus of all the activities of the consultants ought to be on the satisfactory accomplishment of the goals of the consumer in a way that is acceptable to that person. Accordingly, if a person needs to keep an appointment schedule, a notebook computer might do this very well, but so might an appointment book and a ballpoint pen, or an electronic notepad with a calendar feature. There are disadvantages to lugging a computer around all the time, not the least of which is the weight and the cost. Even though prices have fallen tremendously, you can still buy a great many pens and appointment books for the price of the least expensive computer.

The final authority as to the appropriateness of AT should always be the person who will be using it.

POWER USERS

A special concern in using microcomputer technology is ensuring adequate power supply and adequate wiring to support the system. Although each device individually may have a small power requirement, a computer system with many peripheral devices, and perhaps other appliances on the circuit, can add up to an overload, which can create a fire hazard or cause equipment damage. For example, if a person with a disability has a microcomputer system at home for work or for school that includes a microcomputer, monitor, printer, modem, and optical scanner and has a refrigerator, an air conditioner, radio, a television, and a powered wheelchair charging its batteries, there could be a serious overload of the electrical system. Modern computers are more energy efficient, but users are advised not to overload the circuitry. Another consideration is that many electrical devices such as refrigerators and air conditioners turn components on and off during normal operation. This can produce fluctuations in the voltage of the circuit that can interfere with computer functioning.

TRAINING

Anyone who plans to use a tool has to learn how. The person with a disability has to learn how to use a computer, the applications for which it will be used, and how to use all the ATDs or software that will be used. Any ATD will have its own training requirements, such as learning how to use a mouthstick or special keyboard to input data into the computer. Training in these adaptive devices is an essential adjunct to the training that may be needed to use the computer and its applications software. Most computers have tutorial programs, and there is a plethora of books written about computers and software programs. Proper and thorough training in each element is essential to the success of AT.

CONCLUSION

Computer technology can be a part of the solution to many AT problems. It is not always the only solution, nor is it always the best solution. It is important to consider the abilities, preferences, and needs of the person being evaluated; to analyze the tasks to be accomplished and alternative ways of accomplishing them, to look at the environment in which the action will take place, and to consider alternative solutions to arrive at the best choice.

In the case of Joan, whose story began this chapter, a speech recognition system is considered as an effective means for Joan to access her computer and perform her work. The AT team evaluated Joan's abilities and the task(s) she needed to perform. A job analysis and a task analysis provided valuable information, which was coupled with a functional evaluation of Joan, an assessment of her work environment, and consultations with others as needed (e.g., her employer, technology suppliers, engineers, ergonomists). The role of the interdisciplinary technology team is to consider each of the components in the BATS—the consumer, the task, the environment, and the equipment—to provide the best solution for the individual user.

CHAPTER 12

BARBARA A. KOLLODGE

Specialized Computer Applications

The purpose of this chapter is to provide information on different systems and different types of systems as an orientation to the wide variety of assistive technology (AT) related to computers available for individuals with disabilities. The specialized computer applications included in this chapter are by no means all-inclusive. Ongoing development in this area provides the AT practitioner or technology team with new and/or improved products on a monthly or perhaps weekly basis. In this chapter, I attempt to provide an awareness of the basic and more popular potential applications. With a better understanding of the products available and the functional characteristics of the specialized applications, a recommendation for appropriate AT will become easier and more accurate.

The system that will be best for an individual with a disability is determined by the results obtained from the evaluation of function and the assessment of needs. Manufacturers' use of universal, standardized connectors has made possible more integration of systems and innovative uses of products that are well established in the field of AT. The number of potential solutions in most cases has at least doubled in the past few years. The process of selection should consider, as a general rule, the simplest solution working toward the more complex and the off-the-shelf solution working toward a customized system.

FUNCTIONAL ASSESSMENT

A functional assessment for computer technology should be multifaceted and synergistic, as described by the Bain Assistive Technology System (BATS). Thought must be given to looking at the specific situation as it relates to four major areas: the consumer's abilities and/or limitations, the tasks desired to be accomplished, the environment(s) in which the task will be performed, and the equipment and/or specialized AT available for use.

CONSUMER ASSESSMENT

A consumer assessment is needed to determine the functional capabilities of the individual and any limitations that may influence the choice or recommendation of technology. The analysis should focus on

- **Positioning**—Is the individual seated in a position that will permit the maximal use of functional motions while minimizing fatigue and stress?
- **Motor control**—What muscle strength, range of motion, and coordination are available for completing the task(s) within the selected environment(s)?
- **Sensory functions**—Are tactile sensation, visual acuity, and hearing adequate for the use of selected AT?
- **Cognition**—Will the consumer have the interest and/or ability to learn new or changed concepts?
- **Medical prognosis**—Is the consumer's medical condition stabilized, or is he or she expected to improve or lose function over time?
- **Needs**—What are the specific task requirements and personal preferences for using computer technology?

THE TASKS REQUIRED

Any and all potential task requirements of the computer system should be explored during the assessment process. This will include any changes to current methods of operating the system, the consumer's desires and goals, and projected changes due to modified status or skill.

The assistive technology team should consider

- **Uses**—Will the computer system be used for running traditional office application software (e.g., word processing, databases, spreadsheets) only? The operational features of the system may need to be supplemented if it is to be used for internet access (to obtain information from databases, to use e-mail, to participate in bulletin board conversations or help lines, to use on-line shopping services, and/or to manage finances). Speakers and "sound cards" may be needed if the consumer will be creating musical compositions or using a CD-ROM. Special game ports or cards may be needed to run some educational or recreational programs. There will be many variations of necessary features depending on the tasks identified and the potential expansion.
- **Integration**—Could the system be used to increase independence through the operation of an environmental control unit (ECU)? Units are available that can operate lighting, fans, call signals, sound systems, VCRs, and/or other electrically powered appliances from the computer keyboard. For the consumer who is nonvocal, the computer system could also, with appropriate planning, be used to augment speech.
- **Telephone functions**—Some consumers will have a need for frequent use of the telephone during computer sessions. Telephone access, with most of its special features, can be achieved through the computer keyboard (or its alternative).

A comprehensive needs assessment will identify the task requirements of the consumer and result in an appropriate recommendation for equipment.

ENVIRONMENTAL FACTORS

Environmental factors will also have an effect on the selection of technology for a specific consumer. Special consideration should be given to

- **Location of use**—Will the equipment be used at home, at school, on the job, or any combination of these locations? The size, portability, and/or transportability may be important considerations.
- **Hardware concerns**—What currently used equipment in the environment(s) (personal computers—PC or Macintosh, mainframe, printers, modems, etc.) must the technology work with? Or are other major technology devices (powered wheelchair, augmentative and alternative communication [AAC] aid, ECU, etc.) currently being used for functional independence? The integration of these other systems with computer technology may be possible. No compromise of function in other areas should be accepted. The choice of computer technology should enhance or improve the current level of functional independence.
- **Software concerns**—What types of computer programs (word processing, spreadsheet, etc.) or specific application programs are being used in the environment(s)? The selection of a computer type (PC or Macintosh) is usually determined by the specific application programs that are required to accomplish needed tasks.
- **Space/surface**—In the setting(s) for use, is there space available for placing the equipment within the consumer's range of reach? When the equipment is positioned within the available work-window, will there be sufficient work surface available for other necessary activities (telephone, writing, etc.)? A keyboard with a smaller foot-print or a monitor holding arm may free valuable work surface for other activities.
- **Other users**—Will other people within the environment need to use the equipment? If so, any deviations from the traditional set-up that are made for the consumer should also consider the needs of other individuals.

EQUIPMENT AND/OR SPECIALIZED ASSISTIVE TECHNOLOGY DEVICES

The equipment and/or specialized assistive technology devices (ATD) have many variations in performance and functional characteristics. Knowing the answers to the preceding questions may not be enough information to adequately recommend equipment. The technology team should know the operational and/or the functional characteristics of the equipment to recommend the system that will be most efficient for a specific individual.

When recommending a computer system, consideration should be given to

- **Computer**—Will the memory (random access memory [RAM] and read only memory [ROM]), be adequate for management of the applications programs and any specialized computer technology that will be used on the machine? A large hard drive system is usually a must to minimize the use of floppy disks. The option for adding additional memory in the future, should it be needed, is always a plus. A system with multiple drives (5 1/4 and 3 1/2 in. and CD-ROM) is helpful for managing software. The size and physical shape of the central processing unit (CPU) may make a difference for the consumer, relative to their space and/or range of motion requirements. It may be more effective to have external disk and CD-ROM drives for positioning purposes. The speed of the machine is usually not as important as large memory capabilities, unless the consumer will be manipulating many large number calculations such as those used on spreadsheet programs or will be using network services extensively. What kind and how many connecting ports are required to accommodate the peripheral equipment (modem, printer, telephone, mouse, or alternate graphic user interface), in addition to any specialized technology?
- **Keyboard**—Will the overall size, shape, height from the supporting surface, or force required to depress the keys meet the consumer's physical needs?
- **Mouse**—Can the consumer effectively use the mouse that is supplied with the machine? Alternate graphic user interfaces are available in the form of trackballs of different sizes, graphic tablets, touch screens, or light pens.
- **Monitor**—Several factors should be considered when selecting a monitor: a monochrome or a color display, the ability to handle graphics, the quality of resolution, and the size of the monitor. Many specialized computer technology systems have specific requirements for the monitor that will be used.
- **Printer**—Will single sheet or continuous feed paper be easier to manage? Some printers can provide both, with single sheet feed from the front of the unit for easy access. Are the operating controls an appropriate style, and are they located in a position for easy access? Laser printers will be faster for consumers who require or prefer a hard copy of information obtained from on-line services, and they provide a better contrast of the printed characters for consumers with visual impairments.
- **Other peripherals (modem, fax, etc.)**—The controls and the method of operation should be easily accessible.

When the assessment findings have indicated that specialized computer technology is required for the individual to achieve efficient use of the computer, the technology team must also consider

- **Available control site(s)**—What functional motions are available for the most effective use of the computer? The control site should be selected with consideration of accuracy and ease of use without fatigue over an extended period of time. Almost any body part can be used to control a computer as long as it has the endurance for repetitive use and is reliable.

- **Method of input**—Which method(s) of input can be used from the chosen control site: direct selection from the standard keyboard or an alternate device, encoding as in the use of Morse code; directed selection as through a joystick; scanning methods using single or dual switches; or voice recognition?
- **Integration of the controls**—Could or should the controls for the computer be integrated with the control of other major ATDs that the individual needs? Systems are currently available or can be assembled to provide operation of the powered wheelchair, ECU, AAC aids, and/or the computer through a single input device.
- **Functional and operational characteristics of the ATD**—How does it work (the input method(s) required)? What input devices can be used (alternate keyboard, switches, joystick, voice, etc.)? Can it be used in conjunction with other technology systems? What are the space requirements and positioning needs of the system? Will the consumer have independent access to the computer with the system (or will assistance be required for beginning and ending a work session)? What can the consumer expect in terms of learning time and practice required for ease in using the device? What are the specific system requirements of the computer? Will the ATD be compatible with the applications programs that will be used? Can the ATD be adjusted to customize its performance in terms of speed, sensitivity, and/or selection of different features to meet the consumer's needs? Will the consumer be able to independently make adjustments to the system if needed? Does it have a record for use over a long period of time (e.g., is it durable?)? Is there reliable manufacturer support available? Is it affordable?

There are many variables and many possible solutions for the achievement of effective computer access by an individual with a disability. Careful and complete assessments of the consumer and the equipment capabilities will help determine a recommendation for technology that will be functional for his or her needs.

Many times off-the-shelf hardware and software applications can be used by persons with disabilities for access and/or improved productivity. Members of the technology team should be well-informed, smart shoppers who use the local computer store to solve many of the problems faced by persons with disabilities at relatively low costs. A good example is the computer mouse. Many individuals with motoric limitations may be able to use a standard keyboard but are not able to manage mouse emulations. Computer stores and catalog retailers have a variety of alternative methods for managing mouse emulation functions. Trackballs or rollerballs are available in a variety of sizes and shapes, with the click and drag button(s) located in different positions in relation to the movable ball. Small graphic tablets can control the selection pointer on the monitor with a movement of a finger. Software programs are available that can alter the use of keys on the numeric pad to direct the movements of the selection pointer. Also available are light pens and touch screens that will work on many computers.

Depending on the consumer's functional abilities, an easy solution may include one of these alternatives.

Manufacturers of computer equipment are consistently changing and improving their products to make them more efficient and easy to use. These efforts, although directed toward the general consumer, will also benefit the consumer with a disability. We can only expect to see more as the current "technology explosion" continues. Computer systems are becoming smaller and more portable and/or movable. For the technology team, this means that computers will be easier to place in a position for function and that they can be used in several environments. Bigger and better message capabilities are being included in major word processing applications as "macro" functions that are intended to increase productivity by automating a sequence of commands or phrases that are used frequently. Development in the areas of artificial intelligence (for industry and the military) has led to improved word prediction systems that can decrease the number of required keystrokes. Voice recognition technology, also being used by industry, has become adequately reliable for functional use by some persons with disabilities as a method for computer character entry. In the busy American's lifestyle, timesaving and efficiency devices have become big business, the benefits of which are very positive for AT users. Furthermore, computer systems are becoming increasingly easier to install and to learn, but best of all, they are decreasing in cost.

SPECIALIZED COMPUTER APPLICATIONS

What are specialized computer applications? They are any method, commercial, custom made, or specially designed for persons with a disability, by which the standard computer entry process can be made accessible and/or more efficient through the use of hardware and/or software. They include low-tech as well as high-tech applications, they are generally available for all types of computers, they are numerous, and they vary greatly in their functional characteristics.

Some general considerations when exploring potential solutions for a specific problem are

- Look for a simple device before considering a complex solution.
- Remember to check for off-the-shelf products before looking for the solution in specialized equipment. The difference in cost can be great.
- Give careful thought as to the type of computer (PC or Macintosh) that will be used and the consumer's software need requirements. Specialized technology that may be efficient for word processing may not be very effective for managing the operating system (used by programmers), and vice versa.
- Check and double check the compatibility of a potential ATD with the specific computer components that are to be used before recommending the technology for purchase. This is especially important when interfacing AT with one of the "compatible" computer

systems. The internal computer chips may be different, the operating system may be different, and/or the keyboard may be different, any of which may affect the intended operation of the ATD.

- Special attention is needed from the technology team when the ATD will interface with a mainframe computer. When a PC is connected to a mainframe system (as in a "work-from-home" situation), several of the current technology applications may not work properly.
- The companies offering internet services have different system and page formats (e.g., size of the "buttons," screen layouts) for accessing the information. Some features may be easier for the consumer using other forms of AT. In any case, the technology team should ensure that the network server is compatible with the ATD being used.
- The increasingly popular use of windows and window-type applications requires the use of mouse emulating functions. This could be an additional problem if the mouse is difficult to manage and/or the potential AT does not operate within this type of computer environment.
- The increased use of graphics in commercial applications programs may limit the versatility of a potential AT. Not all AT will work within a graphics-dependent environment.

I classify the many types of specialized computer applications into three major groups that are discussed below: keyboard assists, enhancements, and emulators.

KEYBOARD ASSISTS

Keyboard assists are usually hardware additions to the computer system that will make the process of character entry easier for the individual. They include

TYPING STICKS

Typing sticks are rubber-tipped instruments that are held on the hand by means of a palmer cuff, rings, or the pocket of a universal holding device. They are a substitute for an extended finger.

KEYGUARDS

Keyguards are grilled plates with holes that are designed to fit a specific keyboard. Keyguards help direct a finger or mouthstick to a specific key while "guarding" other keys from unwanted key presses. They are most frequently used for individuals who have poor motor control.

MECHANICAL KEY LOCKING OR LATCHING DEVICES

Locking or latching devices are hardware devices that through a lever or spring-loaded mechanism will hold down a specific key (usually the shift key) until released. They are designed to permit simultaneous dual key strokes when only one finger (or a mouthstick) is used for character entry. These devices have also been found to be useful for one-hand typists, especially those with small hands.

KEYBOARD HOLDING DEVICES

These are adjustable platforms that have been designed to maintain a keyboard in an alternate static position when the height or angle of the table surface is not adequate for the user. They are available for attachment to a work surface or to a wheelchair and are usually adjustable in height and/or angle.

WRIST GUARDS

Wrist guards are positioning devices, usually static, that are intended to support the wrist during typing. Many styles and sources are currently available following a recent interest in ergonomic positioning secondary to medical findings regarding cumulative trauma disorders and carpal tunnel syndrome. They are available in a variety of heights, depths, shapes, and surface coverings, all of which deserve consideration before selection. A few dynamic wrist guards are available that permit lateral movements with a minimum of friction.

ARM SUPPORTS

Arm supports are table-mounted devices that offer an articulated resting surface for the forearm. They were originally designed for industry to relieve stress of shoulder and neck muscles during repetitive assembly jobs at a table or work station. These arm supports permit dynamic movements in a horizontal plane, and the height of the supporting forearm trough is adjustable. These devices have been found to be very useful positioning tools for individuals with weak shoulder musculature.

ALTERNATE MOUSE EMULATORS

Alternative methods for achieving mouse emulation functions were discussed earlier in this chapter as an example of off-the-shelf AT. These trackballs, graphic tablets, light pens, and touch screens are all considered to be assists to keyboard access.

WORK SPACE ARRANGEMENTS

The desk height and size as well as the arrangement of tools and peripheral devices can have an impact on effective computer use. A variety of adjustable height desks, copy holders, monitor support arms, and other accessories are commercially available for use by the consumer and technology team.

ENHANCEMENTS

Enhancements are usually software programs that provide a special function to make character entry and/or the use of a computer easier and/or more efficient. They include

ABBREVIATION EXPANSION

Sometimes known as productivity software, abbreviation expansion is a computer "shorthand" feature. Two or more key strokes can be defined to invoke a longer sequence of character entries. They are used to enter frequently used long words and/or phrases (some up to 250 characters) or to simplify complicated or repetitive command sequences. Abbreviation expansion is available as commercial application software, as the macro feature in popular word processing programs, or as one of the features of specialized computer application programs (hardware and software) designed for an individual with a disability. *Note:* Whenever the number of keystrokes is decreased, regardless of the method used, the efficiency of computer usage is improved.

PREDICTED WORDS

Predicted words is a feature in which the computer seems to anticipate the consumer's next word. When the consumer enters the first character of a word, a "pop-up" list of words beginning with that character is displayed on the monitor that may then be selected with an additional keystroke. Most programs will also add a space after the word. Thus, a word such as *anywhere* (nine keystrokes with the space) could be typed with two keystrokes ("a" and the additional designated key—usually a number) at a savings of seven keystrokes. The dictionary of words to be displayed can usually be edited to include the words used most frequently. Some software features an "adaptive" word prediction program that learns the word patterns of the consumer. When a word is selected from the predicted word box, the program will put the most likely next word in the box regardless of the initial letter. It becomes more accurate in its predictions the more it is used, because unused words are automatically replaced by the words used by the individual. Automatic word endings (-ing, -ment, -ly, etc.) are also included. *Note:* This type of enhancement program can be very effective, but because it is a modified method of character input, it will require the user to reorient his or her patterns of character entry. For some consumers, the flashing on the monitor as the "pop-up" boxes change may be a distraction or a potential problem for the visual system. Some therapists have used word prediction methods to help consumers who have "word finding" or spelling difficulties.

POP-UP UTILITIES

Software applications, commercial and/or specialized, are available that permit the user to access and dial telephone numbers, use a calculator, take messages and notes in a separate window for use later, access a calendar or appointment book, and more. *Note:* Many pop-up utility programs are available commercially that have features useful to a person with a disability. Check the compatibility of these programs with the other specialized technology being used. Also, the key codes required to pop-up the utility may be the same as key codes used in the specialized technology.

ENLARGED CHARACTER IMAGERY

For people with visual limitations, the size of text presented on the monitor can be magnified from 2 to 12 times normal size through specialized programs sold separately or as a feature of other specialized applications. The cursor, which is usually a blinking line, can also be changed to a block either through a special program or within the set-up options of many popular word processing programs. *Note:* For individuals requiring only minimal magnification, easier methods for enlarging the characters can be achieved by purchasing a larger monitor or using a larger font size in the word processing program. Check the system specifications for both the applications program and the computer system for compatibility. Some applications for enlarged imagery require large amounts of memory and/or specific video systems. The shape of the characters (squared/jagged edges versus rounded edges) will vary with the different programs.

Visual Cues

For individuals with hearing impairments, several companies offer visual cues or "warning beeps" (a flashing symbol or screen flashing) to substitute for the normal warning beeps of the computer.

Key Latching/Locking

This type of application was discussed earlier as a mechanical keyboard assist that would work on an individual key (usually shift). As an enhancement, the latching function (often known as "sticky keys") is accomplished through software and will usually affect the shift key as well as other control keys of the computer. For example, more than one key can be latched at a time, making possible a "soft boot" (simultaneously pressing CTRL, ALT, and DEL on the PC-type computer) with one finger. *Note:* Some programs may not work on older or "compatible" machines. Also, some programs remain active once installed on a machine, which could make accurate character entry difficult for another individual using the computer in the traditional manner. To solve this potential problem for the traditional typist, most latching programs can be easily disengaged whereas others will automatically disengage when the computer receives a signal of any simultaneous key press.

Mouse Keys

Some people may be able to manage a standard keyboard but, due to difficulty with coordinated movements and/or grasp, cannot effectively use a computer mouse. Enhancement programs are available in which the mouse functions can be controlled through the keys of the numeric keypad. *Note:* The sensitivity or speed of the cursor movements and the "click" speed or preferred click buttons can be adjusted from the windows control panel or the specific mouse driver.

Adjustable Keyboard Responses

When an individual has difficulty with the "feel" or "touch" response of a standard computer keyboard, there are several enhancements that can adjust the response of that keyboard including

1. The timing of the auto-repeat rate can be decreased to prevent unwanted repetitions of a character when a key is depressed a little too long.
2. The accept time of a key press can be increased, requiring a longer press before the key character is accepted to help prevent entry of key characters if a key is bumped.
3. Adjustments can instruct the computer to accept only one character unless there is a slight delay before a signal is received from the same key, when an unwanted second character is accepted because the user has a tendency to "bounce" on a key.
4. A program is available that adjusts the keyboard so that no signal is sent to the computer until pressure is released from that key. This is useful for people who have difficulty lifting off a key.

Computer hardware and software manufacturers have assisted persons with disabilities by providing enhancement programs with their products. Macintosh and Apple IIgs computers have Easy Access, a utility that includes Sticky Keys and Mouse Keys; Close View, an enlarged character adjustment; adjustable repeat rates; and visual signals for the hearing impaired. The makers of IBM computers offer AccessDOS, a program that includes StickyKeys; MouseKeys; ToggleKeys (which indicates the on/off status of CAPS LOCK, NUM LOCK, and SCROLL LOCK); a Keyboard Response Group that includes RepeatKeys, SlowKeys, and BounceKeys; SerialKeys, which permits connecting an alternate input device through the serial port; ShowSounds; and TimeOut, which automatically disengages AccessDOS when unused for a period of time to prevent confusion if another person uses the computer later. The Microsoft Corporation has created an Access Pak for Windows, with special features that are built into the Windows 95 program. All these functional features are available for free or at a low cost to consumers with disabilities.

EMULATORS

Emulators are external devices and/or software programs that provide an alternate method for input of a character selection (e.g., the computer "thinks" that the keyboard is in use and is sending it a signal when actually an alternate method of character entry is being used. Specialized devices in this category are numerous and proliferating. They are generally available for all types of computers, but many products are computer specific (e.g., they work only with PCs or only Macintosh). Products with similar functional characteristics may be available from a different company. Shopping through vendor catalogs and equipment fairs will be very helpful in learning the extent of what is currently available.

For clarification, the category of keyboard emulators will be discussed in four general groupings: alternate keyboards displayed on the computer monitor; alternate keyboards presented on a separate monitor; alternate keyboards that are a separate peripheral device; and no alternate keyboard, only a different signal that is sent to the computer.

"On-Screen" Keyboards

Alternate keyboards displayed on the computer monitor or "on-screen" keyboards are a pictorial representation of the computer keys (Fig. 12-1). Some are presented as the standard QWERTY keyboard, while others are a different arrangement of key characters that the developer designed and arranged for efficiency when using the intended input device or switch. Some on-screen keyboards have several different layers of key characters and others have built-in functions such as predicted words. Regardless of the style, most on-screen keyboards are overlays that sit on top of the application program being used (e.g., they MUST occupy space on the monitor display). Some can be relocated to a different section of the display and/or be miniaturized for viewing the contents of the entire monitor display.

The QWERTY-style on-screen keyboard is usually accessed by a direct selection method using a specialized cursor emulator. These cursor or mouse emulators are most often controlled by a joystick or by head movements. The mouse "click functions" may be automatic when the cursor is held on the selected key, or it may be accomplished through an

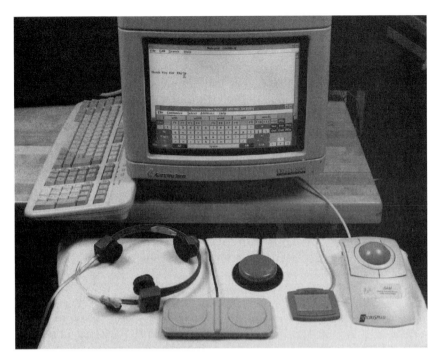

Figure 12-1. An alternate keyboard display on the computer monitor that is accessed with a variety of switches. (Copyright 1996 Tony Velez.)

alternate switch. This is usually a fast method of character input. These QWERTY-style keyboards are often large, and some may cover a significant portion of the monitor display, leaving little visual working space for the document.

The on-screen keyboards with specially arranged character keys are usually designed for a scanning method of input (row-column, directed, step scanning, etc.). The scan and the character selection are achieved by a switch operation (single, dual, or multiple switches). Most of these keyboards are smaller in size, and the characters/functions are displayed on two or more levels. To access the keys used less frequently (numbers, function keys, etc.), the user must first go to a different level, which would involve an additional switch activation. *Note:* Most on-screen keyboard systems are compact and generally portable. Many of them work effectively on portable/laptop computers. If the keyboard display is limited to only one location on the monitor, it may cover the status line or the "cue bars" of some software applications. This type of keyboard emulator is generally NOT very adaptable to difficult positioning because the computer monitor must always be positioned within a clear line of vision.

KEYBOARDS ON A SEPARATE MONITOR

Alternate keyboards that are displayed on a separate monitor usually do not resemble the standard QWERTY keyboard but are arranged for efficiency when using the intended input device (most often a joystick-type switch) (Fig. 12-2). Like the previous grouping of on-screen keyboards, the method of input is usually direct selection, although some do work with scanning methods. *Note:* This type of keyboard is usually large (the full size of the second monitor), and it may be a good choice for individuals with visual limitations or those with minor coordination difficulties (it allows for a larger target area). Some individuals may not adapt well to the extra eye or head movements required to check work that will be displayed on a separate monitor. Space requirements for this type of system are greater than usual and should be considered in the selection process.

PERIPHERAL KEYBOARDS

Alternate keyboards are a separate peripheral device and include (Fig. 12-3)

1. *Mini keyboards* that have an average "foot-print" of approximately 8 × 8 in. Character access is by direct selection using a finger, mouthstick, or special metal wand. Mini keyboards are often a good choice for individuals who have a small functional "work-window" or when work space is a premium.
2. *Enlarged keyboards* are approximately 24 × 18 in. They also use a direct selection method of input. These applications are useful for individuals with poor coordination or those who need a larger target area for character selection.

Figure 12-2. Alternate keyboards displayed on a separate monitor so that they can be arranged for efficiency when using the intended input device (most often a joystick-type switch). (Copyright 1996 Tony Velez.)

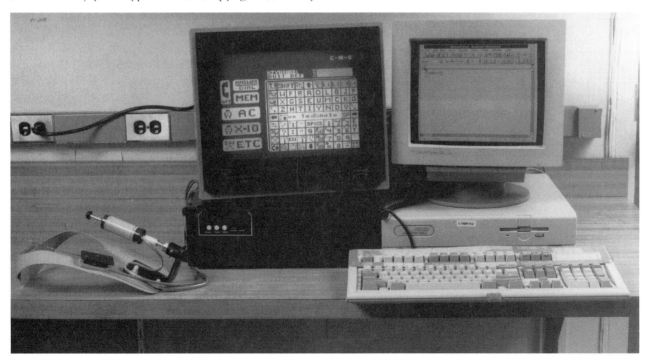

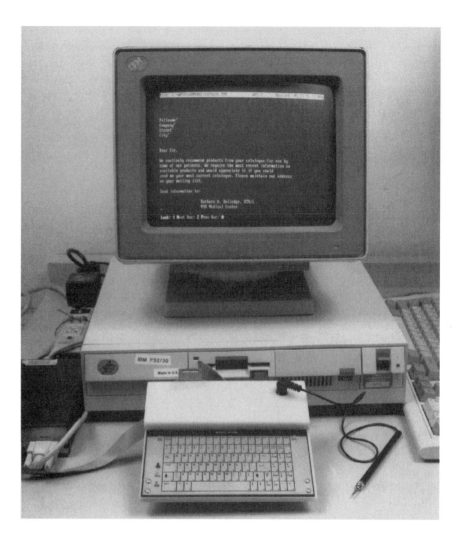

Figure 12-3. Peripheral keyboards.
(Copyright 1996 Tony Velez.)

3. *Peripheral keyboards* are also available that use different types of scan methods (row-column, step scan, etc.). The input devices for these peripheral-type keyboards are most often mechanical single, dual, or multiple switches.

4. Other peripheral keyboards are available that use a *direct selection method* of input using a light pointer that is usually worn on a head band.

Note: This grouping of keyboards, with the possible exception of enlarged keyboards, are relatively small and usually more versatile for difficult or unusual positioning demands such as those required for use while lying in bed.

ALTERNATE INPUT WITHOUT A SPECIALIZED KEYBOARD

The last grouping of emulators have no alternate keyboard, but the signals are sent to the computer from a different source (Fig. 12-4).

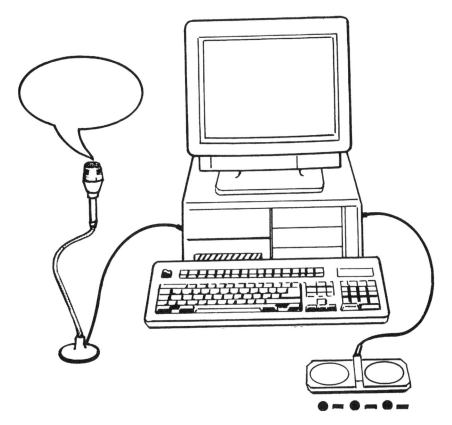

Figure 12-4. Alternate input methods.

These include encoding methods such as Morse code or the use of voice recognition technology. Both of these methods of input require extra learning/ training time to become proficient. Applications that use Morse code are available for all types of computers, and the codes can be sent to the computer via the use of single or dual switches used in a variety of patterns. Once the codes are learned, this can be a fast method of character input.

Voice recognition technology has improved greatly in recent years and has been found to be an effective method of character/word input. An evaluation of speech patterns, voice consistency, and the health of the speech mechanisms should be completed when this technology is being considered for computer access. Training the system to a level of proficiency is a great time investment. The more the system is used, if used properly, the more accurate it becomes. Using the voice for communication (with the computer) is thought to be very natural; however, the method of speaking (one word at a time) is quite unnatural and could be stressful for the speech mechanisms and may be confusing to the consumer. However, these systems could provide a means of access when no other control site is available except the voice. Voice recognition may also be an appropriate choice as an adjunct method of character entry, when the person has very weak upper extremity musculature with poor endurance.

The preceding discussion of emulators covered only the primary function of character entry on a computer. Most of these emulators have many other features that should be considered in the selection process.

- Most systems will operate with several different types and styles of switches. Choose the one that is most efficient or is preferred by the consumer.
- Adjustments are usually available for rate of access, sensitivity, and user responses. Explore the entire program when assessing the functional capabilities of any system.
- Many of the emulators include utility packages that may have useful features for a specific client.
- More than one type of specialized application may be required to meet the client's needs. Specialized application programs that are made by the same company are generally compatible with one another, but this should not limit your thinking. If achieving the necessary functional features requires mixing technology from several sources, try it, but be sure to check the compatibility.
- An increasing number of emulators are now designed for easy integration of their functions with other major technology systems (ECU, AAC aids, etc.).
- In general, most of the specialized computer applications are more complex than described in the manufacturer's flyer. Review the literature from the company, and if the application seems appropriate for the client, contact the manufacturer and request a demonstration disk or a loaner device for trials.
- Keep an open mind when exploring the different systems. Just because the features are stated to have been designed for a specific disability or a particular use does not mean that it is the only possibility. Be creative! If you think it may work for the person you are evaluating, with minor modifications, try it, or consult with the manufacturer for their opinion. The developers of this equipment are always interested in receiving comments and feedback from technology teams and consumers.

CONCLUSION

Chapter 11 began with the case of Joan who had a carpal tunnel syndrome problem. After Joan had a functional evaluation by an occupational therapist, all of her job tasks were analyzed by her vocational rehabilitation counselor, and her work environment was assessed by an ergonomist. In addition to a voice recognition system proposed in Chapter 11, another option for Joan is a computer with a split keyboard. Joan tried a split keyboard, was trained on its application, and enthusiastically agreed that it would solve her problem. A commercially available split keyboard allows a person to use computers with the hands in a vertical position, perpendicular to a desk rather than parallel. This vertical position minimizes the strain on the wrist muscles, which is a major cause of carpal tunnel problems. Joan's employer agreed that she was a valuable employee and purchased the keyboard.

When the split keyboard was delivered to Joan's office, an occupational therapist and ergonomist reevaluated Joan's work site to ensure that she could efficiently use the new keyboard. Six months later, Joan no longer has the carpal tunnel pain, and she continues to be a vital employee.

SUGGESTED READINGS

Anson D: Finding your way in the maze of computer access technology. Am J Occup Ther 48(2):121–129, 1994

Church G, Glennen S: The Handbook of Assistive Technology. Singular Publishing Group, San Diego, CA, 1992

Cook A, Hassey S: Assistive Technologies: Principles and Practice, CV Mosby, St. Louis, 1995

Deterding C: Computer access options. In Hammel J (ed): Technology and Occupational Therapy: A Link to Function. Lesson 6. pp 1–35. American Occupational Therapy Association, Rockville, MD, 1996

Lee K, Thomas DJ: Control of Computer-based Technology for People with Physical Disabilities: An Assessment Manual. University of Toronto Press, Toronto, 1989

Wright C, Nomura M: From Toys to Computers: Access for the Physically Disabled Child. 2nd Ed. Wright, San Jose, CA, 1990

Resources

PUBLICATIONS

Apple Computer Resources in Special Education
and Rehabilitation
DLM Teaching Resources, Inc.
Allen, TX 75002

Beginner's Guide to Personal Computers for the
Blind and Visually Impaired
National Braille Press
Boston, MA 02115

Closing the Gap Resources Directory
(Yearly Update)
Henderson, MN 56044

MAJOR MANUFACTURERS

Apple Macintosh Special Needs
(408) 974-7910

IBM Special Needs Center
(800) 426-4832

Dragon (Dictate) Systems Inc.
(617) 965-5200

Don Johnston
(800) 999-4660

IntelliTools, Inc.
(800) 899-6687

Madenta Communications, Inc.
(403) 450-8926

Microsystems Software, Inc.
(800) 828-2600

Words+, Inc.
(800) 869-8521

CHAPTER 13

AMY G. DELL

Computer Use in Schools

Bernie is a high school junior who loves computers. Despite not being able to walk or use his hands due to athetoid quadriplegia (cerebral palsy), Bernie has succeeded in regular school and is looking forward to attending college. He has been able to demonstrate his intelligence and complete his schoolwork by using a computer equipped with a special adapted input device—a custom-mounted joystick that he operates with his cheek and chin. Coupled with an on-screen keyboard, Bernie uses this adapted joystick to write papers, take tests, and his favorite, create his own personal *HyperCard* stacks. He has also begun keeping in touch with friends through e-mail and "surfing the Net" for fun and information gathering using only his cheek, chin, and joystick.

Todd has learning disabilities that severely impair his ability to organize his thoughts and express them clearly. His handwriting, like many youngsters with learning disabilities, is illegible, even to himself. Without a computer, Todd would have failed most subjects in school. With a computer, he was able to complete high school, attend college, graduate, and get a job as a special education teacher. Todd's most important technology tools were a word processing program, a spell check, and a grammar check program.

Different disabilities require different assistive technology (AT) solutions. These two profiles demonstrate the remarkable ability of computers to transform the school experience of children with disabilities. In the past children with disabilities were often excluded from school activities, relegated to sitting on the sidelines while their classmates experienced "real school." Today, children with disabilities can harness the power of computer technology to increase their independence and become active participants in school activities. Computers have actually changed the meaning of having a disability from not being able to do something to finding new ways to get them done.[1] By creating new abilities, computers have enabled young people with disabilities to learn, to produce, and to succeed in that paramount environment of every childhood—school.

Just as there are multiple uses of computers in the workplace, computers can be used in schools in a variety of ways. As discussed in Chapter 12, computer technology can provide a voice for children who are unable to speak due to conditions such as cerebral palsy or aphasia.

This chapter begins with a discussion about how computers can enhance teaching and learning in schools by serving as a writing tool for children who are unable to grasp a pencil or write legibly. It will then focus on how computers can serve as a motivating instructional tool for all students but especially those who have learning disabilities, behavior problems, attention deficits, and cognitive disabilities. The last section focuses on specific examples of how AT can provide alternative access to schoolwork for all children with disabilities.

THE COMPUTER AS A WRITING TOOL IN SCHOOL

From the early grades on, schoolwork places considerable writing demands on children. They must write to learn new things (e.g., math worksheets to practice math facts), to demonstrate their mastery of the subject matter (tests and papers), and to express themselves (creative writing). How can a child participate in these important learning activities if they cannot hold or manipulate a pencil? You have already read how Bernie completes his school assignments with a computer by operating an adapted joystick with his cheek and chin. Lori, a third grader who has a rare form of muscular dystrophy that causes her to fatigue easily and limits the range of motion in her arms and hands, is able to produce written work with a mini keyboard that she uses in place of the standard keyboard and mouse. Minimal strength, reach, or dexterity is required to use a metal pen-like "wand" that makes contact with metal leads on a tiny keyboard. To reduce the number of keystrokes required, Lori also uses a word prediction program. With this combination of AT, Lori is able to complete all school assignments and homework and to be an active member of her regular third-grade class.

David, a young man who has cerebral palsy, provides an interesting perspective on the computer as a writing tool. He believes that not being able to write using his hands is simply a "minor inconvenience" because of the availability of computer technology. David uses a voice recognition system for writing. This high-tech system allows him to talk to his computer; it essentially enables the user to write with his or her voice. This adaptive input bypasses all his motor impairments and has enabled him to meet the heavy writing demands of college, from which he has graduated.[2]

USE BY STUDENTS WHO ARE BLIND

Computers are also useful writing tools for children who are blind or have visual impairments. To complete her school assignments, Serena, a 12-year-old girl who is blind, uses a laptop computer equipped with a screen reader and a refreshable braille display. The laptop can be connected to both a braille printer and a regular printer. After touch-typing her papers or lecture notes on the laptop using speech and/or refreshable braille as feedback, she can print a braille copy for herself and a regular hard copy for her teacher or fellow students. This set-up affords Serena a flexibility that blind children in precomputer days did not have. Because her classroom teacher and classmates do not need to be able to read braille, Serena can attend her neighborhood school and be fully included. In 3 weeks, she learned to touch-type at the end of second grade—shortly after finishing her basic braille training—using speech output. Some blind youngsters use a portable braille device for input into the computer, but Serena and her parents chose the laptop computer because it allows her teachers and peers, who do not know braille, to have access to what she is writing.

FACILITATING THE WRITING PROCESS FOR STUDENTS WITH LEARNING DISABILITIES

In addition to providing solutions to problems with the mechanics of writing, computers offer invaluable assistance with the process of writing. People with learning disabilities, attention deficits, and neurologic impairments report significant improvements in the quality of their writing when they have access to a computer.[3,4] Often characterized as having "poor reading skills," "weak organization skills," and "difficulty in written expression," these students have tremendous difficulty organizing their thoughts, remembering the rules of grammar, spelling words correctly, and mastering the mechanics of handwriting. Their weak reading skills exacerbate the poor writing because they interfere with the process of editing and rewriting. This combination of problems makes the writing process extremely frustrating and unpleasant, and many youngsters give up trying.

Todd, the young man described above, found a way around these frustrations. First, he solved the problem of illegible handwriting by typing his assignments with a word processing program. After working hard on an assignment, he was able to produce an attractive final copy to submit to his teacher, and the appearance of his papers no longer embarrassed him. Second, with a few clicks of the mouse, Todd could have the computer highlight all his spelling errors so he could correct them before submitting the paper, instead of having to face all those red circles indicating misspelled words. Third, a grammar checking program did the same for common grammatical problems such as capitalization, punctuation, and verb tense agreement. Lastly, the ability to manipulate text quickly and easily allowed Todd to revise his work without starting over from scratch. For students with learning disabilities, this is more than simply a timesaving feature of word processing programs. A simple word processor has the power to unlock intelligent ideas and enable individuals with disabilities to express themselves and participate in educational, work, and community activities.

Two other categories of software programs—organization tools and writing composition programs—offer additional means for students with learning disabilities to experience success in writing. Organization tools assist with generating ideas, creating concept maps, and organizing those ideas into linear outlines. For example, there are software programs for project planning that takes users from the prewriting tasks of brainstorming and developing idea "webs" to organizing their ideas into linear outlines and, finally, into written documents. Some word processing programs contain an easy-to-use outline feature that helps students organize their thoughts before writing. These tools are excellent choices for students such as Todd who have impairments in sequencing and organization. They improve the quality of the students' writing while increasing their independence in completing school assignments.

Composition programs facilitate creative writing and motivate reluctant writers. They combine the fun of graphics and multimedia programs with the power of full-featured word processors, so students can elaborately illustrate their stories, add sound effects and music, and produce a rather impressive document. In addition to providing numerous choices for background scenes and a huge library of clip art for placement in those scenes, some provide a good selection of "story starters" for those students who are apprehensive at the sight of a blank page. For example, one story starter begins with a tropical beach scene, complete with palm trees, and a submarine in the water. The text reads "We found a submarine at the beach. It didn't seem to belong to anyone, so we took it for a ride. What a mistake!" (*Storybook Weaver Deluxe*, MECC).

Some software programs take this idea one step further by linking such story writing programs to the use of theme-based learning. In this approach, the teaching of traditional school subjects is integrated by being organized around central themes. For example, when upper elementary grades study the rain forest, their science, social studies, spelling, and reading activities all revolve around the rain forest. In such a classroom, Imagination Express—Destination: Rain Forest provides a beautiful structure for writing activities. It also contributes to students' research because each "destination" includes an extensive on-screen reference guide that explains all the items in the graphics library. (Other "destinations" in this series include Neighborhood, Ocean, Pyramids, and Time Trip, USA, which offers six different time periods to choose from.) Students with writing problems can compensate for their weak spelling skills by using a labeling feature that provides the correct spelling of a word with a simple click of the mouse on a desired graphic.

SPEECH OUTPUT AND WORD PREDICTION

Many children with learning disabilities benefit from special software. Talking word processors "read aloud" text written by the user. In such programs, auditory feedback can be provided for every keystroke, for complete words, for sentences or paragraphs, or at all these levels; the user chooses which option works best for him or her. Some individuals find that feedback after every keystroke slows them down and interrupts their thought process; others—especially young children—find the immediate feedback helpful. Being able to hear their compositions allows children to check their writing and to hear if they actually wrote what they thought they had written and if they have written it correctly. The speech output feature also helps students identify mistakes that they might otherwise have overlooked, such as misspelled words, incomplete sentences, and run-on sentences. Many of the story writing programs described above include a similar "read aloud" feature.

Word prediction software, although originally developed for people with physical disabilities, is proving to be an effective spelling aid for children who have severe learning problems. These programs can generate a list of possible words after each keystroke and, instead of having to type (and therefore, spell correctly) an entire word, the user can select the desired word from the list. The program automatically inserts the selected word into the text. Word prediction is a useful adaptation for children whose spelling is so poor that they cannot benefit from a spell checking program. It has the added advantage of providing choices for a child who has a poor vocabulary or word finding problems. Brian, a 9-year-old boy with Fragile X syndrome who is included in a regular classroom, uses word prediction with a children's word processing program to complete his daily journal. While the other students in the class write in their journals, Brian uses his laptop computer to compose his entry for the day. To add a handwritten touch, he draws his picture under the printed entry.

BEYOND WRITING: MULTIMEDIA PRESENTATIONS

The ability of computers to manipulate text, graphics, sound, and video has changed the writing process and presents new options for students with disabilities. Research papers and creative writing projects no longer need to be limited to typed words on a page. Instead, students can gather information from a variety of media and, using one of the many hypermedia software programs available, organize it all together into a unique multimedia presentation. This alternative to simple text has several advantages. Students—especially students with learning disabilities, behavior disorders, and attention deficits—find it highly motivating and are able to keep working until they have produced meaningful presentations that demonstrate their new knowledge. For students with physical disabilities, this form of research provides them with access to sources and an ability to share their work, which they otherwise would not have. For example, Bernie has created several *HyperCard* stacks in place of simple writing assignments. He adds clip art and digital photographs to illustrate his work and highlights it with spoken narration and sound effects. These multimedia projects have enabled him to make presentations to the entire class for the first time in his life.

COMPUTERS AS TEACHING TOOLS

PRACTICING ACADEMICS

Many children with multiple disabilities, learning disabilities, attention deficit disorder, mental retardation, and autism are highly distractible and difficult to motivate. At the same time, they need intensive practice to master new skills. How can teachers provide needed repetitions without losing students' interest? Software that is sometimes called "drill and practice" fills this specific need. Math, for example, is a subject that requires a great deal of repeated practice; therefore, it lends itself to computer-assisted instruction. There are numerous math programs that teach basic math facts (addition, subtraction, multiplication, and division), fractions, time telling, money skills, word problems, and even advanced math such as algebra and geometry. What these programs have in common is that they motivate students to practice their math skills by providing many opportunities for success, gradual increases in difficulty, and entertaining, nonjudgmental feedback. Many students with attention problems who cannot handle typical "worksheets" are able to sit at a computer for long periods of time working on their math skills. An effective teacher will permit such students to complete their daily math assignment using one of these software programs in place of the assigned worksheet. By using the software's customizing options, the teacher can set the program to provide the number of problems and kinds of problems he or she wants the student to complete. For example, if the class is working on two-digit multiplication, the teacher can customize the program to provide 10 two-digit multiplication problems. This arrangement also works for students with physical disabilities who cannot write but can access a computer.

Early learning is a subject area for which there are hundreds of well-designed software programs. Software that addresses sensorimotor-level skills such as attending or cause and effect are especially appropriate for toddlers and children with severe multiple disabilities. More advanced programs provide enjoyable practice on matching, identifying, and sorting colors, shapes, opposites, objects, letters, numbers, and early vocabulary. All these programs offer a way to get young children with disabilities interested in—not frustrated by—learning activities. When they experience success early on, they are more likely to believe in their ability to learn, rather than to develop "learned helplessness" as many children with disabilities have tended to do. They also learn fundamental computer skills at an early age so they will be prepared for more sophisticated computer-based learning later in their education. These programs are also effective for older children with cognitive disabilities such as mental retardation or autism who need to master these basic skills.

Spelling and phonics are two other subject areas that lend themselves to drill and practice software. Some programs engage children in the repetitious task of practicing spelling words, which is particularly appropriate for students in special education because users select from several difficulty levels and the program includes a speaking feature. A popular group of programs is available to help children master phonics skills that are considered essential for reading. As in math, these software programs match most elementary curricula and can be used as a complement or an alternative to conventional worksheets.

HELPING DEAF STUDENTS IMPROVE THEIR SPEECH

A quintessential example of computer technology providing students with disabilities intensive practice to master new skills is the use of a "speech viewer" by deaf students to improve the quality of their speech. A primary education goal for many deaf students—even those for whom sign language is their main mode of communication—is to improve the intelligibility of their speech with hearing communication partners. Learning to speak clearly is a challenging task for deaf students because so many speech sounds that they must learn, including vowels, pitch, and volume, are not visible and therefore are difficult to imitate. IBM has developed a program that solves this problem by providing visual representations of correct speech and of a student's speech production. The student speaks into a microphone that is connected to a computer, and the IBM *Speech Viewer II* provides visual feedback on the accuracy of his or her sounds in the form of entertaining graphics and animations. What was previously a tedious and frustrating task is turned into a motivating and productive learning experience through this special application of AT.

FACILITATING EMERGENT LITERACY

Emergent literacy—that period between infancy and the time when children are able to read and write conventionally[5]—has become the focus of much research and intervention in the past few years. It has been recognized as having particular importance for children with developmental disabilities and those with severe communication impairments who use augmentative and alternative communication (AAC) aids. These children often do not acquire conventional literacy skills at the same time as their nondisabled peers; therefore, professionals need to provide multiple opportunities for them to experience early reading and writing. This section discusses how computer technology can provide emergent reading materials.

Electronic storybooks offer children with disabilities the chance to listen to stories independently and "play" with words and pictures with a simple click of the mouse. These programs put favorite children's books and stories on CD-ROM, making them accessible to all, and are especially valuable for those children who cannot hold a book or turn pages independently (adaptations can be used by children who cannot manipulate a mouse). These programs add an interactive component to early reading that tends to capture students' interest and to make reading irresistible. Children can choose to have the entire story read to them (in English or Spanish), or they can click on individual words to hear them pronounced. Clicking on objects in the pictures causes such funny and unexpected things to happen that children cannot wait to enjoy.

Emergent literacy is also a concern for deaf students, many of whom learn written English as a second language (sign language being their first form of communication). At the Texas School for the Deaf, Dr. Gerald Pollard has taken the idea of using electronic storybooks to support early literacy and added a sign language feature.[6] In *Rosie's Walk*, his first CD-ROM, the pictures and text accompany clear video images of a sign language interpreter. Deaf children can now have the story read to them in sign language or can have individual words clarified in sign language by simply clicking on the word. Dr. Pollard's second sign language-enhanced storybook will be a version of *Aesop's Fables* for middle school students.

PROVIDING OPPORTUNITIES FOR PROBLEM-SOLVING AND CRITICAL THINKING

Current leaders in educational technology and educational reform urge school personnel to look beyond drill and practice and word processing when they plan for computer use in their schools. The computer, they point out, offers us an opportunity to transform the traditional curriculum and to completely change the way teachers teach and the way children learn.[7] Rather than relying on rote learning, the computer frees us to involve children in active problem solving and decision making, thereby teaching them the critical thinking skills that are deemed so important in Western industrialized countries. The numerous software programs that have been designed around this approach get students deeply involved in the subject matter while motivating them to continue working until they have solved a particular problem. The main subject taught by these programs is usually science and/or social studies, including history and geography, but their integrated approach requires students to read, think, and problem solve, often cooperatively.[4] There is a popular software series of this type in which students experience another time and/or place and get to talk to historical figures of the past while they are pursue a specific goal. For example, *Oregon Trail* depicts traveling west in a covered wagon during the mid-1800s, and requires students to calculate the amount of supplies needed, to hunt for food, and to forge rivers and lakes. In *Yukon Trail*, students learn about life as a prospector in the Alaskan Gold Rush of the 1890s. In *Amazon Trail*, students learn to identify all kinds of animals and plants that live in the rain forests of South America (while trying not to die of a tropical disease). In *Africa Trail* (MECC) students plan and participate in a cross-country bicycle trek across modern-day Africa.

What is particularly exciting about these critical thinking activities, in addition to their being very effective as a teaching method, is their potential to include children with disabilities. More traditional learning activities, such as completing worksheets on rain forest animals or labeling a map of Africa, frequently exclude students with disabilities. These problem-solving programs, however, are accessible to anyone who can use a computer, no matter how severe their disabilities. Although reading is required, it is never time-limited, and students can take as long as they need to understand the text. Some of the latest programs include speech output to decrease the reading demands even further. Most important, the multimedia quality of these programs—their clever graphics, animations, music, and sound effects—are so engaging that even students with behavior disorders, reading difficulties, and severe attention problems are successful using them. This means that they are participating actively and appropriately in classroom activities and that they are learning the subject matter, thereby meeting their academic goals.

THE INTERNET

Involving children in active problem solving and decision making is taking on new meaning with the advent of the internet and on-line learning opportunities. Simply having access to a computer now means that children with disabilities have access to all of cyberspace and the incredible educational opportunities available "there." A resource room for students with learning disabilities in a suburban New Jersey elementary school, for example, found an exciting context for the teaching of reading and writing skills in an unusual internet project called Balloonin' USA. Billed as "the world's first interactive hot air balloon trek," the project involved having classes across the country follow the balloon's flight through daily e-mail messages and photos posted on the internet. The students with learning disabilities were motivated to write letters and e-mail messages to the balloon's pilot, asking him many questions about hot air ballooning, the weather, and his trip and inviting him to land the balloon in their school yard (which he eventually did). They worked on vocabulary, following directions, and creative writing skills by designing and naming their own hot air balloon, creating an advertisement for a fictitious hot air balloon business, and creating their own Balloonin' USA T-shirts. All this occurs while the students are learning U.S. geography by tracking the balloon's flight on a wall map (and incidentally, learning how to navigate on-line). This internet project is just one of many that actively involves students in exciting memorable learning experiences that teach critical thinking skills, reading and writing skills, and knowledge in specific subject areas. As school districts across the country are wired for internet access, this use of computer technology in schools is expected to mushroom, and students with disabilities will be able to be full participants.

All these innovative uses of computers as a writing and teaching tool are beneficial only if they can be accessed by all students, even those who cannot use the standard keyboard or monitor. Chapter 12 provided an overview of adaptive inputs and outputs that can be used to make computers accessible; this chapter provides specific examples of how these adaptations can be used in schools to enhance teaching and learning.

The task of writing requires access to the entire alphabet and special characters such as punctuation marks and command keys. Children with physical disabilities who cannot isolate a single digit but have control over hand movements can sometimes type using an expanded keyboard with an appropriate overlay. Young children, students with mental retardation, or students who are easily confused by visual stimuli are more successful with a simpler overlay that has the letters arranged alphabetically and contains only a few essential special characters (Fig. 13-1). Beginning writers do not need semicolons, brackets, ampersands, or tab keys, and because they are usually first learning the alphabet, and alphabetical array is easier for them than the standard QWERTY keyboard.

Children who have no reliable control over their hands but good control over their head can access the entire keyboard like Bernie, using an on-screen keyboard and an adapted joystick or with a trackball, head-pointer, or an optical pointer. Children who have only one or two reliable movements—whether it is with their hand, foot, head, elbow, or knee—usually need to use a single switch for input, either through scanning or Morse code. These three access methods—on-screen keyboard, scanning, and Morse code—are made possible by special interfaces that have considerable flexibility built into them. Teachers and therapists can set the speed at which a set-up will work, the kind of feedback (speech, auditory beep,

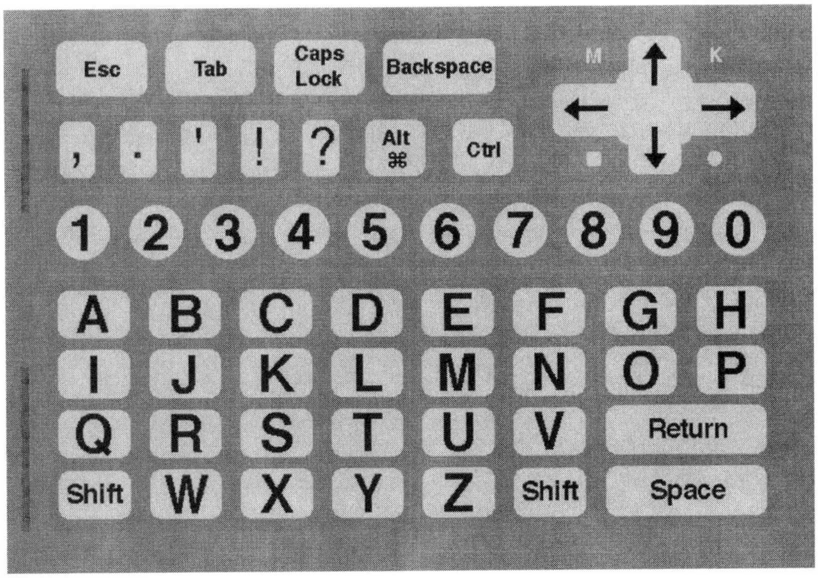

Figure 13-1. A simple keyboard overlay that has the letters arranged alphabetically and contains only a few essential special characters.

or visual only) the user will receive, and the set-up that will automatically be loaded at start-up. These options are important because the goal must always be making the student as efficient and independent as possible in writing tasks. Often, this will mean providing special training to students on using their adaptive input and arranging for them to have additional time to complete writing assignments. Scanning especially is much slower than direct selection, so efforts must be directed at decreasing the number of keystrokes required by using such tools as macros and word prediction software. Many students use scanning arrays that have been specially designed to work with word prediction programs. Using these access methods, students with physical disabilities can benefit from all the computer-based writing tools discussed above.

Adaptive inputs are most powerful when they are customized to match a particular curriculum or activity. Scanning places heavy cognitive demands on users and is very slow if the user has to use a full keyboard scanning array. However, if a customized scanning array is designed, the speed and efficiency of scanning is greatly increased. For example, if the other students in the class are taking a test on the countries of Europe, a custom scanning array can be designed in which each key contains the name of a country followed by a return. Then, instead of having to spell out the name of each country, the student who accesses the computer with a single switch has only to make one selection for each test question. With the motor demands decreased, the student is free to focus on the content of the test.

Another population who can derive similar benefits is students who have learning disabilities, attention deficits, and/or mental retardation. If a student needs to take a test on the multiplication tables, for example, but has difficulty writing, a custom overlay can be designed that requires minimal keystrokes. A single keystroke can result in the multiplication problem being presented on the screen, and all the student needs to do is type the right answer by pressing the appropriate numerals. So, the problem $4 \times 4 = 16$ can be typed with a total of three key presses (the left side of the equation, a 1, and a 6). Another single keystroke will result in the document being printed. Such custom overlays can offer speech output for each key press, a helpful feature for students with visual impairments, learning disabilities, and attention deficits.

Using assistive technology devices (ATDs) to solve access problems is especially easy for some of the most popular educational software series because custom set-ups have been made available by the makers of the ATDs. For example, the Early Learning series from Edmark teaches the skills involved in early math, reading, and science, thinking skills, time and calendar skills, and beginning story writing skills. Each program has an attractive graphic main menu that features the title character, and a series of activities are offered that are accessed with a simple click of the mouse. Customized overlay packages are available that include overlays for each activity and a computer set-up that automatically loads when a specific program is opened (Fig. 13-2). These packages of custom set-ups are convenient for teachers and therapists while providing opportunities for active participation by students. They are a perfect example of AT being used to enhance the school experiences of students with disabilities.

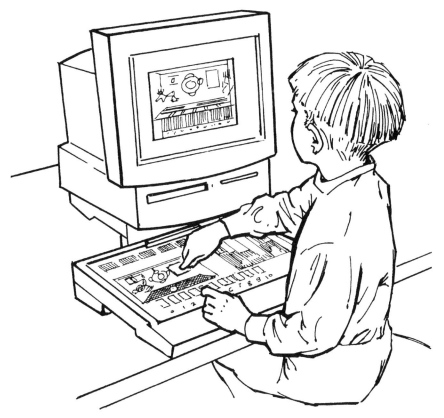

Figure 13-2. Child using a custom overlay for a commercially available software program.

MAKING IT HAPPEN

This chapter summarizes the opportunities for children with disabilities created by innovative applications of computer technology. It is important to recall the Bain Assistive Technology System (BATS), in which the consumer, the environment, and the equipment are each assessed according to the desired task. This is a synergistic system in which each element is dependent on and contributes to the other—one in which the total effect is greater than the sum of the individual parts. In this chapter, the physical and cognitive abilities of the children to perform school tasks vary, the environments are both the school and the home setting, and the equipment is the computer software and hardware and their adaptations (input and output devices). An AT assessment must be performed for each task that the child must perform, because writing is different from reading and is also different from mathematics. Homework may be done in a very different environment than the school setting, and the AT assessment must take this into consideration. Each child has specific school tasks to accomplish in specific environments; the appropriate ATD (computer hardware and software) depends on the physical and cognitive abilities of the child.

Unfortunately, too many children with disabilities are not receiving the AT services they need.[8] This is because many teachers and therapists have not been trained in appropriate applications of AT and do not have the extensive skills or ongoing support needed to integrate technology into their daily work. Additionally, the cost of purchasing, maintaining, and updating hardware, software, and ATDs is considerable and presents another obstacle. Attitudes also play a part: technophobia among administrators, teachers, and therapists is still common, contributing to a lack of appreciation for the benefits of AT and, consequently, a lack of will to do anything about it.

This is where advocacy enters the picture. It is essential that parents, teachers, and therapists are aware of children's rights under the law and learn the strategies they need to make technology integration happen. The federal law that mandates a "free appropriate public education" for all children with disabilities—originally P.L. 94-142, now with several amendments called the Individuals with Disabilities Education Act (IDEA)[9]— includes ATDs and AT services as related services that may be part of a child's appropriate education. If in the development of a student's individualized education plan (IEP), AT is listed as a needed service that will enable the child to benefit from his or her education, then the school district must provide the appropriate technology at the district's expense. It is the intent of IDEA to ensure that a school district cannot categorically deny AT to any student. The provision of AT and all rehabilitation services rests entirely on what is deemed appropriate for an individual child.

The key for the rehabilitation team is getting the specific AT needs delineated in the IEP document. This should be done in a way that clearly shows the link between the technology and a child's educational goals. It is not enough to include a generic statement such as "a computer will be used"; rather, the IEP should delineate how it will be used and for what purpose (e.g., "Brian will use a laptop computer equipped with word prediction software to write his daily journal entry and other writing assignments" or "Jessie will use *Math Blaster Plus* to practice her basic math facts and *Spell It 3* to practice her spelling words using *IntelliKeys* and large-print overlays"). This is the first crucial step in pressuring school districts to integrate AT into a child's curriculum.

Being knowledgable about integrating AT into the IEP is essential for rehabilitation professionals and parents. Parents will also need to be aware of their rights under the law to disagree with a school district and the strategies they can use to resolve differences. They may need to take advantage of training opportunities offered by the parent training and information centers that are located in every state (funded under IDEA). With parents serving as advocates and skilled professionals working to use AT to enhance teaching and learning, school districts will find the will and resources to fully integrate computers into the curriculum, and AT will finally fulfill its promise for children with disabilities.

ACKNOWLEDGMENTS

I thank students at The College of New Jersey (formerly Trenton State College) for their contributions to TECH-NJ that were included in this chapter and member families at the Center for Enabling Technology in Whippany, New Jersey.

REFERENCES

1. Alliance for Technology Access: Computer Resources for People with Disabilities. Hunter House, Inc., Alameda, CA, 1994

2. Clark D: A personal view: the power of technology. TECH-NJ 4(2):3, 1992

3. Dwyer DC: The imperative to change our schools. pp. 15–33. In Fisher C, Dwyer DC, Yocam K (eds): Education and Technology: Reflections on Computing in Classrooms. Jossey-Bass/Apple Press, San Francisco, 1996

4. Male M: Technology for Inclusion: Meeting the Special Needs of All Students. Allyn & Bacon, Boston, 1994

5. Blackstone SW: Augmentative Commun News 9(3):1–12, 1996

6. Pollard G: Rosie's Walk (CD-ROM). Texas School for the Deaf, 1995

7. Sheingold K, Hadley M: Accomplished Teachers: Integrating Computers into Classroom Practice. Center for Technology in Education, Bank Street College of Education, New York, 1990

8. Hutinger P, Johanson J, Stoneburner R: Assistive technology applications in educational programs of children with multiple disabilities: a case study report on the state of the practice. J Special Ed Technol 13(1):16–35, 1996

9. Individuals with Disabilities Education Act (IDEA) of 1990. PL 101–476, Title 20, U.S.C. 1400 et seq: U.S. Statutes at Large, 104, 1103–1151, October 30, 1990

Resources

BOOKS AND JOURNALS

Alliance for Technology Access: Computer Resources for
People with Disabilities. 2nd Ed. Hunter House, Inc.,
Alameda, CA, 1996

*Written for parents, consumers, and professionals, this guide
presents a process for readers to follow in selecting the AT tools
that will meet their specific needs. Informative section on selecting
access methods.*

Closing the Gap: Annual Resource Directory.
Closing the Gap, Henderson, MN

*A comprehensive and up-to-date listing of numerous products—
hardware, software, peripherals, and AAC aids—with brief
descriptions, prices, and vendor information.*

Exceptional Parent. 13th Annual Technology
Issue 25(11), 1995

*Each annual technology issue is filled with helpful resources
and personal stories about how AT is changing the lives of
children with disabilities.*

Learning and Leading with Technology: The Journal of the
International Society for Technology in Education (ISTE), Eugene, OR

*This journal for technology-using educators publishes successful
uses of computers in schools, often arranged by subject area.*

Male M: Technology for Inclusion: Meeting the Special Needs
of All Students. Allyn & Bacon, Boston, MA, 1994

*With a third edition about to be published, this is the best
text available on integrating computers into the curriculum
in schools.*

SOFTWARE PUBLISHERS AND ATD MANUFACTURERS

Apple/Macintosh
(800) 600-7808 or (408) 974-7910

Educational and special needs programs

Broderbund Software
(800) 521-6263

Living Books Series. School editions include helpful teacher's guides

Claris Corporation
(800) 325-2747

ClarisWorks

Davidson and Associates, Inc.
(800) 545-7677

Spell It 3, Math Blaster Plus

Don Johnston Developmental Equipment
(800) 999-4660

Ke:nx, Co: Writer, Write: OutLoud, and other easy-to-use access products and special software

Dragon Systems
(617) 965-5200

Dragon Dictate

Edmark Corporation
(800) 426-0856

*Imagination Express series; Destinations: Rain Forest, Neighborhood, Ocean, Pyramids, Time Trip USA
Early Learning series: Millie's Math House, Bailey's Book House, Sammy's Science House, Thinkin' Things 1, Trudi's Time and Place House, Stanley's Sticker Stories
School editions include helpful teacher's guides*

Educational Resources
(800) 624-2926

Excellent selection and discount prices on educational software

Inspiration Software (available from
Educational Resources,
(800) 624-2926

*Inspiration—a "brain storming" and project
planning program*

In Touch Systems
(914) 354-7431

Magic Wand mini keyboard

IntelliTools
(800) 899-6687

*IntelliKeys, customizing software for all platforms,
and special software. Overlay packages for popular
Edmark and Broderbund software programs*

IBM; Independence Series Products
(800) 426-2133

*Speech Viewer II—speech modification/therapy program
Thinkable/DOS—attention and memory program*

Screen Reader—text-to-speech conversion

Laureate Learning Systems
(800) 562-6801

Software for language development

The Learning Company
(800) 852-2255

The Writing Center, The Reader Rabbit series

McIntyre Computer Systems
(810) 645-5090

Wordwriter (on-screen keyboard)

MECC
(612) 569-1500

*Storybook Weaver Deluxe, a popular story writing program
"Trail" series: Oregon Trail, Yukon Trail, Amazon Trail, Africa Trail
Many innovative educational software programs, especially learning
adventures, problem-solving journeys, and creative writing tools*

Prentke Romich
(800) 262-1984

HeadMaster

Roger Wagner Publishing
(800) 421-6526

HyperStudio—multimedia presentation software

ORGANIZATIONS

Alliance for Technology Access
(415) 455-4575

Call to locate the center(s) in your state.
A national network of community-based computer
resource centers that offer information and assistance
in choosing AT solutions for people with disabilities

Parent Training and Information Centers

Call your state Department of Education to find the center
in your state. Funded under IDEA, these centers provide
information and training for parents on exercising their
child's right to a free, appropriate public education

Mobility

A Fortune 500 company has invited members of various departments to a meeting to confer on transportation guidelines for their works sites to meet the Americans with Disabilities Act (ADA) regulations.[1] One member, Sue, will take a kneeling bus in her powered wheelchair, Harry will drive his modified van from his powered wheelchair, Marion will drive her powered scooter from the building where she works to the conference site, Bill will walk two blocks from the subway using his laser long cane, Cris will fly a commercial airline and then use his standard wheelchair adapted with a power pack, and Wendy will lead the conference in her standing wheelchair, which she has transferred from the adapted hand-control car she drove to the meeting.

Members of this committee are using mobility devices that have been developed in the past 20 years as a result of the technological advances of materials such as improved batteries, light-weight metals, electronic circuits, and switches. Another factor is that as more architectural barriers are removed, more people with mobility limitations are able to participate in work, recreational, and community life activities. In addition, knowledgable consumers have collaborated with manufacturers of wheelchairs, cars, vans, and transportation systems to improve and develop new mobility devices.

This chapter presents general concepts of mobility, including how to assess persons with disabilities for powered mobility. In this chapter, we consider physical limitations due to spinal cord injuries, progressive neuromuscular conditions (e.g., multiple sclerosis [MS], muscular dystrophy [MD], amyotrophic lateral sclerosis [ALS]), degenerative musculoskeletal conditions (arthritis, aging), amputations, and the sensory limitation due to loss of vision.

Powered mobility needs to be considered as an integrated technology system that includes the abilities of the consumer, the tasks that the consumer and/or the caretaker need the mobility aid to perform, all the places where the device will be used, and the device or devices required for a total system to meet the needs and goals of the user all day. Usually, a consumer will need a powered mobility device due to limited motor function of both legs and arms, limited coordinated motions of all extremities, low level of endurance, limited range of motion in the lower and upper extremities, and a combination of any of the above.

The tasks that a mobility device should be capable of are transverse mobility over a variety of surfaces indoors and outside, ranging from smooth linoleum floors to gravel roads; vertical mobility for ascending and descending curbs, ramps, stairs, buses, trains, and airplanes; and rotational ability for maneuvering in restricted areas such as elevators, bathrooms, and confined office spaces and around machines or equipment. All environments in which the device will be used, including the home, work site, school, and the community, as well as the climatic conditions in each, are important factors in the total mobility system.

The salient characteristics that are desirable for powered mobility devices include safety, comfort, dependability, portability for long-range transportation, light weight that requires minimal effort for lifting into a car or van or any other form of transportation, ease of maintenance, ease in operation for the consumer as well as the caregiver(s), compatibility with other devices (ventilators, augmentative and alternative communications [AAC] aids, environmental control units [ECUs]), and personal acceptance by the consumers. The reader is referred to three major sources: articles on abandonment by Phillips,[2] evaluating criteria for powered wheelchairs by the Rehabilitation Engineering Center at the National Rehabilitation Hospital,[3] and American National Standards Institute (ANSI)–RESNA Wheelchair Standards[4] for specific characteristics of powered and standard wheelchairs, which is beyond the scope of this book. The intent of this chapter is to present mobility that will enhance the ability of persons to move about their homes, travel to work or school, and be mobile in the community. Of all assistive technology devices (ATDs), power mobility is the most complex system and requires close team effort in selection.

ASSESSMENT FOR A POWERED MOBILITY SYSTEM

The assessment process for a powered mobility system should begin with proper seating and positioning (see Ch. 4). Powered mobility is a means of preserving vital energies for productive pursuits, to improve the quality of life for many persons with physical limitations of function, and to enhance the user's independence. Therefore, each part of the system must be carefully evaluated before a composite assessment can be made to select the most appropriate device or devices for a total mobility system. In this section, the evaluation of the salient characteristics of the consumer, the tasks to be accomplished, all environments, and various devices are presented, with the recommendation that the reader review the nine-step problem-solving assessment in Chapter 3.

The evaluation of the consumer's physical abilities should include muscle power, as well as physical endurance, range of motion, and coordination, which will assist in selecting the best control site. Visual perception must also be evaluated, especially figure-ground, spatial relationship, and the body's position in space.

When evaluating the tasks to be accomplished with a mobility system, all tasks required in the home, at school, on the job, and in the community must be analyzed. For example, a powered scooter might be effective in a small kitchen when the user's task is preparing a meal and he or she needs maneuverability. When the task is traveling to work or school, the person will need to be able to access public or private transportation and negotiate the passage from home to a vehicle, and vice versa. Once at the school or work site, the person must be able to perform desk and other activities that may alter their mobility requirements. Furthermore, all personal hygiene tasks must factor into the mobility system.

The most crucial area of a mobility evaluation is the careful analysis of all environments including the terrain and climate. To illustrate this point, consider a farmer with limited function in his or her lower extremities, who may use a powered wheelchair around a barrier-free home environment with smooth floor surfaces. When the farmer goes outside to work where the ground may have sand, gravel, mud, or loose soil and the climate is wet or icy, any wheelchair will be difficult to propel. He or she may also need hand controls on a truck, tractor, or all-terrain vehicle.[5]

The further afield a wheelchair user travels, the more obstacles he or she may encounter. For example, when the consumer is planning to travel in an airplane, he or she should know that a powered wheelchair with wet or acid batteries is not allowed in an airport environment because wheelchairs are stored in the baggage area. Furthermore, when a powered wheelchair user arrives at his or her destination, the user may find that local taxicabs may not accommodate a wheelchair and a special van will be needed to transport the powered wheelchair user from the airport to a barrier-free and accessible hotel or friend's home. Careful planning is required when traveling in different environments. Some suggestions are for the consumer to call the airlines or train or bus companies, ask very specific questions, and ask for literature; if possible, do a practice run before the need to travel; travel with a friend or caregiver the first time the transportation system is used; and allow extra time for emergencies and so as not to be rushed. With the passage of the ADA, more environments are becoming accessible.

Powered mobility devices can be used to enable consumers to travel to school, to work, and around the community. These include powered standing wheelchairs, powered wheelchairs, powered scooters, golf carts, kneeling buses, modified cars and vans, and trains with accessible platforms and space for wheelchair users. As with any device, the characteristics of the input, throughput, output, and feedback should be considered. The most common input for powered wheelchairs is usually a joystick or four-point head pressure switch (Fig. 14-1). Most scooters use hand controls similar to those used to operate motorcycles. Golf carts, cars, and vans are modified with special hand controls and switch panel boards. Some municipal transit authorities provide access to kneeling buses; more are becoming accessible as the ADA is phased in. To access many train or subway systems, the user should obtain a map to determine which stations have accessible platforms and elevators and for information about key access, if necessary.

The throughput of scooters and powered wheelchairs is gel/dry or acid/wet batteries; some golf carts use batteries, some use gasoline; cars, vans, airplanes, and buses use gasoline; and trains usually use electricity. It should be noted that both gel and acid batteries require routine recharging. Chapter 5 contains detailed information about different kinds of batteries and their uses. When selecting a mobility system for a person with weak strength in their arms, the problem of transferring from a wheelchair to a vehicle is an important factor and may require a hydraulic lift or assistance from another person. In addition, the heavy weight of scooters and powered wheelchairs prohibits lifting by the user, although some fold up or break down for easier transportability.

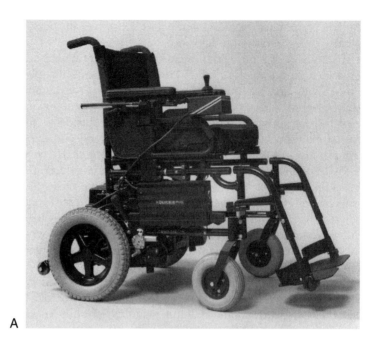

A

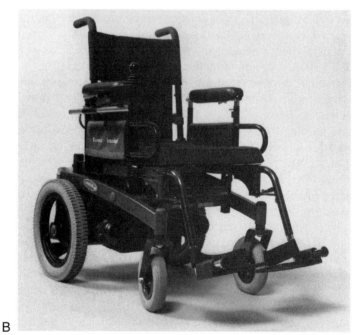

B

Figure 14-1. **(A & B)** Powered wheel-chair access with a joystick. (Copyright 1996 Tony Velez.)

As stated in the introduction, the purpose of the mobility system is to enable the user to move (the output) (1) transversely or horizontally, (2) vertically, and (3) rotationally to maneuver around in small spaces and (4) to travel long distances over (5) various terrains in different climatic conditions, (6) conserving as much energy as possible. The output of powered wheelchairs and scooters will meet the criteria of items 1, 3, 4 (many blocks), 5 (limited terrains), and 6 but not 2 (vertically). The exceptions include a powered wheelchair on the market that will climb stairs, and some scooters that can climb a 6-in. curb. Golf carts, tractors, cars, and vans do meet all six points of the criteria except item 3, for they are restricted from entering most buildings because they have combustion engines. Usually the output of a complete system will require both manual and powered wheelchairs and/or a scooter for short distances at the work site or school, plus a car, van, golf cart, or bus, train, subway, or tractor for longer distances when traveling to school or work or in the community. Therefore, an assessment of the complete mobility system's outcome must include both short- and long-distance travel.

Besides the obvious feedback of motion, the feedback for powered wheelchairs and scooters are visual battery lights indicating the battery status and auditory sounds from horns. All other forms of mobility have dials and horns, and some special cars even have a voice that talks to the driver.

Most vendors have assessment forms or equipment checklists; however, the evaluation of the user's abilities, needs, and environments are the responsibility of the professionals in the rehabilitation technology team. When assessing the complete mobility system, other factors that the team must take into consideration are the integration of the system with other assistive technology (AT) equipment (including ECUs and AAC aids), funding, routine maintenance, and repairs. Before the consumer tries a powered wheelchair (and then every month after acquisition of a mobility system), the following items should be checked:

- Check the pulleys for tightness or laxity
- Check the belts and clutches for proper adjustment
- Check cables
- Check joystick or access switch and mounting apparatus
- Test wheelchair in all directions and all speeds
- Check level of fluid in batteries (add distilled water every 6 to 8 weeks per manufacturer's directions)
- Check wheel brakes and locks for tightness and adjustment
- Clean the upholstery monthly, and check wear on tires, footplates, armrests, cushions, and/or adapted seating materials

When seeking reimbursement, consideration should also be given to the time and energy savings for the caregiver as well as the increased independence of the user. Some car and van manufacturers allow a discount or rebate to persons with a disability, and most state offices of vocational rehabilitation pay for some car and van modifications, especially if the vehicle is used for educational or job-related activities.

MODIFYING CARS OR VANS

Safety is the primary concern in the design of all vehicles but especially in the design of those driven by the persons with disabilities or those used to transport people in wheelchairs. It is imperative that all vehicle modifications are performed by authorized car dealers. Some individuals

Equipment	Right Arm	Left Arm	Right Leg	Left Leg	Right Arm and Leg	Left Arm and Leg	Both Arms	Both Legs (Para)	Arms and Legs (Quad)
STEERING Spinner knob	x	x			x	x		x	
Tri-pin								x	
U-shaped cuff								x	x
Quad cuff									x
Amputee ring	x	x			x	x		x	
Deep dish wheel								x	x
Tilt wheel								x	x
Horizontal									x
Low effort								x	x
Zero effort									x
GAS/BRAKE Hand brake			x	x	x	x		x	x
Left foot gas pedal			x		x				
Hand controls Push/pull								x	x
Push right angle								x	x
Push/twist								x	
Low effort								x	x
Zero effort									x
Vacuum									x
ACESSORIES Large key holder									x
Left gear shift	x				x				
Right directional		x				x			
Hand dimmer switch			x	x	x			x	x
Hand parking brake			x	x	x	x		x	x
Chest harness								x	x
Wheelchair lockdown								x	x
Lift								x	x
Raised roof								x	x
Power pan									x
Console for accessories									x
FOOT CONTROLS							x		

Figure 14-2. Needs for persons with specific loss of function—adaptive driving equipment. (Chart courtesy of Louise Stasik.)

will be driven to their school or workplace by a caregiver or friend; however, many persons with disabilities drive themselves in cars or vans that are equipped with special doors, lifts, and hand controls developed by technology mainly from the automobile industry. Most of these vehicles are custom designed for the specific needs of each user (Fig. 14-2). When designing these special vehicles, technical and human factors were considered: how the person would transfer from wheelchair to vehicle; how the person could be seated securely; where the wheelchair could be stored during the trip; and what alternate controls and emergency back-up systems must be available for safety. Some of these devices, such as the tilt-away steering wheel, had been developed for standard automobiles; others, such as the wheelchair lift and hand controls, had to be developed specifically for the driver with physical limitations.

TRANSFER FROM WHEELCHAIR TO VEHICLE

If a person with a disability has strong arms but weak legs, he or she can readily transfer from a wheelchair to a car; if his or her arms are weak or if he or she is overweight, it may be necessary to use a beveled or swivel transfer board. However, when transferring to a van seat, which is higher from the ground, a ramp or lift may be required. Ramps are metal platforms that can be portable or connected to the side or rear doors of the van and folded for storage during transport. Lifts are often installed inside or under the vans and are electrohydraulically operated by the wheelchair user or by someone else. The control switches for a lift are located both inside and outside the van, and for safety, a key is used to activate the lift. There are many configurations of lifts to accompany many types of vehicles. For example, in some designs, after the powered doors are opened, a platform is lowered to ground level, then the person with a disability rolls the wheelchair onto the platform and locks the chair in position. Next, the person in the wheelchair activates another switch, which is located on the lift, to raise the lift and rotate it into the van. Once the wheelchair is inside the van, it is unlocked and rolled off the lift. The lift is then automatically folded for storage, and the van doors are closed. Some "kneeling" vans are available that facilitate easier access for wheelchair users.

At this point, some wheelchair users will transfer from their wheelchairs to the driver's seat; others will drive their van while sitting in their wheelchairs. Technology has also developed a six-way power seat that provides easy transfer from the wheelchair to the driver's seat. This seat can move forward and backward, up and down, and it can swivel 90 degrees. In addition, some vans are equipped with tilt-away steering wheels that enable a person to transfer into and out of the driver's seat with great ease. Other vans are adapted to allow the driver to remain in a wheelchair that is locked in place while driving. In such vans, the regular driver's seat is removed and the car's controls are mounted on a panel board located at a height readily accessible to the driver; the van floor is lowered to accommodate the wheelchair. Maneuverability is an important concern for users of specially equipped vehicles and must be taken into consideration when selecting the best configuration for a specific consumer.

SAFE AND SECURE SEATING

A research project on crash testing of wheelchair passengers and drivers was conducted at the Highway Safety Research Institute at the University of Michigan in Ann Arbor.[6] As a result of this research, they recommend that the wheelchair restraint system should (1) keep the chair and passenger from moving in any direction; (2) include a lap belt and shoulder harness that would hold the person independently of the wheelchair and be attached directly to the floor; (3) provide for the wheelchair tie-down and belts to be fastened through the floor with hardened bolts and nuts and large washers; (4) not require that the wheelchair tie-down's main point of attachment be the wheelchair's crossbrace center bolt; (5) position lap belts across the pelvis and not soft tissue such as the stomach; and (6) require all passengers to face forward. This safety restraint system should be required for all vans that transport persons in wheelchairs. Most automobile manufacturers recommend that individuals should not be transported in wheelchairs but placed in suitable automotive seats and secured with seat belts.

ALTERNATE CONTROLS

After World War II, mechanical hand controls for cars were designed for the numerous veterans who had low or no functional use of their legs. Conventional hand controls consist of two long rods attached to the standard brake and accelerator, running parallel to the steering column and terminating in hand bars, which are at a convenient height so that the controls can be activated by squeezing the hand bars, similar to the controls of a motorcycle. These conventional hand controls are simple to install and are designed for most cars, vans, light trucks, and farm equipment. (See Ch. 16 for a detailed discussion of alternate controls.)

Today, there are pneumatic hand controls that provide effortless acceleration and braking, with feedback to ensure sensitive control. These pneumatic controls are designed for most cars, vans, and light trucks equipped with power steering, power-assist brakes, and automatic transmissions.

For the person who has limited arm strength or range of motion, there is now a horizontal steering system that eliminates arm lifting motion. It can be installed on any tilt or nontilt steering column, and the wheel is fully adjustable in all planes and has a telescoping feature. In addition, for the person with weak arms, a special knob control system can be attached to a standard steering wheel that allows a rotation of 10 degrees and reduces the manual power required of the driver.

Because there is an increasing demand for adapted cars and vans, more rehabilitation equipment companies are designing and developing modifications that will increase the consumer's independence and mobility. Many lifts and safety devices that have been adapted by wheelchair users may also prove useful for the cardiac and elderly population. The predominant factor to be considered when modifying a car or van is the safety of the driver and any passengers. If the technological advances of the space program can adapt the Space Rover to be driven by persons who have no functional use of their legs and minimum use of their hands, the future technological advances for the people with disabilities seem endless.

MAJOR TECHNICAL ADVANCES
OF MOBILITY DEVICES

WHEELCHAIRS

There have been significant technical advances in the following three categories of wheelchair design: repositioning the user from sitting to standing or reclining, development of a variety of new control systems, and providing special attachments to convert a standard wheelchair to a powered wheelchair.

REPOSITIONING

There are several standing or lifting wheelchairs commercially available. There is also a powered wheelchair that enables the user to stand and move. It has rear steering that provides a short turning radius and is narrower in width than most powered wheelchairs; however, it is very expensive and requires special technical skills for service and maintenance. The above-mentioned devices assist the person with a disability to rise to a standing position and securely support him or her in the process of standing to reach for objects or to work at a higher level. Furthermore, medical research indicates that when persons with disabilities passively stand, they not only increase their functional reach from 18 to 60 in. but they also improve the physiologic and metabolic function of their skeletal, muscular, and urinary system.[7]

In addition to these standing wheelchairs, multiadjustable chairs have been developed that allow the user to sit, stand, recline, tilt, and change leg position (Fig. 14-3). Presently, most basic adjustable chairs allow the

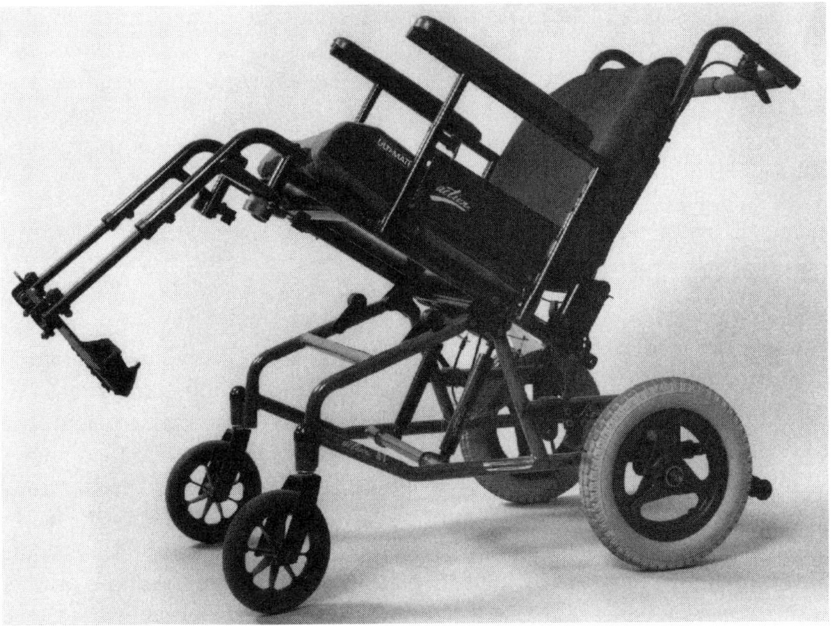

Figure 14-3. Multiadjustable wheelchair. (Copyright 1996 Tony Velez.)

wheelchair user to semirecline by lowering the back section and raising the leg rests. In the past, these adjustments frequently caused the wheelchair to tip; the new multiadjustable chairs are stable enough to transport a 300-lb person lying down.

CONTROL SYSTEMS

In the past 20 years, the most significant refinement of the standard manual wheelchair has been the addition of an 80-lb battery power source. This advancement has significantly increased the independent mobility of persons with severe impairments and persons who have limited muscle power and/or coordination in their arms. Today, the powered chairs can be activated by a variety of control systems including a joystick, a head rest or chin control, or a pneumatic (sip-and-puff) control.

The most frequently used control system is the joystick, which is usually attached to the arm of a wheelchair for the person who has some functional use of his or her hand or even of one finger. Some joystick control systems can also be activated by chin or head movements. Another frequently used control system is pneumatic, which requires the person to perform hard puffs and sips to control forward and backward motions, and soft puffs and sips control proportional turns. Powered wheelchairs are usually controlled by proportional or microswitches. Chapter 6 presents additional information about switches for powered wheelchairs and other control systems.

CONVERSION DEVICES

To compensate for the added weight of batteries and the difficulty of bringing battery-operated mobility devices on public transportation, special add-on devices are available. One such device is designed to convert a manual wheelchair to a power-driven wheelchair by mounting a 24-V power pack and a portable battery-driven power pack motor unit on the back of a standard wheelchair (Fig. 14-4). This power pack drives the back wheels and enables the wheelchair to travel more than 10 miles on a single charge. Furthermore, it can be transferred from one wheelchair to another and is readily removable for storage in a compact transport case, which can be stored in the overhead compartment of an airplane. The economics of converting a standard wheelchair to a powered wheelchair is significant; however, add-ons are not suitable for a person who needs a powered wheelchair more than 50 percent of the time or who requires special power seat functions.

SCOOTERS AND OTHER MOBILITY AIDS

POWERED SCOOTERS

With the increasing number of people who need mobility while working in small areas and the increase in the elderly population, there has been an escalation of technological advances in powered scooters. The most significant recent changes are (1) the bucket seating that allows stronger back and side support and allows modification for limited correction of positioning; (2) the base of some new models has four wheels, rather than three, which increases the scooter's stability and allows some to be converted to wheelchairs; (3) an adjustable telescopic handle or tiller with improved hand controls that allows for one-arm operation; (4) the

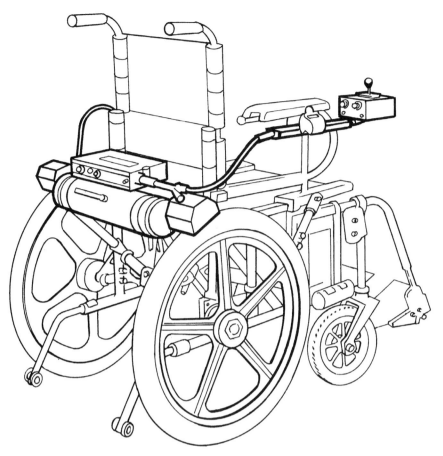

Figure 14-4. Device to convert a manual to a powered wheelchair.

front- or rear-wheel drive option; and (5) the ability to easily disassemble and reassemble that requires less lifting energy and increases the possibility for storage when transporting the scooter. Furthermore, some armrests can be flipped up for ease in transferring, and some seats can swivel for transfer and to allow the user closer access to work surfaces.

When evaluating a person for a scooter, it is recommended that careful attention be paid to the user's seating balance, hand coordination, and visual ability and that all environments and possible scooters be evaluated carefully. For example, if the user will be maneuvering in tight spaces and over hard surfaces, a scooter with a small front-wheel drive may be the best choice. If the user will be maneuvering over grass, dirt, gravel hills of 10 degrees or less, or heavy carpeting, then a scooter with rear-wheel drive that has greater traction may be the best choice.

Scooters have many advantages because they are lighter in weight, look cosmetically less "disabling," are easy to maneuver, and cost less than powered wheelchairs. Scooters should be considered after a careful evaluation that includes a trial period and an interdisciplinary team recommendation.

VERTICAL MOBILITY AIDS

Besides the need for making wheelchairs and scooters more efficient physically and more maneuverable, there is the need for upward mobility to climb curbs and to ascend and descend stairs. Manual wheelchair users with powerful arms can tilt their chairs backward on the large rear wheels and bump up to climb a curb; however, climbing a flight of stairs remains a problem for powered wheelchairs and scooters.

PORTABLE RAMPS, PORCH LIFTS, AND ELEVATORS

The technological advances of metal alloys and the development of stronger fiberglass have resulted in the design of new portable ramps. Most portable ramps are constructed of metals: aluminum, expanded metal, or heavy-duty steel. They have a nonslip surface and a smooth finish. Metal ramps are available in 24- to 36-in. widths and various lengths from 5 to 7 ft, or in 3-ft sections, which can be interlocked to achieve the desired length. Most portable metal ramps of 3 ft or more are heavy and require considerable strength to remove from a car or van and then to position near an entrance. Some of these have carrying handles and small casters to facilitate transport. By contrast, fiberglass ramps are lighter in weight than comparably sized metal ramps, but few have the convenient interlocking feature of the metal ramps. Fiberglass ramps are constructed with a commercial-grade nonskid finish and are available in 2- to 5-ft lengths. The major advantage of portable ramps, especially in the workplace, is their versatility. For example, they could be used for access from the outside of a factory, office, or school in the morning and evening and moved during the day to provide access to a conference or lunch room.

Portable ramps are one functional means of providing entrance to some buildings, but where weather conditions present a problem or where the grade of the stairs is so steep that it does not allow for the standard 1- to 12-in.-grade ratio, various lifts have been permanently installed and successfully used. Mainly through industrial technology, porch lifts or porch elevators have been developed. Most of these lifts have a compact 12-square-ft platform for the use of one wheelchair or scooter at a time and therefore can be installed adjacent to a flight of stairs (Fig. 14-5). They can also be used indoors and are available in various models. Many are constructed of aluminum and resemble a box, which lowers the front 5-in. section for use as a ramp during entrance and then raises it 90 degrees to close during the ascent. Most have keyed call/send controls, are powered by 12-V batteries, and have a backup system. For many older buildings, these are economical and cost a fraction of permanent ramps or standard elevators.

Ramps and porch lifts provide most wheelchair and scooter users with vertical mobility for entrance into many buildings; however, once inside, many older or three-story buildings have only stairs or small freight elevators. In these buildings, the wheelchair or scooter user has the option of staying in the wheelchair and using a wheelchair lift or transferring to a chair lift. In some chair lifts, the passenger is carried in the wheelchair or transferred to a seat. One lift is available for straight and curved staircases. It ascends up to three stories with intermediate stops and requires few or no building modifications. It is electrically operated from a single unit and has a manual backup. The platform and seat fold up easily to keep the

Figure 14-5. Porch lift.

stairway free. In the event that a chair lift is used, arrangements must include a means to transport the wheelchair up and down the stairs and to facilitate transfer between the chair lift and the wheelchair. Also available for vertical mobility are small vertical elevators for open or in-shaft operation between two or more floors. Most are large enough for a standard-sized powered wheelchair or scooter and an additional person. These special devices should be installed by a licensed reputable company that will also provide service and maintenance.

To summarize, in the past 10 years technology has developed a variety of portable ramps and lifts that increase vertical mobility for many persons. Now that there is a variety of devices available, the selection must be determined by carefully analyzing the needs of most mobility users, the space that is available, the cost per device, and the financial resources of the consumer. As in all building renovations, the administrators will need a committee to consult with architects to ensure proper building codes are being observed, various distributors of rehabilitation equipment to select the best device, persons with disabilities to learn what they have found most practical and economical, and organizations of persons with physical disabilities, to use their practical experience and knowledge about the problems of limited vertical mobility.

Creative teams will seek alternative solutions for powered wheelchair or scooter users who live in multiple-floor homes. These would include rearranging rooms so that the user can sleep, eat, bathe, and recreate on a single level. Similar accommodations might be necessary at school or work, where luncheon and bathroom facilities might not be located on the same floor as the office or classroom. In such cases, portable ramps can be used effectively.

DOOR OPENERS

Another technological device that increases the independence of persons who use various mobility devices is the powered door opener. Electric-eye door openers, similar to those used to open supermarket doors, have been installed at many work sites and in some schools. These electric-eye door openers can be prohibitively expensive and can be problematic because they require a flat 5-ft lead path in front of the door. These two problems can be addressed by the installation of an infrared door opener. This is a small control box ($7 \times 10 \times 2$ in.) attached to the upper portion of any door that is then connected to a 3×5-in. switch placed at wheelchair level or controlled from a wheelchair. When the switch is activated by the operator of a wheelchair or scooter, the door opens slowly and remains open for a predetermined time to allow the user to pass through, and then it automatically closes. This electric door-opening device can be installed by any electrician for less than $1,000, compared with $3,500 for an electric-eye-type door opener. It can be installed on either an inside or outside door and does not detract from the entrance to a building or the interior of the building. Door openers can also be operated by a control mechanism from the wheelchair or incorporated into a general ECU system that operates lights and other appliances.

SUMMARY

Besides moving transversely, vertically, and manually in small spaces, most people have to travel to their jobs or schools, requiring public or private transportation. The next three chapters discuss driver training programs and public transportation.

ACKNOWLEDGMENT

I thank Adrienne Bergen for her professional comments and review of this chapter.

REFERENCES

1. Americans with Disabilities Act of 1990 (Public Law 101–336), 42 U.S.C. 12101, 1990

2. Phillips B: Technology abandonment from the consumer point of view. NARIC Q 3:3–11, 1992

3. Rehabilitation Engineering Center: Evaluating Powered Wheelchairs. National Rehabilitation Hospital & ECRI, Washington, DC, 1993

4. American National Standards Institute—Rehabilitation Engineering Society of North America: ANSI–RESNA Wheelchair Standards. RESNA, Washington, DC, 1991

5. Freeman S, Brusnighan D, Field W: Selecting mobility aids for farmers and ranchers with physical disabilities. Technol Disability 4:63–67, 1992

6. Jones K: Can you survive a crash? Accent on Living, Fall:48–52, 1983

7. Abramson A: Advances in the management of the neurogenic bladder. Arch Phys Med Rehabil 52:143–149, 1971

SUGGESTED READINGS

Axelson P, Minkel J, Chesney D: A Guide to Wheelchair Selection: How to Use the ANSI/RESNA Wheelchair Standards to Buy a Wheelchair. Paralyzed Veterans of America, Washington, DC, 1994

Deitz J, Jaffe K, Wolf L, et al: Pediatric power wheelchairs: evaluation of function in the home and school environment. Assist Technol 3(1):24–33

Furamaso J (ed): Childhood Powered Mobility. 2nd Ed. RESNA Press, Arlington, VA, 1997

Kangas K: Assessment and treatment strategies for pediatric powered mobility. In: Proceedings of the Ninth International Seating Symposium, Memphis, TN, 1993

Taylor SJ: Powered mobility evaluations and technology. Top Spinal Cord Injury Rehabil 1(1):22–36, 1995

Trefler E, Kozole K, Snell E (eds): Selected Readings on Powered Mobility for Children and Adults with Severe Physical Disabilities. RESNA Press, Washington, DC, 1986

Warren CG: Powered mobility and its implications. pp. 74–85. In Todd SP (ed): Choosing a Wheelchair System. Veterans Health Services and Research Administration, Washington, DC, 1990

Resources

INFORMATION ON MOBILITY EQUIPMENT

National Registry of Rehabilitation
   Technology Suppliers
Lubbock, TX
(806) 797-7299

National Association of Medical
   Equipment Suppliers (NAMES)
Atlanta, GA
(703) 836-6363

Annual show of medical equipment

European Conference on the Advancement
   of Rehabilitation Technology (ECART)
Conference and proceedings
Uallingby, Sweden 4686201700

MAJOR MANUFACTURERS OF POWERED WHEELCHAIRS

Everest & Jennings
St. Louis, MO
(800) 235-4661

Invacare
Elyria, OH
(800) 333-6900

LA BAC System
Lakewood, CO
(303) 914-9914

Permobil
Woburn, MA
(617) 932-9009

Quickie
Fresno, CA
(800) 456-8165

MAGAZINES

Team Rehab Report
Malibu, CA
(301) 317-4522

Monthly for professionals in assistive technology

Accent on Living
Bloomington, IL
(309) 378-2961

Quarterly for people with special needs

New Mobility
Malibu, CA
800-543-4116

Special international travel issue December 1996

CHAPTER 15

Predriving Evaluations

The ability to drive increases the independence of persons with disabilities as it enables them to obtain employment and participate in community life. This chapter discusses clinical and on-the-road assessments for driver training using assistive devices that allow persons with disabilities to operate motor vehicles safely and efficiently. Adaptive driver training is required as well as the assistive devices to create a safe and independent driving environment. Chapter 16 details the behind-the-wheel training component for driver education programs.

Not all persons who undergo driver evaluation and/or training will obtain their operator license. It is imperative to understand that a driver's license is a privilege and not a right; therefore, it must be earned. A thorough evaluation must take place before any prescription or training with adaptive driving equipment. An adaptive driver evaluation should be completed by a professional who understands disabilities, medications, and the implications of these for driving. Clinical evaluation or a predriving evaluation (PDE) can be completed by a physical therapist or occupational therapist. A Certified Driver Rehabilitation Specialist (CDRS) can provide the clinical and behind-the-wheel evaluation and training.

Program content varies. Some programs provide evaluations, training, and escorting the consumer to obtain his or her driver's license. Others offer refresher courses to help persons prepare for the written examinations. There are also programs that provide evaluation and education for van modifications for persons who will be passengers. The Association for Driver Educators for the Disabled (ADED) is a good starting point for locating adaptive driving programs throughout the United States and Canada. ADED is an international organization that also provides guidelines for clinical evaluations or PDEs.

Many persons with disabilities may benefit from adaptive training and assistive devices. (See Ch. 14 for more information about mobility.) Such disabilities include but are not limited to traumatic brain injury, cerebral vascular accident, spinal cord injury, spinal bifida, cerebral palsy, muscular dystrophy, multiple sclerosis, diabetes, arthrogryposis, and visual and hearing impairments. Consumers who are mentally or cognitively challenged, with mental retardation, learning disabilities, attention deficit disorders, and/or psychiatric impairments, may also benefit from compensatory techniques to operate motor vehicles safely.

The clinical evaluation and initial interviews are fairly consistent among all consumers with disabilities. The clinical evaluation should consist of an initial interview and assessment of the person's physical abilities and deficits, including limitations of range of motion and grasp. The evaluator will also discuss with the consumer the type of vehicle the consumer should purchase, insurance coverage, the state licensing laws for medical clearance, funding for driver training, and the specifics for that consumer's disability. The predriving screening should address the consumer's visual, cognitive, perceptual, physical, emotional, and behavioral abilities.

VEHICLE RECOMMENDATIONS

A two-door vehicle is usually recommended for those who will be loading their own manual wheelchairs into the car. For individuals using powered wheelchairs, full-size vans or minivans are strongly encouraged. Power brakes, power steering, and automatic transmission are required when adding adaptive driving equipment. Tilt steering, power windows, power locks, power mirrors, and a rear defroster are recommended. Certain adaptive devices only interface with certain vehicles; therefore, education regarding appropriate vehicles must be provided. There are a variety of wheelchair loaders, ramps, lifts, and tie-downs that must be discussed with the consumer depending on the individual's needs. It is helpful to provide the consumer with materials on vans and adaptive equipment. Consumers are strongly encouraged to try the assistive devices to be sure they can understand and manipulate all the controls. This can be completed after the clinical evaluation and before the test drive.

INSURANCE ISSUES

Most consumers should not have difficulty obtaining insurance coverage. The Americans with Disabilities Act does not allow insurance companies to discriminate due to disability. Consumers should obtain insurance for any assistive devices installed on their vehicles as well as the vehicle itself. The consumer must inform the insurance agent about the adaptive equipment on the vehicle. Most states also require that the consumer and/or the physician inform the medical review board of the driver licensing agency about the adaptive equipment on the vehicle.

MEDICAL CLEARANCE

Licensing laws vary from state to state. Some states require medical clearance from a physician before driver training that may involve the completion of mandated forms. Consumers with progressive disabilities may need to complete yearly examinations. Persons with past history of seizures or drug/alcohol abuse need to be seizure-free or free of any substance abuse for 3 months to 1 year before returning to operation of a motor vehicle. Again, a good driver rehabilitation specialist will know the individual state laws.

FUNDING

Resources must be located to pay for the vehicle and its modifications and maintenance. Some manufacturers provide rebates or deductions for the purchase of a new car that will be adapted for use by a person with a disability. Most third-party payers consider driving to be a luxury that is not "medically necessary," so that driver evaluations and training may not be reimbursed. If the consumer is school age, PL 94-142 may help secure partial payment for the driving assessment but not the driver training. Usually, driver evaluations and training are paid for by the state's vocational rehabilitation programs or worker's compensation fund.

SPECIAL CONSIDERATIONS

Each disability and prescribed medication present specific implications for driving. Certain medications can make one drowsy, slow processing, and can even blur the vision. The rehabilitation professional or CDRS may need to explain dysreflexia to persons with spinal cord injuries or tell the person who has lost sensation in the lower extremities to use the defroster and not the heater. Rear air conditioning is a must for persons riding as passengers in full-size vans if they have problems regulating their body temperatures.

CLINICAL AND VISUAL ASSESSMENT

A visual assessment should be included in any evaluation for assistive technology (AT). The technology team must have an understanding of how the optical muscles work before the consumer will be able to effectively manipulate the AT. The visual system is especially important for driving, because of the need to track activities in the environment. The eyes are the means for information to get to the brain, where it will be processed. There are muscles around the eyes that must be evaluated. It is very important to listen to what consumers disclose when they say, "My eyes get watery; my head hurts when I read; or I lose my place when I am reading." These can show subtle changes in the visual system. If the technology team or driver education professional does not feel comfortable in this area, the consumer should be referred to an optometrist, ophthalmologist, or behavioral optometrist.

   When evaluating the ocular system, the evaluator must consider the legal standard for visual acuity and horizontal vision of the state in which the consumer resides. The eyes should be examined together and individually. The consumer needs to be tested for near and distance acuity. Peripheral vision (superior, inferior, temporal, and nasal fields) should also be evaluated. Some states allow bioptic/telescopic driving for persons who have macular degeneration, albinism, or retinitis pigmentosa. Other areas of the visual system that need to be addressed are the consumer's scanning and tracking skills, eye range of motion, convergence and accommodation skills, saccades, and alignment of the eyes. The alignment is especially important for understanding if the eyes work together or separately to assess depth perception. There are standardized tests to see if the consumer suppresses one eye when using both eyes together. For clarification, scanning skills are needed to identify objects in the driving environment (road signs, people, etc.). The ability to track allows the driver to maintain lane position. Accommodation skills allow the individual to look in the driving area and then back down at the vehicle controls to check car speed. Rapid eye movement is necessary to allow a driver to look quickly from the rearview mirror to side mirrors, as well as track the speedometer and other indicators on the dashboard. When visual deficits interfere with driving skills, adaptations such as panoramic rearview mirrors or spot mirrors may be added. Some states allow prism glasses to be worn while driving to increase the driver's field of vision. Other compensatory strategies are also available from the driver rehabilitation specialist.

PERCEPTUAL ASSESSMENT

The ability of the brain to understand and process what the eyes are seeing is imperative. Assessing spatial relations, figure-ground, visual closure, and visual memory is needed during the predriving assessments. Figure-ground deficits may not allow the individual to locate the correct road sign in a cluttered city environment. Consumers with visual closure deficits may not perceive the entire driving environment around a construction site or a traffic accident. Consumers must be able to quickly identify, remember, and follow road signs and road markings.

Depth perception should be assessed as it is needed when overtaking vehicles, passing vehicles, or parking between vehicles. Color perception is also usually assessed, to ensure that the driver can distinguish between traffic signals. The reader needs to understand that persons may have deficits in any of the mentioned areas. There is training in compensatory techniques to enable the consumer to be a safer driver.

COGNITIVE ASSESSMENT

Adequate attention skills, arousal level, and the ability to initiate and inhibit behaviors are a must for the operation of a motor vehicle. Shifting of attention and mental flexibility are important. Decision-making and good judgment skills are imperative, as there are few safe ways to compensate for the loss of these cognitive abilities.

PHYSICAL ASSESSMENT

Strength, range of motion, coordination, sensation, endurance, and hearing are all necessary components of a clinical evaluation. Reaction and processing times are evaluated through standardized testing.

There are numerous ways to evaluate all the above areas. Standardized testing is performed for visual, perceptual, cognitive, and physical abilities. Most rehabilitation professionals are familiar with the tests. There are driving simulators and even virtual reality in the driving field. However, most evaluators use the simulators and PDEs as screening tools for predicting how a consumer may perform on the road.

The clinical screenings also give the evaluator/trainer ideas for where the consumer needs extra help with compensatory strategies. Of course, not all disabilities are the same nor are all people with the same disability alike. Therefore, the evaluation can be individualized to meet the needs of the consumer (e.g., a person with diagnosis of paraplegia may not need an in-depth cognitive and perceptual evaluation, which is recommended for a person with a traumatic brain injury). The PDE needs to be holistic, in the same manner as the Bain Assistive Technology System (BATS), in which the consumer, the device, and the environment are assessed according to the task that will be performed. The professional should have knowledge of adaptive methods and assistive devices. Basic hand controls for joystick driving and voice input for accessory controls (lights, horn, dimmer switch, signals, etc.) are available. Not all evaluators will feel comfortable with all types of AT devices, so the consumer should feel free to check professional references and consult with other centers.

Most consumers do not stop at the predriving assessment unless legal standards are not met. Not all persons will be able to handle a vehicle. A complete understanding of what the consumer can and cannot do will be demonstrated when the client is evaluated behind the wheel of a car.

SUGGESTED READINGS

Jones DG: Assistive devices for driving. pp. 641–653. In Goldberg B, Hsu J (eds): Atlas of Orthoses and Assistive Devices. 3rd Ed. Mosby-Year Book, St. Louis, 1997

Digman GH: Driver rehabilitation programs. Lesson 4, pp. 1–47. In Hammel J (ed): Technology and Occupational Therapy: A Link to Function. American Occupational Therapy Association, Bethesda, MD, 1996

Resources

American Automobile Association
1000 AAA Drive
Heathrow, FL 32746

Association of Driver Educators for the Disabled
P.O.Box 49
109 West Street
Edgerton, WI 53534

As-Tech Inc.
8 Shovel Shop Square
North Easton, MA 02356-1445

The Braun Corporation
1014 S. Monticello
P.O. Box 310
Winamac, IN 46996

Bruno Independent Living Aids, Inc.
1780 Executive Drive
P.O. Box 84
Oconomowoc, WI 53066

Crow River Industries, Inc.
14800 28th Avenue N.
Minneapolis, MN 55447

Doron Precision Systems, Inc.
P.O. Box 400
Binghamton, NY 13902-0400

EMC, Inc.
2001 Wooddale Boulevard
Baton Rouge, LA 70806

Mobile Tech Corporation
P.O. Box 2326
Hutchinson, KS 67504-2326

National Mobility Equipment Dealers
    Association (NMEDA)
909 E. Skagway Avenue
Tampa, FL 33604

Assistive
Technology:
An
Interdisciplinary
Approach

CHAPTER 16

RICHARD W. NEAD, JR.

Behind-the-Wheel Driver Training

Independence through mobility is the absolute goal of all driver rehabilitation programs (DRP) and their participants. One aspect of a DRP is determining the consumer's fitness for driving as related to his or her disability. Another is the determination of the appropriate vehicle type and potential assistive technology (AT) required for vehicle modification and/or adaptation. A driving candidate or someone seeking transportation should explore the options through a comprehensive evaluation in a DRP.

In this chapter, we examine behind-the-wheel (BTW) strategies and techniques as deployed by the driver rehabilitation specialist (DRS) in the DRP. We include the identification and implementation of available AT with regard to diagnostic requirements.

DRIVER REHABILITATION PROGRAM

Participation in a comprehensive DRP ensures proper assessment, education, and preparation. Assessment is normally a team approach. Potential players in assessment can include physicians, psychologists, occupational therapists, physical therapists, and DRS. The more reliable DRP will employ DRS, certified through the Association of Driver Educators for the Disabled (ADED). The certified driver rehabilitation specialist (CDRS) will have had the benefit of exposure to workshops, seminars, and other forms of education pertinent to driver rehabilitation. These experiences (some ADED approved) will have prepared the specialist to take ADED's certification examination. The examination is a minimum-competency examination ensuring the specialist of having the base core of knowledge to perform in this specialty.

Driver rehabilitation is a medically oriented program based on the medical requirement and necessity to remain independent in mobility. Referral into a program is done by prescription of a physician of any specialty. A program can consist of several progressions including predriving or clinical assessment, simulation, BTW training, driver rehabilitation/training, licensure issues, prescription development, transportation alternatives, and follow-up services. Predriving evaluation (PDE) is discussed in Chapter 15.

TRAINING, LICENSURE, AND FOLLOW-UP SERVICES

After a thorough PDE that results in the creation of a mobility plan, training strategies and methodology are commenced and licensure issues addressed. The potential operator shall be capable of driving at or above the level of efficiency enjoyed before medical compromise. Repetition will be required to familiarize the consumer with his or her new driving situation. Through this repetition, the objectives are to develop a competent and confident level of performance. While dealing with individuals of different backgrounds and disabilities, the training format must be flexible, yet remain with specific and realistic objectives. The DRS must be capable of training both inexperienced and mature drivers. The time frame for driver training will vary. Generally, new drivers and those using high-tech systems will require greater repetitions in comparison with those involved with low-tech AT.

In many states, individuals using adaptations of the primary controls for vehicle operation are required to possess a classified or endorsed license. In New Jersey, for example, potential drivers must complete an application and undergo testing for a classified license. For new drivers, this is accomplished when they successfully complete their initial road examination. For the previously licensed operator, an examination that includes a vision screening and a road test is required. The individual enrolled in a comprehensive DRP is prepared and should encounter little difficulty in meeting different state requirements. The DRS should ensure that the candidate meets the specific requirements of the home state.

On completion of the assessment, training, and licensure process, the DRS will remain involved with the individual through various stages. When adaptation and modification processes are involved, prescription development or amendment is completed and implemented. In instances of high-tech van conversion, the DRS may be required to work with the mobility equipment installer during the initial and final fitting process to ensure that a proper interface of the driver and the controls is achieved. On completion of the vehicle, the DRS should conduct a driver check-out session that will include an inspection of the vehicle for adherence to the prescription, static driver interface with the controls, dynamic interface with controls, and driver training of various duration in the adapted vehicle.

When involved with individuals whose diagnosis is progressive in nature, consideration to medical status change is imperative. Progressive diagnosis should be considered for assessment on a yearly basis or sooner if status change occurs. This can ensure continued appropriateness for driving with regard to both medical and equipment issues.

In instances in which individuals do not present as appropriate driving candidates, alternative transportation means should be discussed. Although mass transportation remains sorely deficient regarding the disabled community, it has greatly improved over the past few years. When living and working close to available mass transit, the option of usage is present. Many state and county transportation programs are currently available when mass transit is not easily accessed. Laws governing public transportation systems are discussed in Chapter 17. Despite the increase in available alternative means, personal transportation remains the most effective and reliable, allowing the individual independent access to the community at his or her convenience.

ASSISTIVE TECHNOLOGY

The advancement in technology related to adapted and/or modified driving conversions has moved rapidly in recent years. The most basic of mechanical hand controls have been redesigned and improved for ease in operation, maintenance, and safety. Power-assisted controls (PACs) are now digital, and most manufacturers have improved the reliability and applications of their products. Unilever driving systems are now available, and voice activation of secondary control functions will be introduced in the near future.

Car drivers who rely on wheelchairs for mobility have found that newer materials and designs have made loading an easier task in the proper vehicle. Even rigid frame chairs with their ease of component breakdown are becoming more manageable.

For those using a van for their mobility needs, the emergence and subsequent refinement of the minivan conversion have become increasingly popular. The minivan can offer some individuals the accessibility of a larger van with the handling and economy features of a car. The improved design, performance, and interior amenities of minivans have increased their popularity among drivers with disabilities (Fig. 16-1).

This advancement and the diversity of such possibilities have introduced many (including those once limited to nondriving options) to the

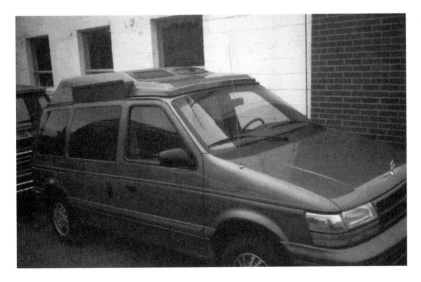

Figure 16-1. Minivan with sport top and raised entry option. (Courtesy of Kessler Institute for Rehabilitation, West Orange, NJ.)

threshold of driving independence. This increase in availability does not come without concerns regarding diagnosis, safety, and finance. With these issues properly addressed in a comprehensive DRP, transportation options have never been more diverse.

LOW TECHNOLOGY DEVICES

This section highlights some of the low-technology adaptations that can be used to modify the interior of a vehicle for use by a person with a disability. Issues of transfer and storage are discussed in Chapter 14. An individual must be totally independent in his or her transfer to and from the vehicle. Once in the vehicle, they must demonstrate adequate seating and trunk stability to operate both within and outside of its confines. Available upper extremity strength and dexterity must be present to allow for loading of the chair and its components.

GRASP ENHANCERS

A grasp enhancer such as a keybar has been designed to assist those unable to manipulate a control due to lack of reliable grip, decreased active range of motion (AROM), or impaired fine motor coordination. These devices can be made of many different materials, with the most common being wood, metals, and plastics. They include off-the-shelf devices and devices customized to meet the needs of a consumer. Many devices are modified and/or created in the occupational therapy clinic or by a rehabilitation engineer. In relation to driving, these devices are most often used to facilitate key manipulation. This can include unlocking and locking doors, key box control centers, or in ignition activation. The devices can eliminate the need for costly high-tech adaptations for both cars and vans. Costs are variable and in most cases insignificant.

DIRECTIONAL AND GEAR SELECTOR: CROSSOVERS AND EXTENSIONS

When a person is unable to access the directional selector with the left upper extremity secondary to decreased function, adaptation must be provided for actuation. When AROM denies any access and the right upper extremity is intact, a directional crossover can be implemented for operation. The unit is of simple design, attaching to the existing activator, extending over the steering column, and relocating the directional selector to the right. If function is present in the left side and access is marginally denied, an extension can be added to the existing actuator. This type of unit can also be used in cases in which the left knee will activate the directional selector.

When a person is unable to access the gear selector secondary to decreased function in the right upper extremity, a crossover or extension can be incorporated with the existing actuator. Extensions are applied when right arm function is marginally affected. The crossover is implemented when function is absent or the right upper extremity is occupied in another primary control function (e.g., acceleration or braking). If the vehicle has a floor-mounted console gear selector, neither device can be considered a reliable solution and high-tech solutions should be considered.

Extensions and crossovers, when properly installed and applied, are functional and cost-effective solutions. Found in both car and van scenarios, the units will allow continued access to the original activators for the able driver.

MANUAL PARKING BRAKE EXTENSION

Vans or cars equipped with foot-operated parking brakes require application using the left lower extremity (LLE). When a person is unable to access the parking brake because of his or her decreased function, a manual extension can be added to allow operation of the existing actuator. Operation is achieved by using the left upper extremity. Release of the brake is accessed by using the existing release mechanism. When unable to apply this unit effectively, high-tech options are available. Successful use of the manual extension will eliminate the higher costs and reliability issues involved with other options. This application allows for operation of the existing actuator by the able driver as well.

SCANNING ASSISTIVE TECHNOLOGY

The degree of success one encounters in driving can be directly related to visual processing skill. A person's success in scanning protocols is directly related to their inherent useful field of vision. Physical dysfunction in the neck or torso or a decrease in the useful field of vision can dramatically impair the information-gathering processes required for efficient motor vehicle operation.

In some instances, the strategic placement of auxiliary mirrors can allow the operator visual access to blind spots to the front, rear, and sides of the vehicle. Mirrors mounted on front fenders can extend the driver's field to include immediate blind spots (left and right) that normally require neck rotation for head checks.

Mirrors mounted on the front bumper, above the hood line, reflection angled inward, will indicate traffic flow coming from left and right at intersections. Convex mirrors can be used both inside and outside to enhance traffic awareness. Four- and five-panel mirrors replace the rearview mirror, granting greater visual awareness of traffic to the sides and rear of the vehicle. Effective use of these devices requires time for the driver to become acclimated and learn to use all the information provided by the mirrors. Repetitions with the DRS are recommended in assisting with the transition. Able operators will find it difficult to neglect these devices, so familiarization is required for them as well. The mirror arrangements discussed can be applied to both van and car situations and are very cost-effective.

STEERING ASSISTIVE DEVICES

Individuals with singular upper extremity impairment will require an assistive device ensuring adequate steering function. The device, operated by using the unaffected limb, allows for the completion of steering sequences without a break from contact with the steering wheel. When evasive actions are required, the unit will allow for continued interface with the wheel while executing the desired maneuver.

Positioning of the device on the wheel will be determined by the limb to be used and comfort zone of the individual. Left-handed operation will usually require placement in the 7 to 9 o'clock position on the wheel, and for right-handed drivers, at 2 to 5 o'clock. Higher positioning on the wheel often leads to instability while maintaining straight away driving for long periods. Position of the limb in an elevated extended plane for even short periods will raise questions regarding endurance. Lower placement on the wheel can create overly stable positioning, where initiation of movement can be hindered.

Steering devices are quite often used in conjunction with hand controls. These two devices will allow for efficient vehicle control under all conditions. The following is a listing of common steering devices and a description of their applications:

1. *Spinner knob.* The most commonly used device, a spinner knob, requires a functional grasp and intact AROM in the limb in most applications. In some applications, the individual with limited AROM and strengths can use the knob in conjunction with smaller-diameter steering wheels and reduced steering efforts if grasp is present. Individuals with postpolio or arthritis are examples.

2. *Single post grip.* Like the spinner knob, functional grasp is a requirement for use of a single post grip. Lengths and diameters of the post will vary pending specific requirements of the user. This is most often substituted for a knob when grasp capacities indicate a smaller diameter, or AROM limitations in the wrist and forearm of the person with a disability inhibit complete pronation.

3. *V-grip, bi-pin, or quad yoke.* Known by differing names, this device requires minimal grasp efficiency. On interface with the unit, the device should fit snugly across the palm and back of the hand. Function requires strong wrist flexion and extension. An example of a potential user could be a C-7 quadriplegic with adequate tenodesis and wrists (Fig. 16-2).

4. *Tri-pin.* As suggested by its name, this unit is a series of three posts in a triangular format. Two of these posts support the wrist on each

Figure 16-2. Quad keybar in use. (Courtesy of Kessler Institute for Rehabilitation, West Orange, NJ.)

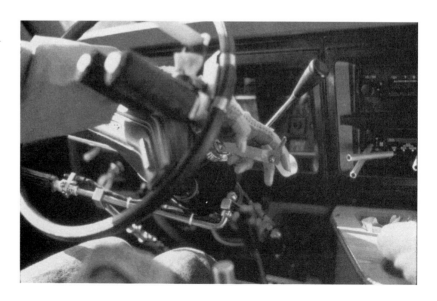

side while the third fits in the palm of the hand with the thumb wrapping around the post near the top. The device is designed for those with unreliable or no present grasp. Positioning of the pin must be precise, allowing for a snug but not overly tight fit. This will allow for firm support in use for steering and independent interface in accessing other secondary control items. The largest population using this device are those individuals with diagnosis of quadriplegia. In some individuals diagnosed with multiple sclerosis, unreliable grasp is present. The tri-pin can create a reassuring and effective result in performing steering sequences for these drivers (Fig. 16-3).

5. *Sierra driving ring.* The driving ring adaptation is used by a person with a prosthesis for steering, secondary to upper extremity amputation. The device interfaces with the hook or pincher surfaces of the prosthesis. Both ring and pincher should be coated with a soft reliable surface, promoting friction during steering sequences. Not prevalent in use, assessment for safer solutions should be explored.

6. *Palm-grip.* Also used with consumers who have limitations in functional grasp, a palm-grip unit requires pronation at the wrist allowing the hand to slide between two curved upright supports. When properly interfaced, support is placed at the metacarpal region as the fingers wrap over the front edge. This provides the stability while attempting required steering sequences. Very often discomfort is experienced during operation, and so the palm-grip is not commonly used for this purpose.

7. *Splints and orthotics.* In some instances, standard issue steering devices will not meet the required need. Consultation with the orthotics department can lead to the development of customized steering devices. This is not uncommon when working with individuals whose upper extremity disability is secondary to burns, in the event of amputation above the wrist and below the elbow, and

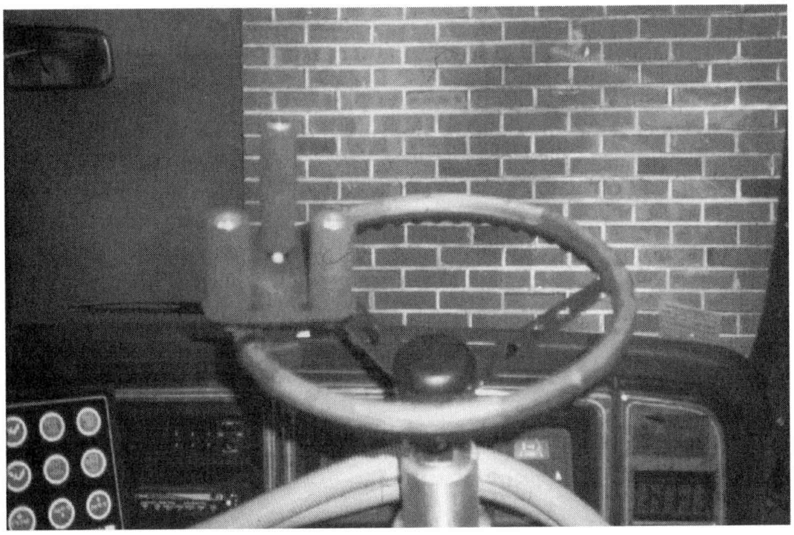

Figure 16-3. Tri-pin steering device. (Courtesy of Kessler Institute for Rehabilitation, West Orange, NJ.)

in some quadriplegic cases. Because the orthosis will likely be used only for driving, independence in access and removal is imperative regarding degree of effectiveness.

As driver side airbags (supplementary restraint systems) have become standard equipment on many vehicles, it is important to ensure that the location of all steering devices is clear of the field of activation. Failure to make this kind of adjustment may result in the propulsion of the device into the operator when it is deployed, with the potential for devastating injury. Incorporating dense foam sleeving with all friction fit devices (posts) will help in alleviating skin complication potentials. This material, capable of moderation with temperature swings, can prevent contact with overly hot or cold devices. Quick release features allow the able driver clear access to the wheel while they are driving. The devices are found in all adapted driving scenarios when prescribed.

LEFT FOOT ACCELERATOR

The left foot accelerator is an extension from the existing actuator down to the floor, across a mount, and up to the left side of the brake pedal. Relocation to the left allows users the capacity to use the left lower extremity for acceleration and braking purposes when impairment exists in the right lower extremity (RLE). When not in use, the unit can be removed from its base or folded back to the floor (depending on the type), allowing the able operator to have unimpeded access to the original activators. Many individuals with right hemiplegia use this adaptation in conjunction with a spinner knob for primary vehicle control operation. Another population that may use this technology are persons with RLE amputation. When amputation is secondary to diabetes, careful screening should take place during the PDE as to its affect on the LLE when considering this adaptation. In instances in which involvement precludes use of the left foot accelerator, hand controls are an appropriate option.

PEDAL EXTENSIONS

When individuals of short stature are unable to activate the existing acceleration and braking controls, extensions are available. Bolting to the existing actuators, these extensions will allow for normal operation of these functions. Some units provide for quick release, moving the pedals out of the able driver's way.

HAND CONTROLS (MECHANICAL)

When a person is not able to use either lower extremity for efficient acceleration and braking function, hand controls are a solution to accessing these operations. In conjunction with a suitable steering device and proper training, driving independence is easily maintained. There are several manufacturers of hand controls that are both low and high tech. In regard to low-tech or mechanical devices, activation is manual without power assist.

When preparing to purchase a vehicle that will be used with hand controls, the vehicle should be equipped with the following features:

1. *Automatic transmission*. With lower extremities unavailable and both arms occupied with primary control, clutch and shifting sequences cannot be accessed. High-tech AT is available for assist with these functions. This costly system will allow the driver using hand controls to operate a standard transmission vehicle. The system is time proven and reliable but not prevalent in use. The gear selector can be either floor or column mounted, depending on transfer and wheelchair loading status.
2. *Power braking*. To facilitate ease of braking resistance, power braking uses the smaller, less powerful muscles of the arm.
3. *Power steering*. Power steering is used to facilitate ease in steering patterns.
4. *Hand-operated parking brake*. When a vehicle is equipped with a hand-operated parking brake, it eliminates the need for a manual emergency brake extension in most low-tech applications.

PUSH/PULL HAND CONTROLS

As with all mechanical hand controls, braking is achieved by pushing the lever toward the dashboard (front of the vehicle). Acceleration is applied by pulling in the same plane, back to the torso. When released, the properly maintained control returns to a neutral position with neither function in operation. Various grasping devices are available, allowing persons without complete function the capacity to activate the control. The easiest control to train on, it is most often found in populations with functional grasp.

PUSH/PULL RIGHT-ANGLE CONTROLS

The second in popularity, acceleration using right-angle controls is accessed with a downward motion toward the thigh region. This will allow for the natural weight of the arm to apply the function of acceleration. On release, a properly maintained unit will return to the neutral position. Return to the neutral position must take place before braking. Without such return, simultaneous acceleration and braking will result, increasing the distance needed to stop safely. This simultaneous operation is suitable for stoppage on an incline but not desirable when occurring in panic stop situations. Proper training is essential on this unit to eliminate the occurrence of simultaneous operation. In most instances, proper training will limit use of this feature. Various grips are available to accommodate most populations. Right-angle controls are often used with quadriplegic populations capable of mechanical control operation. These controls are also desirable when working with persons with multiple sclerosis, for whom a pulling motion is fatiguing and grasp is unreliable. In some minivan applications, access is difficult due to space restrictions between the driver's leg and the unit (Fig. 16-4).

PUSH/TWIST CONTROLS

Acceleration using this control is achieved by twisting the actuator in the same manner as in accelerating a motorcycle. Release of the control will return operation to the neutral position. This control also permits

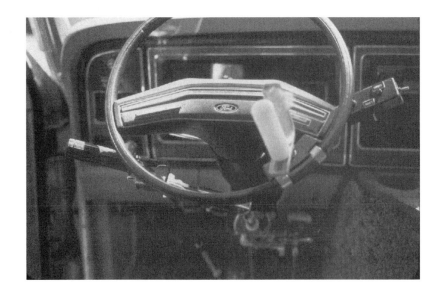

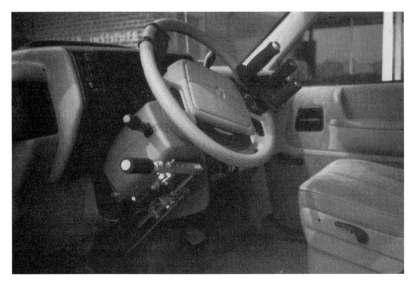

Figure 16-4. Two views of a steering device with right angle/push-pull hand control. (Courtesy of Kessler Institute for Rehabilitation, West Orange, NJ.)

simultaneous acceleration and braking. These types of controls are available but not prevalent in use.

PUSH/LEVER PULL DOWN CONTROLS

Acceleration is accessed by pulling an upright lever (similar to a single post steering device) downward at a right angle to the dashboard or torso. Release returns the control to the neutral position. Simultaneous acceleration is achievable.

FLOOR MOUNT PUSH/PULL CONTROLS

Found mostly in full-size van applications, the activator extends upward from the floor mounting bracket, into the user's AROM. In some instances known as a quad push/pull, the control is useful to individuals who are unable to use standard column-mounted mechanical devices and PAC units. The most costly and space-consuming of the mechanical units, it remains more cost-effective than a PAC unit. When proper interface is achieved, activation and control are quite simple and effective. These units are often found with a tri-pin grasp device when directional function can also be accessed.

One of the major advantages to the use of mechanical hand controls is their cost-effectiveness. Other desirable features are reliability, ease of maintenance and capacity to be moved to another vehicle with minimal change. The purchase of these types of controls can be considered a once-in-a-lifetime expense.

HIGH TECHNOLOGY DEVICES

High-tech assistive technology devices (ATDs) are usually reliant on auxiliary electrical activation. These ATDs may be used in conjunction with other forms of activation. When relying on auxiliary power sources for activation, reliability and cost issues will be raised. Although readily available for use, they should be considered only after all manual and mechanical possibilities have been exhausted.

STEERING SYSTEM MODIFICATION

Persons who are unable to operate standard power steering system arrangements can obtain modifications to the steering column and steering resistances and adaptation to the steering wheel. Extensions to the steering column are usually available for persons using a wheelchair when access directly to the driving station is hindered by available space limitations. As mentioned earlier, the column can be modified to allow for the horizontal placement of the steering wheel when limitation does not permit vertical operation. Limited AROM, strength, and dexterity at the shoulder and arm regions will likely require this type of modification. Small-diameter steering wheels are often used in conjunction with column modifications, enhancing performance capacities with similar deficits. It is not uncommon to see wheel diameters of 4 to 6 in. in high-tech driving systems. When wheel diameter size is reduced, steering resistance is increased.

Factory power steering efforts, when not operable for a driver with a disability, can be modified to a reduced or low effort or to a zero or minimal effort. In considering factory effort as 100 percent, classification of reduced effort would be between 25 and 50 percent of that resistance. Minimal effort would be classified as from 20 percent of factory effort on down. Although most steering reductions are achieved by modifying the existing steering column and box, auxiliary systems that are both digital and hydraulic/electric are available, allowing for the most flexibility in placement and resistance reduction.

Whenever providing a reduced resistance system, a back-up system is imperative for safety in the event of system failure. On activation, the system will allow the driver complete steering function, permitting the driver to safely move to the side of the road and out of traffic. This is imperative when the vehicle is being operated by a person whose disability requires the use of modified resistance systems, who otherwise would not have enough available strength to maintain vehicle control. Systems are available to modify most cars and vans.

ACCELERATION AND BRAKING SYSTEMS

PACs are classified as high tech and are required by those individuals with limited AROM strength and dexterity in the upper extremities. Similar to the steering systems, placement can be achieved within the individual's most advantageous access points. The units require 6 in. or less of AROM, both front to back or side to side in function access. Operation can be done with either upper extremity. The efforts for effective application of the desired function are reduced, with newer systems adjustable to within 2 oz or less. Systems available include those electrical/digital, electrical/ hydraulic, and electrical/pneumatic in nature. As with the steering systems, these modifications are found widely in van applications and are also available in many cars.

UNILEVER DRIVING SYSTEMS

Commonly known as joystick-operated systems, acceleration, braking, and steering functions are all accessed through the activation of one lever or, in one system, a small-diameter wheel. Left and right movement controls steering, forward acceleration, and backward braking in most applications. Required AROM can be as little as 4 in. in some systems. An individual with intact fine motor control in the applied upper extremities will find mastering of the joystick systems easier. Those with only gross motor function will find the mini wheel more user-friendly than the joystick in most applications. The mini wheel system also provides for single-lever operation for those without sufficient grasp. The system in this form requires adequate supination and pronation at the wrist, applicable to a person with the diagnosis of quadriplegia. The mini wheel would be useful for a person with muscular dystrophy (Fig. 16-5).

Figure 16-5. Unilevel steering drive system. (Courtesy of Kessler Institute for Rehabilitation, West Orange, NJ.)

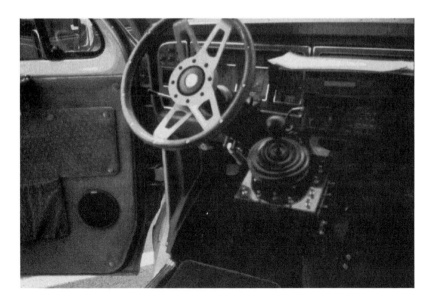

PRIMARY AND SECONDARY CONTROL REMOTES

Persons requiring high-tech primary control modifications and others operating a vehicle from a wheelchair may not have access to other controls related to vehicle operation. Controls in which access is required while in motion are considered primary to safe vehicle operation. These can include the light dimmer, wiper functions, directional signals, horn, and cruise control. Other functions in which access is not essential while driving can include ignition, gear selector, parking brake, climate controls, head lamps, radio, and other auxiliary controls. Low-tech access methods may include dash extensions and keybars. High-tech adaptations are electric console systems. Consoles can be located anywhere within the user's AROM. They can be of singular function or multifunction, with several consoles or pads linked together to provide the desired arrangement. The more common designs are command or multifunction, mini, elbow, headrest, and dash mounted. Activation can be achieved through the operation of toggle switches, extended toggles, rocker switches, singular button, and membrane or raised activator membrane switches. Recent additions to these options are auditory and voice-activated systems. All systems allow for the operation of controls otherwise out of the AROM of the driver (Fig. 16-6).

When consideration is given to any high-tech driving system, affordability must be discussed. Costs can run thousands of dollars in excess of their low-tech, mechanical counterparts. Proper assessment in a comprehensive DRP will ensure that the individual does not receive equipment he or she does not require. The cost of driving a van from a wheelchair will average from $30,000 to $40,000 using low-tech primary controls. When using high-tech primary control options, the cost can run as high as $70,000.

High-tech primary control systems are normally accessed by those persons with advanced physical dysfunction diagnosis. Requiring consistent attention and reaction to the task, individuals with disabilities that include cognitive or perceptual involvement are not good candidates for these

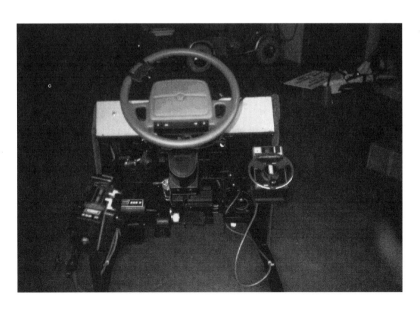

Figure 16-6. Digital steering, acceleration, and braking mock-up. (Courtesy of Kessler Institute for Rehabilitation, West Orange, NJ.)

adaptations. When properly assessed in a comprehensive DRP, trained, licensed, and interfaced, persons with disabilities can find expanded opportunities to remain independent in the community through personal transportation.

SUGGESTED READINGS

Brooke MM, Questad KA, Patterson DR, Valois TA: Driving evaluation after traumatic brain injury. Am J Phys Med Rehabil 16(3):149–161, 1992

Cook CA, Semmler CJ: Ethical dilemmas in driver reeducation. Am J Occup Ther 45(6):517–522, 1991

Digman GH: Driver rehabilitation programs. Lesson 4, pp. 1–47. In Hammel J (ed): Technology and Occupational Therapy: A Link to Function. American Occupational Therapy Association, Bethesda, MD, 1996

Digman GH, Lewis D: Psychosocial considerations in driver rehabilitation. Presented at the Association of Driver Educators for the Disabled Annual Conference, Tampa, FL, 1994

Johnson CA, Keltner JL: Incidence of visual field loss in 20,000 eyes and its relationship to driving performance. Arch Opthalmol 101:371–375, 1983

Nouri FM, Tinson DJ: A comparison of a driving simulator and a road test in the assessment of driving ability after a stroke. Clin Rehabil 2:99–104, 1988

Sipajlo JC: Driver education for the physically disabled. pp. 815–822. In Goodgold J (ed): Rehabilitation Medicine. Mosby, Washington, DC, 1988

Resources

ORGANIZATIONS

American Automobile Association
Traffic Safety-Disabled Driver Programs
1000 AAA Drive
Heathrow, FL 32746
(407) 444-7962

Provides training and information for the adapted driver

American Occupational Therapy Association
4720 Montgomery Lane
Bethesda, MD 20824
(301) 652-AOTA

Resource guide and list of driving courses for persons with disabilities

Association of Driver Educators for the Disabled
P.O. Box 49
Edgerton, WI 53534
(608) 884-8833

Professional organization providing education, conferences, networking, testing for certified driver rehabilitation specialist

National Mobility Equipment Dealers Association
  (NMEDA)
909 E. Skagway Avenue
Tampa, FL 33604
(813) 932-8566

Association of dealers that provides information, conferences, and workshops on installation and use of adaptive transportation equipment

Society of Automotive Engineers
400 Commonwealth Drive
Warrendale, PA 15096
(412) 776-4841

Develops recommended standards for adaptive devices, practices, and vehicle modifications

223

Behind-the-Wheel
Driver Training

CHAPTER 17

LORI PETRUCCELLI-SAFER
BEVERLY K. BAIN

Public Transportation

The Americans with Disabilities Act (ADA)[1] was signed into law on July 26, 1990, and basically extends civil rights protection to the more than 43 million Americans with disabilities. The ADA mandates and specifically ensures equality in the areas of employment, state and local government services, public transportation, privately operated transportation available to the public, places of public accommodation, and telephone services offered to the general public.

This chapter presents an overview of Title II of the ADA that prohibits discrimination on public transportation and Title III that prohibits discrimination in public accommodations operated by private entities. Transportation is the vital link that is necessary to allow the individual to use the newly accessible structure. For instance, if a factory becomes fully accessible yet the disabled worker is unable to get to work because all bus and subway lines are inaccessible, what good is the accessible building? A poll of persons with disabilities conducted in 1985 by Louis Harris found that 67 percent of Americans with disabilities between 16 and 64 years of age are unemployed and only 25 percent are employed full-time. Comparatively, 88 percent of nondisabled Americans are employed full-time in the same age group. Fifty-six percent of people with disabilities say that their disability limits their mobility, which affects the possibility of employment. In the past 20 years, great accomplishments have been made in the areas of educational and vocational training of the disabled. With this increase in skilled disabled individuals, transportation to prospective work sites has not increased.

Subtitle B of Title II of the ADA states that all buses, trains, and any other entity that operates on a fixed or prescribed route system and schedule must become accessible to individuals with disabilities, including wheelchair users. Key issues include

- New public transit buses and rail cars ordered after August 26, 1990, were to be accessible to individuals with disabilities.
- All new rail and bus stations constructed after that date were to be fully accessible.
- Existing rail systems of at least two vehicles in length must make one accessible car per train by July 26, 1995.
- One-car trains, such as streetcars, are not required to become accessible.

- Key stations in rapid and commuter rail systems were to be made accessible by July 26, 1993, with extensions up to 20 years for commuter rail.
- Alternative systems must be offered by state or local government for any disabled person who is unable to independently board, ride, or disembark from any vehicle on a fixed system (examples of these paratransit services are vans that can be built or retrofitted to accommodate persons who cannot access or live too far from fixed route systems).
- All bus and rail stations must become accessible with existing facilities renovated.
- By the year 2000, all Amtrak passenger coaches must have the same number of accessible seats as would have been available if every car were built accessible (one car must become accessible for every two in existence).
- All existing Amtrak stations must be accessible by the year 2010.

Aircraft and historic vehicles are excluded from ADA provisions. Airline transportation is included under the Aircraft Carriers Act, and historic vehicles are included in the National Register of Historic Places.

Title III of the ADA states that all public transportation provided by private entities must be made accessible. Generally, within 30 days after the enactment of the bill, all new purchases or leases of vehicles must be accessible. Such private entities may not purchase or lease a new vehicle, other than an automobile or a van with a seating capacity of less than eight passengers, unless that vehicle is accessible. After August 26, 1994, private entities that operate a fixed route system and purchase new vehicles with a seating capacity of more than 16 passengers must all be accessible. The same one car per train rule applied to trains operated by public entities with the same effective date of July 26, 1995. Alterations to existing facilities operated by private entities were to also become accessible by July 26, 1993, with some allowance up to 30 years.

New York and New Jersey provide examples of the impact and new accessibility in transportation. The New York City Transit Authority (NYCTA) and New Jersey Transit have continued to make changes that should enable commuters with disabilities greater access. In 1988 and 1989, NYCTA completed six new accessible subway stations, four in Queens and two in Manhattan, in anticipation of the new ADA laws. Twenty New York City subway stations are now accessible to persons with disabilities including wheelchair users, providing accessible subway service for the first time to Manhattan from the Bronx, Brooklyn, and Queens. The E line is the first accessible subway route that is entirely accessible, with accessible stations at Jamaica Center, Sutphin Boulevard, Jamaica-Van Wyck, 42 Street/8 Avenue, and the World Trade Center. All accessible stations have elevators or ramps or are at street level.

Many of these subway stations have also been changed to accommodate persons with visual impairments. The first step and base of many stairways are painted a bright color to help passengers with visual impairments. Guide strips have been placed on all platforms to allow visually impaired passengers to identify the platform edge. These strips are painted a color designed to be easily distinguishable by the partially sighted and have a special texture that can be felt with a guide cane. Graphics were changed several years ago to make signs easier to read. Recently, Baruch College has made available a topographic map for commuters with visual impairments in New York City.

NYCTA began to purchase wheelchair-accessible buses in the 1980s. They now operate more than 6,000 wheelchair lift-equipped buses. Virtually all Transit Authority buses are now accessible, and the NYCTA offers a half-fare for passengers with disabilities that is not a requirement of the ADA. New York City has initiated a pedestrian ramp program that has installed more than 600 wheelchair ramps to assist in accessing subway and bus stations.

In New Jersey, the PATH train, which runs rail cars between New Jersey and New York City, has accessible stations at key locations including Hoboken and Journal Square in New Jersey and 14th Street and 33rd Street in New York. All six accessible stations have elevators and ramps. Graphics and lighting have been changed to assist the visually impaired as well. By the completion of their project, there will be seven accessible stations and all trains will be accessible. New Jersey Transit has more than 500 accessible buses available on its 152 routes throughout the state. New Jersey Transit has 12 rail lines that have more than 400 accessible rail cars. Nearly all stations are either accessible or undergoing renovations at this time.

These changes in New York and New Jersey are reflective of the changes that are occurring throughout the country. These changes will bridge the gap for qualified persons with disabilities to access a desirable job and to be able to commute to work in a dignified way.

REFERENCE

1. Americans with Disabilities Act (ADA) of 1990. PL 101-336, Title 42 U.S.C. 12101 et seq: U.S. Statutes at Large, 104, 327–378, July 26, 1990

SUGGESTED READINGS

Betty Bacharach Rehabilitation Hospital: Driver Education at Betty Bacharach Rehabilitation Hospital. Betty Bacharach Rehabilitation Hospital, Pomona, NJ, 1982

Cheever RC: So you want to learn how to drive. Accent on Living, Winter: 75–77, 1991

Kessler Institute for Rehabilitation: The Adapted Driver Education Program. Kessler Institute for Rehabilitation, Inc., West Orange, NJ, 1980

Sipajlo JC: Driver education for the physically disabled. pp. 815–822. In Goodgold J (ed): Rehabilitation Medicine. Mosby, Washington, DC, 1988

Walsh E: Driver evaluation program—putting clients back in the driver's seat. Occup Ther Forum, October 23: 3, 1993

Resources

ASSOCIATIONS

U.S. Department of Transportation
400 Seventh Street, S.W.
Washington, DC 20590
(202) 366-9305
(202) 755-7687 (TDD)

Architectural and Transportation
   Barriers Compliance Board
1331 F Street, N.W.
Washington, DC 20004-1111
(800) USA-ABLE
(202) 272-5434 (voice)
(202) 272-5449 (TDD)
(202) 272-5447 (fax)

CHAPTER 18

Ergonomics

Olivia was diagnosed with multiple sclerosis; her symptoms included visual impairment and weakness exhibited in the extremities. She was employed as a receptionist and loved her job, although it was becoming difficult to perform the many tasks. To allow her to maintain her current level of duties, a professional was called in to look at her workplace. Olivia's capabilities in reach, eyesight, and grasping, carrying and holding strengths, and endurance and mobility were observed, as were her job tasks and environment. As a result, several modifications were recommended to reduce her energy expenditure, minimize reaches and weights, and improve her ability to read and write in terms of visual ability. After a period of adjustment to these modifications, Olivia was revisited to determine that the modifications truly made the positive difference for which they were intended and to ensure that they did not cause any additional stresses.

This chapter deals with the definition and application of ergonomics, which is primarily associated with tasks undertaken in a work environment, either at home or in the "workplace," a factory, office, or commercial facility. The concepts discussed herein, although usually applied to a "worker," can also be applied to any assessment of a person with a disability who wants to use assistive technology (AT) to accomplish a task. Many of the tools discussed in this chapter can be used in conjunction with other evaluative methods used by occupational therapists, physical therapists, and others working with consumers of AT.

DEFINITIONS

The term *ergonomics* is derived from the Greek words *ergos,* meaning work, and *nomos,* meaning laws. Consequently, the field of ergonomics is based in work-related topics such as job task analysis and product or work station design. However, as the essence of ergonomics is an analysis of the relationship between the individual and the activity he or she is performing, the term *ergonomics* often extends beyond the typical work activities to be associated with activities of daily living such as meal preparation, seating, or mobility.

The National Institute for Occupational Safety and Health defines ergonomics as "the discipline that strives to develop and assemble information on people's capacities and capabilities for use in designing jobs, products, workplaces, and equipment".[1] This definition is continued in the goal to "establish through job design, a 'best fit' between the human and imposed job conditions to ensure and enhance worker health, safety, comfort and productivity."

HISTORY

Although ergonomics was introduced into the literature by a Polish educator and scientist, Wojeiech Jastrezebrowski, nearly 125 years ago,[2] it is still a relatively young and evolving field. During the turn of the century, Frank and Lillian Gilbreth, as well as Frederick Taylor, began work with time and motion studies, which are considered by some to be the first formal use of ergonomics in the workplace. However, it was not until World War II and the apparent need to optimize human performance and safety that this field gained momentum.[3] In the 1990s, ergonomics has also become a marketing and media buzzword to redefine comfort through product and work station design.

IMPORTANCE

The benefit of ergonomics lies in its systems approach to matching the demands of the task (and the related tools and environment) to the abilities and limitations of the worker. This is a concern for both the worker and industry. In today's growing global economy, businesses must cut waste, increase sales, and boost productivity to stay competitive. In turn, legislation such as the Occupational Safety and Health Act of 1970, the Americans with Disabilities Act of 1990,[4] and state worker's compensation laws give rise to additional employer concerns. These issues highlight the need for safe and efficient design of the workplace.

The costs associated with workplace injuries are borne by employers and society as a whole. In 1989, an estimated $34.3 billion was spent in worker's compensation. Beyond this, the 1992 edition of *Accident Facts* records wage losses, medical expenses, insurance administration costs, and uninsured costs of an estimated $26,000 per disabling injury, for a total of $63.3 billion in 1991.[5]

Many of these dollars reflect cumulative trauma disorders, or overexertion injuries, such as back injuries. Of the total percentage of illnesses and injuries resulting in days away from work, 27 percent are caused by overexertion injuries.[6] Back injuries in particular have been reported by the Bureau of Labor Statistics as a leading cause of absenteeism, second only to the common cold. Cumulative trauma disorders are discussed in greater detail in Chapter 19.

To reduce injuries and provide nondiscriminatory hiring practices, a closer look at the workforce is necessary. The 1990 U.S. Census records an increasing percentage of an older working population. This translates to an average of 3 percent of the working population being age 65 or older in 1996.[7] Concomitant to this is an increase of women in the workplace, such that 46 percent of the U.S. labor force is female.[8,9] When these workers interact with the tools and work environments that were previously designed for a young, healthy, male workforce, difficulties arise that lead to a demand for ergonomic assessment and modification of the job.

Changes are also being observed as a result of increased advocacy by and for persons with disabilities. This advocacy has changed people's perceptions about the abilities of persons with disabilities. It has also given rise to changes in legislation, such as the Americans with Disabilities Act, which mandates that employers must make reasonable accommodation for workers with disabilities who are otherwise able to meet the requirements of the job.[4] These may include the installation of access features such as ramps or sensor-activated entrances and/or the acquisition of AT to meet the special needs of the employee.

WHO DOES ERGONOMICS?

As part of its evolution, there is much confusion about who is qualified to work in the field of ergonomics and how it differs from similar disciplines such as human factors, engineering psychology, or biomechanics. This confusion arises from the differences in the applications or outcomes being sought and, consequently, in the need for different expertise in the health, science, and design fields. The term *human factors* is often used synonymously with ergonomics but is more commonly associated with products, whereas *ergonomics* is associated with processes. The discipline of human factors focuses on human beings and their interaction with products, equipment, facilities, procedures, and environments used in work and everyday living.[10] Engineering psychology is a combination of experimental psychology, which is behavior oriented, and human factors. It involves basic research on human capabilities and limitations.[11] Biomechanics is the application of physics, engineering, and biology to determine forces placed on the musculoskeletal system.

Although there appears to be a capaciousness about ergonomics, the different expertise and various applications all focus on a central theme of the interactions between the work and the worker. It is paramount that with each goal or application area, the necessary expertise is recognized and made an integral part of the process.

Professional areas involved in ergonomics include industrial design, engineering, occupational therapy and physical therapy, psychology, and related health and safety areas.

The information being presented in this chapter is for readers interested or involved with AT to familiarize themselves with the role of ergonomics and ergonomic professionals in designing workplace, home, and school settings. It is not intended as a training course to develop such expertise, which requires specialized education and training. However, the principles of ergonomics should be taken into consideration when undertaking any form of assessment or task analysis in which the consumer, the assistive technology device (ATD), and the environment must all be taken into consideration. Ergonomic analysis works in conjunction with the Bain Assistive Technology System (BATS) used throughout this text. Ergonomics is more than a static concept or end result, it is a process that

- Identifies needs, risk factors, and barriers
- Implements solutions
- Assesses the result of intervention

JOB ANALYSIS

A balance between the demands of a job and the abilities of each worker is critical for optimal functioning in the workplace. However, this can be a multifaceted challenge with any of a variety of goals being targeted. These goals may include injury prevention, increased productivity, accommodations for job entry or return to work, or meeting the needs of a changing workforce that includes aging workers or people with disabilities, to name a few. To understand all the factors involved in these goals, information in the following areas is required:

- Capabilities of the worker
- Components of the tasks to be performed
- Tools or equipment used in the job
- A broader picture of the working environment
- Influence of related standards and legislation that affects the job and potential recommendations

These components are often referred to as the man-machine environment, or human work system, and are based on a system model approach used in the engineering field for functional planning. Similar to this is the person-environment fit described by Grandjean[12] that suggests that the fit between the worker and the environment influences his or her health and performance.

The first step is identifying what the actual needs and ultimate goals are. This usually begins with the nature of the request: is it to make a job site more accessible for a person who uses a wheelchair, to return an injured worker back to his or her old job, or to design a work station to prevent or alleviate cumulative trauma disorders? This type of review will help set the parameters for who the players are, what resources will be needed, and what information needs to be collected.

The information collected needs to completely describe the system and the relationship of its components: the worker, the tasks, the tools, and the environment. This information may be general or specific, depending on what needs to be described. For example, the information needed to employ a law clerk who uses a wheelchair may not require the collection of data on the clerk's information-processing capabilities. A facility architectural access evaluation would not be a priority when the objective is to set up a computer work station for an individual with a visual impairment. Similarly, it may be necessary to draw on the expertise of someone qualified to measure strength capabilities when looking at reentry into a job with lifting requirements but not necessarily so when looking at a microscopist's work station to prevent cumulative trauma disorders.

Before this type of identification, a preliminary review is undertaken that points to areas for intervention, such as injury reports, complaints, or vocational placement considerations. In short, the problem needs to be defined such that all the parties concerned can outline the goals for ergonomic intervention from which potential data-gathering techniques and resources can be identified. From this framework, a process can be initiated to investigate the variables in the human work system.

Once the groundwork has been laid on where to focus ergonomic efforts, the next step is to take a more detailed look at the components that make up the work system. The goal is to identify incompatibilities between what is expected of the worker and how the worker is able to perform. This type of information typically points to risk factors that must be eliminated or reduced, such as lifting requirements that exceed the limits of the worker. Sometimes there are not risks associated with a job but barriers such as architectural obstacles that limit an individual's capabilities. Examples may include controls that cannot be reached by a person who uses a wheelchair or door handles that cannot be turned by someone with severe arthritis.

TOOLS AND TECHNIQUES

There are two basic focal points for investigating job demands: the requirements presented by the work, and the capabilities of the worker in meeting those demands. Among its many definitions, *work* is a sustained physical or mental effort to overcome obstacles and achieve an objective or result.[13] The ability to perform such work is influenced by the task, tool, and environment that comprise it. To match the individual and the job, more information is needed about each of these system components. This information is usually gleaned through on-site visit(s) to observe the tasks, tools, and/or environment, as well as direct contact with the individual(s) concerned. The actual methods of data collection may range from physical stress surveys to postural evaluations to comfort ratings. In many cases, it will be necessary to use several techniques to provide a complete picture. Techniques of data gathering may include one or more of the following: interviews, observation, surveys, and measurement.

Data collection may include, but is not limited to, such tools as

- Force gauge
- Heart rate monitor
- Electromyography equipment
- Electrogoniometer
- Environmental and skin temperature-sensing devices
- Noise and vibration instruments
- Video camera
- Computer/software (e.g., for strength prediction)
- Tape measure
- Motion-sensing equipment

Due to advances in technology, there is an increasing number of tools to aid in data collection and analysis. Computer software in particular is available so that an investigator can simulate a work situation along with characteristics of the worker to observe fit or potential risk factors. This type of software can create three-dimensional views of the worker and the work space to observe postures, reach, maneuverability, or other design features. Strength demands can also be observed by programs that match lifting loads with assumed postures and travel distance. Additional technologies are available that aid in gathering of forces, awkward postures, or repetitions by directly recording a worker's movement and positions. The purpose of such technologies is to provide objective measurement, but in many cases the validity and reliability of these tools are unknown.

TASK ANALYSIS

The actual tasks to be performed greatly dictate the human requirements. Therefore, being able to detail this information makes it much easier to match specific subtasks with a worker's strengths and limitations. It is typical to look at work demands in terms of responses of the individual under a work load. This may be broken down as physical, psychological, or mental/perceptual demands, from indirect metabolic measures of the body's response that evaluate energy expenditure.

Metabolic measures include heart rate, blood pressure, respiration, metabolism, body temperature, and/or muscle activity; physical work load can be measured by biomechanical, motion, and/or timed activity analysis[14]: mental/perceptual work loads are typically reflected by sensation, information processing, and effectoral/motoric or cognitive analysis; and psychological measures typically look at stress or satisfaction.

What confronts the person investigating job tasks is determining what information to record. Under the Americans with Disabilities Act, essential duties are recorded as necessary features of a job that a worker must perform. This process is continuously changing, as new techniques for task analysis are tested and used in the field. Nonetheless, there are several features that are common to such data collection, such as a description of the tasks to be performed and the expectations placed on the worker. Salvendy[15] characterizes task analysis as a "formal methodology . . . which describes and analyzes demands made on the human element of a system."

Different sources will have different background information to be recorded, but task information usually documents the specific task description and sequence, frequency, duration, duty cycle, and specific skills.

Assessments looking at specific issues such as cumulative trauma disorders will typically look for particular risk factors, or factors that when present are associated with an increase in the potential for injury. This includes, but is not limited to, awkward posture, mechanical stress, force, repetition, duration, and recovery time. However, the mere presence of a risk factor may not result in injury, due to varying characteristics of individuals.

EQUIPMENT ANALYSIS

Many of these risk factors are associated with tool usage, which gives credence to the need to evaluate work demands imposed by tools or equipment as well as the task. Characteristics to note can consist of reaches, clearances, weight, controls, operating forces, and assumed postures. Tool selection can influence the ease, safety, and productivity of a particular task, and often simple modification of tools can assist an injured or disabled worker in performing his or her job. If a tool requires excessive force to be operated or controlled, an injury may result. The improper selection, installation, or use of a tool may require the worker to exert excessive force over a short or long period, leading to muscle fatigue or injury.[16] A job analysis that leads to the selection of alternative hand tools can greatly reduce the likelihood of injury in the performance of a task and allow differently abled individuals to participate in a wider range of employment opportunities.

ENVIRONMENTAL ANALYSIS

An analysis of the working environment is often performed in conjunction with task and tool investigation. This provides information about environmental components that could influence task performance and could include both physical as well as organizational and social parameters. Typical physical characteristics of the environment to examine include lighting, noise, vibration, ambient temperature, maintenance, and safety.

In addition to these characteristics, the investigator should consider psychosocial issues that may not be as apparent. These are usually administrative issues and commonly affect the stress level of workers. Stress can occur when the demands of the situation exceed an individual's ability to cope with it. These demands may be related to job demands such as work pace or error rates, job control, social support, and/or job satisfaction.

WORKER CHARACTERISTICS

Last, but certainly not least, are the abilities and limitations of the worker. Inherent to modifying a workplace is knowing what parameters define such specifications. Anthropometry is a branch of science that deals with the measurements of the human body. Its contribution to ergonomics lies in the knowledge gained of physical dimensions that can be transferred to workplace and product design. Basic body dimensions include length, breadth, girth, and weight. This information can then be applied to reach distance, body clearance needed, or application of force.

In most cases, a specific range that represents a percentage of the population is chosen as a model of a particular work environment or tool. However, certain situations demand tolerances that account for the extremes in the population. Such would be the case when trying to provide light switches to be reached by an employee who uses a wheelchair. Placing the switch too high would prevent access for a person in a wheelchair, but placing the switch within his or her reach envelope would still be a usable solution for an ambulatory person.

Anthropometric data are a good source of information for the available ranges of motion of workers. Other design criteria include principles such as strength, endurance, balance, coordination, and aerobic capacity of workers. These activities are frequently reflected in a functional capacity evaluation (FCE). An FCE is a comprehensive objective test of a person's ability to perform work-related tasks[17] that is administered by health professionals such as occupational therapists, physical therapists, vocational counselors, or psychologists.

WORKPLACE MODIFICATION

Ergonomic intervention may take the form of physical changes in the work space, tools, or work organization. Intervention may be solutions that remove barriers to employment or eliminate or reduce risks associated with certain jobs; it may correct existing problems or prevent potential problems.

The idea behind using ergonomic principles in making work site modifications and identifying appropriate AT is to look at the whole picture to provide a comprehensive and successful solution for everyone concerned. Such modifications must be prescribed responsibly. The final product not only needs to meet the goals originally identified but should be the most cost-efficient and least stigmatizing solution for both the employer and the worker. In light of this, a general hierarchy should be kept in mind when making accommodations:

1. *Look at the task for possible modification:* If a job consists of repetitive work that could stress a particular group of muscles, wherever possible it would make more sense to vary the tasks so that the worker could take breaks and provide rest and recovery time for those muscles than to engineer a new work station. This approach does not draw attention to the worker and is usually a quick and economical solution.

2. *Use commercially available solutions:* When it is not possible to change the task, the next option would be to look for what modifications are readily available to solve the problem. There is no need to waste time and money recreating the wheel when something is currently available to meet the need. Many catalogs and databases are available that list products for a variety of user needs. The Job Accommodation Network, established by the President's Committee for the Employment of People with Disabilities, has set up a service to provide information on a variety of accommodation issues, including commercially available products and modifications. The Thomas' Register is also a valuable source of information to search for products. This lists information both by product and by vendor and is primarily for products used in industry such as fatigue mats, office furniture, or lift carts. Additionally, products once considered specialty or rehabilitation products—such as tub grab bars—are finding their way into the mainstream.

3. *Modify commercially available solutions:* Although there is a great variety of products available to improve work sites, there is also a great diversity among workers. Therefore, it is important to look for products and modifications that are adjustable to meet a variety of needs. When working with an individual, this often means that there may be technology available that slightly misses the mark. This gives rise to the need to look at commercially available products that can be modified to make the match. Because a worker does not have the pinch grip to hold a pencil does not mean he or she cannot write; it means that the pencil diameter needs to be enlarged. If a secretary develops neck pain using a computer, it

does not mean that he or she must discontinue typing; but the secretary perhaps needs to raise or relocate the monitor for a proper viewing angle.

4. *Design and develop new technology:* Not every modification need can be met with commercial solutions, but to develop new technology means research and development as well as material costs. This also presents the potential for drawing unwanted attention to the worker using specialized technology. The introduction of new products or processes must not distract from the main work goals or present new problems. However, the provision of such customized technology may be integral to making employment a reality. In such cases, measures must be taken to ensure a useful solution.

From a study on technology abandonment, the National Rehabilitation Hospital reported four important features for AT[18]: effectiveness, affordability, operability, and dependability.

These objectives were taken from consumer feedback but apply to general design principles as well. Accommodation is more than products and modifications. It must also incorporate training and information to introduce the worker to safe and effective use of new technologies or work strategies. Providing a new "ergonomically designed" chair for a worker may be meaningless if he or she does not know how to adjust it for a proper fit. Similarly, a voice-output word processing program may be purchased for a worker with visual impairments, but if he or she does not know how to use the computer, the technology is not effective.

Occupational rehabilitation (formerly known as work hardening) is an interdisciplinary program that uses a simulated work environment to facilitate recovery and return to work of injured workers.[19] These programs are staffed by a variety of personnel and use a wide variety of materials to re-create a work environment that closely proximates the target of the individual client. To standardize occupational rehabilitation programs and protect consumers, the Commission on Accreditation of Rehabilitation Facilities developed standards for treatment with which organizations must comply to be accredited.[20] (Occupational rehabilitation programs are discussed in Chapter 20.)

FOLLOW-UP

The ergonomic process of workplace modifications cannot be complete until the initial goals have been achieved. Without a review of such modifications a priori, this is not a given. This type of review is similar to previous evaluation of the human work system but with reference to the changes made. If the goals originally identified have not been met, it is the mission of the investigator to locate where the breakdown exists and to step back in the process to instigate the changes necessary to correct the situation.

The follow-up to ergonomic intervention relies on an organizational mechanism to sustain its effect. Acceptance of modifications and a willingness by all to use ergonomic principles on a consistent basis is crucial to the success of maintaining the health and productivity of employees, in addition to nondiscriminatory employment practices. The most effective ergonomic interventions will involve the active participation of labor and management; often the "work organization" issues are as important as physical factors in creating poor work environments. These issues include job satisfaction and work stress levels; the presence of an ergonomic intervention team or committee can go a long way to improving the psychosocial stressors in a work environment. The active participation of the consumer and health care team is an essential component in the holistic approach to ergonomics.

ACKNOWLEDGMENT

The author acknowledges Manny Halpern, M.A., for his comments and review of this chapter and David Goldsheyder, M.A., for research assistance.

REFERENCES

1. National Institute of Occupational Safety and Health: Comments from the National Institute of Occupational Safety and Health on the Occupational Safety and Health proposed rule on ergonomic safety and health management. Comments DOL S-777: 1–63, 1993

2. Monod H, Valentin M: The predecessors of ergonomy (in French). Ergonomics 22: 673, 1979

3. Anderson MA: Ergonomics: analyzing work from a physiological perspective. pp. 3–39. In Isernhagen SJ (ed): The Comprehensive Guide to Work Injury Management. Aspen Publishers, Gaithersburg, MD, 1995

4. Americans with Disabilities Act (ADA) of 1990. PL 101-336, Title 42 U.S.C. 12101 et seq: U.S. Statutes at Large, 104, 327–378, July 26, 1990

5. National Safety Council: Accident Facts. NSC, Chicago, 1993

6. Bureau of Labor Statistics: News: Characteristics of Injuries and Illnesses Resulting from Absences from Work, 1994. BLS, Washington, DC, 1996

7. Bureau of Labor Statistics: Data: Labor Force Statistics from the Current Population Survey. BLS, Washington, DC, 1996

8. Bureau of Labor Statistics: News, USDL-94-213. BLS, Washington, DC, 1994

9. Chaffin DB: Ergonomic advances as a science with applications in health and safety. Occup Health Safety 61(1): 38, 1992

10. Saunders M: Human Factors in Engineering and Design. McGraw-Hill, New York, 1993

11. Wickens CD: Engineering Psychology and Human Performance. Harper Collins, New York, 1992

12. Grandjean E: Fitting the Task to the Man: An Ergonomic Approach. Taylor & Francis, London, 1988

13. Webster's Ninth New Collegiate Dictionary. Merriam-Webster, Inc., Springfield, MA, 1991

14. Eastman Kodak, Human Factors Section: Ergonomic Design for People at Work. Lifetime Learning Publications, Belmont, CA, 1983

15. Salvendy G: Handbook of Human Factors. Wiley, New York, 1987

16. Radwin RG, Oh S, Carlson-Dakes C: Biomechanical aspects of hand tools. pp. 466–479. In Nordin M, Andersson GBJ, Pope MH (eds): Musculoskeletal Disorders in the Workplace: Principles and Practice. Mosby-Year Book, Philadelphia, 1997

17. Isernhagen SJ (ed): Work Injury: Management and Prevention. Aspen Publishers, Gaithersburg, MD, 1988

18. Phillips B, Zhao Hongzin Z: Predictors of technology abandonment. Assistive Technology 5(1):3, 1993

19. Darphin LE: Work-hardening and work-conditioning perspectives. pp. 443–462. In Isernhagen SJ (ed): Work Injury: Management and Prevention. Aspen Publishers, Gaithersburg, MD, 1988

20. Commission on Accreditation of Rehabilitation Facilities (CARF): Standards Manual for Organizations Serving People with Disabilities. CARF, Tucson, AZ, 1992

SUGGESTED READINGS

Astrand PO, Rodahl K: Textbook of Work Physiology. McGraw-Hill, New York, 1977

Burke M: Applied Ergonomics Handbook. Lewis Publishers, Boca Raton, LA, 1992

Chaffin DB, Andersson GBJ: Occupational Biomechanics. John Wiley, New York, 1991

NASA: Anthropometric Source Book. NASA Reference Publication 1024. 3 vols. NASA, Washington, DC, 1988

Pheasant S: Bodyspace: Anthropometry, Ergonomics and Design. Taylor & Francis, Philadelphia, 1986

Tilley AR (ed): The Measure of Man and Woman. Whitney Library of Design, New York, 1993

Wilson JR, Corlett EN (eds): Evaluation of Human Work. Taylor & Francis, Bristol, PA, 1990

Resources

ASSOCIATIONS

The Job Accommodation Network (J.A.N.)
918 Chestnut Ridge Road, Suite 1
P.O. Box 6080
Morgantown, WV 26506-6080
1-800-ADA-WORK (1-800-232-9675)
    Voice & TDD

Americans with Disabilities Act Accessibility
    Guidelines (ADAAG)
Architectural & Transportation Barriers
    Compliance Board
1111 Eighteenth Street N.W., Suite 501
Washington, DC 20036
1-800-USA-ABLE (1-800-872-2253)

Standards Manual for Organizations Serving
    People with Disabilities
Commission on Accreditation of Rehabilitation
    Facilities (CARF)
101 Wilmot Road, Suite 500
Tucson, AZ 85711

CHAPTER 19

DAWN LEGER
MANNY HALPERN

Cumulative Trauma Disorders

Cumulative trauma disorders (CTDs) are disorders of the muscles, tendons, peripheral nerves, or vascular system. They can result from, be precipitated by, or be aggravated by a variety of mechanical factors. These factors include intense, repeated, or sustained exertions on a specific body part, motions of that body part, vibration, exposure to cold, or insufficient recovery from these stresses. Although this definition extends to the entire musculoskeletal system, including low back problems, in this chapter we focus on the upper extremity. CTDs can also be called repetitive motion injuries, repetitive stress injuries, or overuse injuries.

CTDs are characterized by the following:

- Many related factors both inside and outside the work environment are associated with CTDs
- CTDs generally develop over periods of weeks, months, and years
- If not detected or treated early, recovery may require weeks, months, or years and, in a few cases, may never be complete
- Most work-related CTDs involve muscles and tendons

Many people associate CTDs with carpal tunnel disorders or other keyboard-related musculoskeletal problems. However, job categories that have particularly high prevalence of CTDs range from construction to clerical, with high worker's compensation claims from food preparation such as meat-cutters and canners, the apparel industry, and other manufacturing services.[1]

The definition and diagnosis of CTD is controversial in the legal and medical communities. There are many distinct types of CTDs, with separate diagnoses, treatments, and implications, but the aim of this chapter is to provide a broad introduction rather than a comprehensive analysis of the phenomenon. For purposes of ergonomic intervention and prevention of CTD, the clinical diagnosis is not critical except insofar as a person has been identified with a problem that needs amelioration.

EPIDEMIOLOGY

The aforementioned difficulty in defining CTD also complicates the analysis of its prevalence in society. Different countries, and indeed, jurisdictions within those countries, use widely different methods for classification of CTD and statistical reporting. Thus, one country may appear to have an epidemic of carpal tunnel syndrome (CTS) whereas the problem can be masked in another by the use of the terms *sprain* or *overexertion* injury. As it is defined in the scientific literature, CTD is used in the United States to describe a class of work-related musculoskeletal disorders associated with highly repetitive and/or forceful activity. In the United States, it is estimated that more than half of all work-related injuries reported are CTDs.[1] Data collected at work sites suggest that CTDs are responsible for a significant amount of lost work time and high labor turnover.[2] Additionally, the incidence of reported cases is increasing at a fast rate, although overall incidence is unclear. The 1988 National Health Survey found that 1.47 percent or 1.87 million workers claimed they had CTS, and 0.53 percent or 675,000 stated that their prolonged hand discomfort was diagnosed as CTS by a medical person.[3]

CTDs appear over a long span of time. Sometimes, the symptoms appear and disappear and the limitations develop slowly over the course of several years. By definition, there is no single event or injury that precipitates the onset of pain, and the disorder may never be reported as such if the worker changes jobs or retires.

Risk factors are those characteristics or activities that increase the probability that a disease or disorder may develop. Epidemiologic studies identified several such factors associated with CTD of the upper extremities. The physical stresses are force, posture, vibration, and cold temperature. These stresses have characteristic dimensions of exposure such as the magnitude of the stress, the repetitiveness or the frequency that the physical stress occurs, and the duration or amount of time that the stress is sustained.

The dimensions of the physical stresses may be the result of organizational factors such as limited and repetitive tasks, machine-paced activities, or pay incentives for high production rates. These may trigger psychosocial stress responses such as job dissatisfaction, boredom, or helplessness that affect the reporting of musculoskeletal pain in some individuals.[4,5] Some of these activities may occur outside the workplace, during participation in recreation that may include woodworking, sports, or handicrafts. Age, gender, and some medical conditions may influence the disposition of a person toward CTD.

Because of the complexity of the relationship between the risk factors, epidemiologic studies have not been done to date that quantify the magnitude, frequency, or duration that place an individual at risk. It is important to note that the mere presence of a risk factor does not necessarily mean that an individual performing the activity is at excessive risk of injury. Generally, it appears that the greater the exposure to a single risk factor or combination of factors, the greater is the risk of CTD.[4,6]

INJURY MECHANISM

Repetition of tasks is often thought to be a common and influential factor contributing to CTD; its other names—repetitive motion injury, repetitive stress injury—place the emphasis firmly on the frequency of task performance as the overriding determinant of injury. However, physiologically, repetitiveness cannot be viewed separately from muscle tension. The repetition of tasks requires rapid and frequent contraction of specific muscles. Muscles develop less tension during rapid contractions than at lower velocities. Consequently, more muscle tension is needed during rapid movements to exert a constant force. Therefore, an object with a constant weight may require more force during fast manual handling movements than during slower movements. When the time to recovery is insufficient to remove waste products from the working tissue, fatigue may ensue.[7]

The tendons of some muscles encounter friction as they pass through narrow spaces such as the wrist (carpal tunnel).[8] The mechanical friction may wear and tear tendon sheaths, resulting in swelling and increased pressure on adjacent nerves. This way, the frequency of movement may contribute to the development of tenosynovitis or nerve impingement syndromes. The use of keyboards (from typewriters to pianos) was thought to be a case in point. Keying does not necessarily require forceful muscle output; it is debilitating because of the repetition of contracting the same muscle groups over a short period of time. Manual typing, which required a greater exertion of muscle force, also involved enforced "microbreaks" for carriage return and insertion of paper and therefore was not as stressful to the wrist and hand as modern keyboard work. However, recent studies observed that although electronic keys respond to light touch, people tend to punch them with a force higher than necessary.[9]

Muscle tension can develop to counter the force of gravity. This is the case when we maintain the body's posture in space. When a posture is sustained for long periods of time, muscles contract isometrically. In this type of contraction, muscles cannot act as pumps to remove waste products from the tissue and are particularly vulnerable to fatigue. Static work is performed by the neck and shoulder muscles in many jobs, which may explain the complaints registered typically by computer workers or dentists.

An awkward posture can be defined as a position in which a body joint is held close to the extreme of its range of motion. Often, the neutral posture is the position in which muscles are relaxed; as the joint moves toward the end of its range of motion, more tension develops in the muscle. The performance of tasks in an awkward, twisted, or constrained posture can cause muscle fatigue, cramping, and strains.[7] This is particularly true for overhead work or work that requires bending the neck, such as microscope use.[2] Finally, the effect of the awkward posture is not limited to the upper extremity. The body is a linked chain system; the maintenance of awkward posture in the upper extremity will have an adverse impact on the trunk and lower extremity as it attempts to compensate.[10]

Muscle tension is also needed to exert forces on a component or tool. Grip requirements must therefore be taken into consideration. If a tool is sharp-edged, ill-fitting, or vibrating, muscles are easily fatigued and other soft tissue injuries can occur.[11,12] Poorly fitting gloves or tools are also important contributors to CTD. The muscles may have to overcome the restraints of the glove, thus exerting excessive forces. Tool handles, such as scissors or pliers, may press directly on vulnerable tissue in the palm of the hand. Even leaning the forearm on hard and sharp-edged work benches may pressure the nerves going through the elbow or the wrist.[12]

The holistic view of the work system is also described by the Bain Assistive Technology System; the task, consumer, device, and environment are interrelated elements that cannot be considered alone. Even seated postures can be stressful if the work station is poorly arranged and tasks badly designed. Every aspect must be considered when performing an evaluation: the worker, the tool, and the environment in which the task is to be performed.

PREVENTION

The National Institute of Occupational Safety and Health (NIOSH) lists four areas of strategies to control and prevent musculoskeletal injury[13]:

- Engineering controls to redesign tools, tasks, and work station design
- Administrative controls including
    Work practices (job rotation or enrichment, limited overtime, work/rest cycles)
    Safe work practice training, including body mechanics
    Worker placement evaluation (employee selection)
- Personal protective equipment (PPE), such as gloves, padding, wrist rests
- Medical management to minimize the impact of the health problems

The goal of NIOSH's hazard prevention and control is to eliminate, reduce, or control the presence of ergonomic hazards. NIOSH supports a tiered hierarchy of controls as an intervention strategy, in which engineering changes are viewed as first preference, administrative changes are a second preference, and PPE is the last choice.

These control strategies are also essential in CTD prevention programs. However, the effectiveness of some of the strategies in preventing CTD (e.g., employee screening or PPE) is far from clear.

ERGONOMIC INTERVENTION

The ergonomic process requires an identification of

- **Where is the problem:** knowledge of the tasks at work in which risk factors are present

- **What is the problem:** the specific risk factors (force, posture, repetitiveness), their magnitude, and the body parts at risk
- **Why is there a problem:** the ergonomic causes (i.e., hazards [tool design, product design, work station design, individual technique] and barriers [work organization, psychosocial factors that may exacerbate the condition])
- **What to do:** prioritize solutions by feasibility

The principles and steps for accommodating individuals with CTD have been outlined in Chapters 2 and 18. As part of a comprehensive multidisciplinary rehabilitation treatment, the ergonomist conducts an on-site ergonomic analysis to identify potential risk factors. The analysis often includes videotaping of the job to which the patient is to return. The job is sometimes broken into tasks and their elements. These job components are analyzed for repeated or sustained exertions, forceful exertions, localized mechanical pressures, and awkward postures. Based on the analysis, suggestions are made to the worker and the supervisor regarding low-cost modifications to facilitate a safe return to work and reduce the likelihood of relapse. This information can also be used in an occupational rehabilitation program that uses work conditioning or simulation to instruct the worker and to facilitate a self-management approach to risk reduction.

Ergonomic interventions are used in accommodating persons with CTD. In principle, ergonomic interventions are designed to control the exposure to mechanical stresses that may aggravate the individual's condition. A few typical examples are provided in the following:

1. *Static force exertions* can be relieved by using various supports and rests that are commercially available (for video display terminal [VDT] users, see Ch. 12).

2. *Awkward postures* can often be relieved by improvised changes in work station layout (e.g., neck pain can be relieved by changing the placement of a VDT monitor); commercially available adjustable furniture is often used for the prevention of musculoskeletal discomfort (e.g., for VDT users, the use of keyboard holders).

3. *Awkward hand and wrist postures* are often imposed by tool design; by modifying the tools, usually the handle, the posture may change. For example, a standard flat keyboard forces the user to pronate the forearm and ulnarly deviate the wrist while maintaining the arm hanging down close to the body and the elbow at a right angle. By splitting the keyboard and inclining the halves sideways, pronation may be reduced; by swiveling the halves horizontally, ulnar deviation may be eliminated (Fig. 19-1). Similarly, many scissors and knives force the hand into ulnar deviation while exerting force; by tilting the handle with respect to the tool, ulnar deviation may be eliminated (Fig. 19-2). These devices are no longer restricted to the domain of specialty rehabilitation products; they are available commercially by hand tool manufacturers.

4. *Forceful exertions* can sometimes be eliminated by mechanization or use of mechanical assists. Repeated removal of fixtures from a work bench can be facilitated by installing a chute; spring-loaded

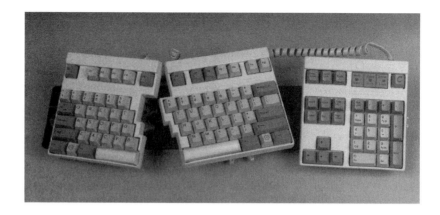

Figure 19-1. Example of a split keyboard.

balancers can be used to suspend power tools such as drills and reduce the force needed to hold them in place (Fig. 19-3).

5. *Braces and splints* are designed to keep joints at neutral position. They should be prescribed and used with caution; NIOSH and the American National Standards Institute view them as therapeutic devices, not PPE.[4] In general, these devices should not be used at work. When used at work, one should check whether they aggravate the task demands because more force is needed to overcome the resistance of the brace. One should also check whether the devices transfer the problem to other joints; occasionally, immobilization of one joint such as the wrist may be compensated by increasing the awkward posture and movement by other joints, typically the upper arm and shoulder.

As with any ATD, the involvement of the person with the disability is important in accommodating CTD cases. Typically, this requires training. When adjustable furniture or accessories are available, the user needs to be trained on when and how to make the adjustments. Ideally, the consumer should be present at the installation of the devices and be able to try them out for a while. For example, work station accessories such as keyboard holders may not be installed properly (e.g., too far away from the edge of the desk), even though they are perfectly sound. Similarly, follow-up and documentation are necessary to check whether the hazard has been effectively removed and whether the device has been acceptable to the user. Abandonment of AT at work is probably as common as in nonoccupational environments.

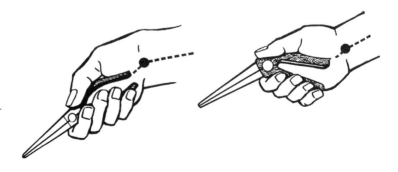

Figure 19-2. Many scissors and knives force the hand into ulnar deviation while exerting force; by tilting the handle with respect to the tool, ulnar deviation may be eliminated.

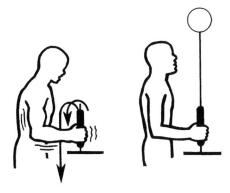

Figure 19-3. Spring-loaded balancers can be used to suspend power tools such as drills and reduce the force needed to hold them.

REFERENCES

1. Bureau of Labor Statistics: Characteristics of Injuries and Illnesses Resulting from Absences from Work, 1994. BLS News. USDL-96-163, BLS, Washington, DC, 1996

2. Lee KS, Waikar WL: Physical stress evaluation of microscope work using objective and subjective methods. Int J Ind Ergonomics 2:203, 1988

3. Tanaka S, Wild DK, Seligman PJ et al: Prevalence and work-relatedness of self-reported carpal tunnel syndrome among U.S. workers: analysis of the occupational health supplement data of 1988 National Health Interview Survey. Am J In Med 27(4):451, 1995

4. American National Standards Institute: ANSI Z-365: Control of Work-Related CTD. Part 1: Upper Extremities (draft). NSF, Itasca, IL, 1996

5. Bongers PM, deWinter CR, Kompier MAJ, Hildebrandt VH: Psychosocial factors at work and musculoskeletal disease. Scand J Work Environ Health 19:297, 1993

6. Silverstein B, Fine LJ, Armstrong TJ: Hand wrist cumulative trauma disorders in industry. Br J Ind Med 43:779, 1986

7. Armstrong TS, Buckle P, Fine LJ et al: A conceptual model for work-related neck and upper-limb musculoskeletal disorders. Scand J Work Environ Health 19:73, 1993

8. Moore A, Wells R, Ranney D: Quantifying exposure in occupational manual tasks with cumulative trauma disorder potential. Ergonomics 34(12):1433, 1991

9. Armstrong TS, Foulke JA, Martin BM et al: Investigation of applied forces in alphanumeric keyboard work. Am Ind Hyg Assoc J 55:30, 1994

10. Parker KG, Imbus HR: Cumulative Trauma Disorders, Lewis Publishers, Ann Arbor, MI, 1992

11. Pfalzer LA, McPhee B: Carpal tunnel syndrome research. pp. 127–192. In Isernhagen SJ (ed): The Comprehensive Guide to Work Injury Management. Aspen Publishers, Gaithersburg, MD, 1995

12. Putz-Anderson V (ed): Cumulative Trauma Disorders: A Manual for Musculoskeletal Diseases of the Upper Limbs. Taylor & Francis, New York, 1988

13. National Institute of Occupational Safety & Health: A National Strategy for Occupational Musculoskeletal Injuries: Implementation Issues and Research Needs—1991 Conference Summary. DHHS (NIOSH) Publication 93-101, 1992

CHAPTER 20

BARRY A. WOLF
JEFF HARTEN
DAWN LEGER

Technology and Occupational Rehabilitation Programs

Occupational rehabilitation programs, also known as "work hardening" programs, are defined as interdisciplinary programs that use graded conditioning tasks to progressively improve the biomechanical, neuromuscular, cardiovascular/metabolic, and psychosocial functions of a person in conjunction with real or simulated work activities.[1,2] These programs provide a transition between acute care and return to work while addressing the issues of productivity, safety, physical tolerances, and worker behavior. Occupational rehabilitation is a highly structured, goal-oriented, individualized treatment program designed to maximize the person's ability to return to work.

Since the inception of work hardening programs in the late 1970s, there have been many changes in the theory, practice, and standards. Originally, work hardening programs were designed for the industrially injured worker.[3,4] Sparked during a period when worker's compensation costs were escalating in the United States, work hardening programs enjoyed tremendous growth in the 1980s. A lack of regulation and enforcement of standards created an atmosphere of confusion, however, and a wide variety of treatment modalities came to be known as work hardening. Some of these work conditioning programs were very successful, but the proliferation of less rigorous programs cast a negative shadow over the practice. The Commission on Accreditation of Rehabilitation Facilities (CARF) established guidelines for the accreditation of work hardening programs that are usually hospital based, medically affiliated, or private facilities.[2] However, these changes did not stop the decline in referrals to work hardening programs, and a major revision of the standards for occupational rehabilitation programs was undertaken, culminating in a new set of guidelines issued in 1996.[1]

The worker who is injured and disabled has become the focus of much attention and concern by the medical and business communities. Worker's compensation and disability costs continue to surge upward.[5] In response to the need for appropriate care for injured workers, the new standard for occupational rehabilitation programs outlines the compensable services to be provided. There is a need for programs designed to return persons who are injured and disabled to work. The 1996 Standards Manual and Interpretive Guidelines for Medical Rehabilitation defines occupational rehabilitation programs as comprehensive, outcome oriented, and designed to minimize risk and optimize the work capacity of the person served.[3] These services are integrative in nature, with the capability of addressing the issues of return-to-work health and rehabilitation. While focusing on identifying and reducing the risks of injury, illness, and disease, programs should encourage the proactive management of workers with injury or illness and their participation in rehabilitation and prevention programs.

PROGRAM CLASSIFICATION

Occupational rehabilitation programs fit into one of three classifications: acute, work-specific category one, and work-specific category two.

- **Acute**—An acute program is usually offered at the onset of injury/illness but may be offered if appropriate at any time throughout the recovery phase. Although focusing on functional restoration and return to work, the goals of the program include improving cardiovascular and neuromuscular function, patient education, and symptom relief.
- **Work-specific category one**—A work-specific category one program may or may not be preceded by acute rehabilitation. This type of program uses real or simulated work to restore physical, behavioral, functional, and vocational skills.
- **Work-specific category two**—Category two programs differ from category one in that they are delivered by a team with expertise in occupational rehabilitation and occupational medicine. Category two requires that an occupational medicine physician be part of the team. This program consists of evaluation, treatment, and management of work-related injury/illness and associated issues.

Common threads throughout all three categories of programs include an emphasis on function, prevention, cost-containment, and collaboration between providers and consumers. These threads reflect the emerging trend as the transition to managed care continues. In the future, technology will play an integral role and have a large impact on occupational rehabilitation programs.

It is important to follow the CARF guidelines describing the four different types of functional capacity evaluations that should be considered when developing a comprehensive treatment plan.[1,2]

1. *A baseline evaluation* is performed to assess the functional ability to perform work activities, including the U.S. Department of Labor's physical demand factors.

2. *Job capacity evaluations* assess the match between the consumer's capabilities and the demands of a specific job.

3. *An occupational capacity evaluation* assesses the match between the consumer's abilities and the demands of an occupational group.

4. *A work capacity evaluation* assesses the consumer's abilities and the demands of competitive employment.

TECHNOLOGY IN OCCUPATIONAL REHABILITATION

The evolution of technology within occupational rehabilitation has been a multidimensional process. Its acceptance and use stems from the following:

1. The tremendous need for objective quantifiable results. Many programs have purchased devices that help to objectively assess such things as a person's physical capacity, amount of progress, and range of motion.

2. Legislation, such as the Americans with Disabilities Act. Reasonable accommodation requirements for workers with a disability have led to the introduction of both low- and high-tech modifications.

3. The documented relationship between a healthy, safe worker and increased productivity, decreased absenteeism, and decreased health care costs. The use of technology is becoming more common in the analysis, implementation, and evaluation of prevention programs and ergonomic interventions.

4. The need to accurately simulate a large variety of occupations.

5. Marketing is becoming more and more important as competition increases not only for occupational rehabilitation programs but for equipment manufacturers and distributors. In a cost-conscious health care environment, programs are under pressure to justify their expenses with well-documented results. Outcomes are the only important measure for hospitals in a cost-cutting mode and for insurance companies setting reimbursement rates.

TECHNOLOGY: PREVENTION, EVALUATION, AND TREATMENT

Innovative evaluation instruments, high-tech equipment, and advanced safety devices have not only stimulated widespread interest in the field but have enhanced the acceptance of occupational rehabilitation and fostered new avenues of scientific inquiry and research. Recent instruments and tools have been developed that objectively evaluate strength, endurance, work skill, work loads, and power. These tools have enabled evaluators to accurately assess an injured or disabled worker's level of physical effort and intensity and make the appropriate intervention to enable that worker to return to a specific job. The increased capabilities of computers have also positively affected the methodology and outcome of testing and treatment, promoting high standards of norm setting, percentile ranking, validity, and reliability. Computers have also increased the accuracy and availability of data used in psychometric test scoring, job matching, and the identification of employment opportunities.

Health care workers should recognize that no single assessment instrument can have the same use for every client or population and must be used with an understanding of the norms to which the assessment has been standardized. Sometimes the best assessment tools in occupational rehabilitation are those that more closely resemble or simulate the essential demands of an injured or disabled worker's job, so that when possible, it is invaluable to perform testing and treatment at the actual job site.

During treatment, technology may be used effectively to monitor progress and objectively quantify work loads. The exclusive use of high-tech equipment versus actual and simulated work may prove better in certain circumstances in which space is limited or a tight budget prohibits access to actual work tools and materials (e.g., brooms, shovels, garbage cans, hammers). No other treatment modality can match the efficacy of purposeful activity, especially as it relates to an injured or disabled worker's job. The desired motivational benefits are enormous and facilitate recovery by convincing workers who are injured that they can, in fact, return to their jobs.

The use of technology within the field of occupational rehabilitation can be classified under three broad headings: prevention, evaluation, and treatment. Although some technology is exclusive to one area, many times it can be used in two to three areas.

1. *Prevention:* As the shift to managed care continues, prevention will increasingly receive more attention. Software packages, educational aids, computer keyboards, ergonomic chairs, lighting systems, forearm supports, furniture, ergonomic power tools, etc., are currently being used to help prevent injury and illness. There are literally hundreds of products on the market.

2. *Evaluation:* Technology is presently being used for the evaluation of patients and their work areas. It includes such diagnostic equipment as treadmills, stationary bicycle ergometers, heart rate monitors, computerized strength and range of motion testing equipment, software packages, work simulation equipment, nerve conduction monitors, and video cameras. A debate rages over some evaluative technology. With the increasing emphasis on function, there are questions as to whether some of these devices truly measure one's functional capabilities.

3. *Treatment:* Much of the technology used in the evaluative process can also be used for treatment, and vice versa. Additional technology includes exercise equipment, biofeedback devices, vibrating seats, etc.

Occupational rehabilitation programs benefit from advances in assistive technology (AT). The areas of ergonomic prevention and evaluation are being developed rapidly, whereas the growth has slowed in the development and adaptation of AT for treatment programs. Treatment programs are established within a specified framework, using proven equipment and treatment protocols. Greater attention is being paid to research into prevention and evaluation methods, also driven in large part by the shifting type of medical referrals. Treatment is also being moved from the rehabilitation facility to the work site.

Known as transitional work programs, on-site occupational rehabilitation programs are generating more and more interest. These are productive, job-specific programs. In many cases, the therapist has input in establishing job functions. The advantages to this approach are that the employee actually works part of the day, receives therapy at the work site, and communicates with both his or her supervisor and the therapist at the work site. Further, the therapist can help with the biomechanics of the job functions and suggest ergonomic interventions while easing the transition back to work. These types of programs will use technology from all three areas listed previously.

CONCLUSION

The use of AT in the field of occupational rehabilitation can be highly effective. It could continue to stimulate much growth, interest, and expertise in the field and ultimately expand its boundaries to incorporate new trends and avenues of discovery. However, to ensure this progress, rehabilitation professionals must continually advance their technological skills and competency. The inclusion of technological competence in educational programs will better serve rehabilitation professionals and their clients (persons with injuries or disabilities).[6]

Technology in occupational rehabilitation can be used successfully when applied with a holistic approach to any person with an injury, illness, or disability. Occupational rehabilitation needs to balance the use of high-tech equipment with "high-touch" therapies (e.g., human interaction, stress management). A work-related injury is not just a medical diagnosis that can be addressed by clinical solutions alone, but it is a complex psycho-socio-economic problem.[3,4,7] Some of the psychosocial considerations are

- Fear of reinjury when returning to work
- Concerns about the response of the supervisor
- Concerns of coworkers about the competency of the injured or disabled worker to do the same job, to carry an equal work load, and to avoid injuring self or others
- Financial disincentives associated with legal and/or worker's compensation cases
- Concerns about job security and the skill acquisition[8]

Cost will always be an issue, not only to occupational rehabilitation programs but to insurance companies, employers, and injured/ill employees who need to purchase the equipment. This must always be weighed against the benefit. Therapists must not succumb to automatically considering and recommending technologically advanced equipment. Creativity remains extremely important and will be crucial in the cost-conscious system of the future.

The future of occupational rehabilitation will be dependent, in part, on its ability to remain evolutionary by responding to change.[9] State and national health care changes have already influenced occupational rehabilitation. Although the entire health care industry faces an uncertain future, it is important to focus on treatment modalities for the whole person, to design rehabilitation programs that will best achieve the goal of returning the injured or disabled person to productive work.

REFERENCES

1. Commission on Accreditation of Rehabilitation Facilities: 1996 Standards Manual and Interpretive Guidelines for Medical Rehabilitation. CARF, Tucson, AZ, 1996

2. Commission on Accreditation of Rehabilitation Facilities: Standards Manual for Organizations Serving People with Disabilities. CARF, Tucson, AZ, 1991

3. Ellexson MT: Work hardening. In Hertfelder S, Gwin C (eds): Work in Progress. American Occupational Therapy Association, Rockville, MD, 1989

4. Isernhagen S: Work Injury Management and Prevention. Aspen Publishers, Baltimore, MD, 1988

5. O'Shaughnessy E: Trends in Work Hardening and Industrial Rehabilitation. New Jersey Rehab, Fairfield, NJ, 1994

6. Jacobs K: Embracing technology. Rehabil Manage 6:2, 1993

7. Ogden-Niemayer L, Jacobs K: Work Hardening State of the Art. Slack, Thorofare, NJ, 1989

8. Taylor SE: Industrial rehabilitation. pp. 248–257. In Hopkins HL, Smith HD (eds): Willard and Spackman's Occupational Therapy. 8th Ed. Lippincott-Raven, Philadelphia, 1993

9. Burgess C: Rehabilitation in the year 2010. Rehabil Outlook, Summer 1996

Assistive
Technology:
An
Interdisciplinary
Approach

CHAPTER 21

BEVERLY K. BAIN

Service Delivery Systems

One Sunday evening, friends were talking on line via their computers and modem. The topic of future work plans was under discussion. Greg wrote that he wanted to complete high school and get a job. "No more of this school stuff for me! (pause) My counselor said I should look into a 'transition program' that was offered at a local college to prepare me for the 'big move' from school to a career. Have you guys heard or done any of this?"

This reply was logged in: "I have been helping a deaf high school friend with the local college transition program, and it has turned him around from being depressed to looking to a positive future."

At this point, James logged in. "I need a job NOW. My counselor was talking about a supportive employment program where I could get a job before I finish high school. Of course, I would need a 'job coach' to train me. I have another and greater problem. I need my own place or a group home where I can make some decisions. Have any of you used the services of an independent living center? I received a brochure that tells how they can help with home management skills, learning the social services system, public transportation, adaptive equipment, and places to live."

Tom sent the following message, "I want to go to college and then to law school. I want to not only make the big bucks in the legal profession, but I would like to become a legal advocate for persons with disabilities. Maybe my legs and hands don't move as they did before my accident, but my brain works over-time! I know the ADA was passed in 1990, but how much of it is being enforced and what can I do about it? Do any of you know which colleges are accessible for a person in a powered wheelchair, who plans to drive his own van to college, while living at home?"

"Sure!" came a reply. "I am blind and know two sources that were valuable to me when I was in college. They are the resource center known as HEATH and a college-wide organization called AHEAD. Both can help you find the best college for you and tell you about the services that you should expect."

"Just a minute guys, can a woman join this discussion? I graduated from college 3 years ago, with honors in computer science, and I haven't found a job yet. I would like to take a computer training program that would prepare me for a job either working mainly at home or in an office. My vocational rehabilitation counselor mentioned a program called 'Lift.' Have you heard of this program?"

"Yes, you are on the right track with Lift. It is a great program. Not only did they train me in computer programming, but they also helped me find a well-paying job where I can work at home 2 days a week and go to the office 3 days."

"Can I interrupt this group?" a new voice entered the conversation. "I noticed that you all seem very familiar with the 'disability system,' and I need some help with my 5-year-old son. He will be attending a local public grammar school next year. He'll need to travel with his wheelchair on a school bus, and he needs a computer for written work and a special communication device to enable him to talk with his teachers and classmates. What can I do to get this special equipment that he needs? Who do I contact? How should I start moving the system?"

"I can give you some suggestions," one of the group replied. "I have struggled through the system for 18 years. First, your child has the right to a free and appropriate education mandated by the Individuals with Disabilities Education Act. But in order to get any services or equipment, it must be part of your child's individualized educational plan, designed to meet your child's needs by the special education school board with your participation. You can appeal their decision if they decide not to provide any part of the plan, so don't be afraid to speak up. You should contact your state department of special education right away to learn about your child's rights. Also, check with your state's advocacy department and let them know you are a concerned parent. Remember that any device has to be relevant to your son's education—anything you need for medical reasons has to come from other sources. Good luck! You're smart to get started early, and I hope your advocacy will help your child to 'make it' in the system."

Work is an important part of independence for most people. Today, through the use of assistive technology (AT), a greater number of persons with disabilities are enhancing their abilities to compete in the workplace and live productive independent lives. Many of these changes are the result of the advocacy on the part of individuals with disabilities, as well as the electronic and material advances developed by science, helped along by the passage of several pieces of legislation, described in detail in Chapter 1.

In the past 15 years, AT has significantly contributed to the successful employment of many severely disabled persons. The next four chapters present information and cite examples of how technology can enhance the possibilities for employment and accessible living arrangements for persons with disabilities. Chapter 22 discusses transition from school to work and cites a program that uses computer training to encourage high school students with disabilities to learn essential future employment skills. Chapter 23 is an overview of independent living centers and their valuable contribution of providing technology information to persons with disabilities. Chapter 24 has resource material on how AT is applicable in postsecondary education. Chapter 25 explains the Lift computer training program and how it collaborates with businesses to hire and mentor persons with disabilities.

The Technology-Related Assistance Acts of 1988 and 1994 (Tech Acts) address both assistive technology devices (ATDs) and AT service for persons with disabilities.[1,2] Previous chapters presented assessments and the application of various devices. In this chapter, we provide an overview of various AT service delivery models, discuss the roles of AT practitioners, and provide examples of how AT services have been administered to enhance the functional abilities of persons of all ages. According to the Tech Act, AT services include the evaluation of needs, the selection and acquisition of ATDs, coordination with therapies or existing education and rehabilitation programs, training or technical assistance to individuals with disabilities and their families, and training service providers.[1,2]

ROLE OF THE ASSISTIVE TECHNOLOGY PRACTITIONER

Many individuals and professions are involved in evaluating an individual's need for AT and in the selection, procurement, adaptation, training, and service for an AT system. The members of a technology team come from different professions and are also known as AT practitioners. Their roles may include

- Screening individuals who may need AT
- Evaluating the needs, capabilities, and potential benefits of AT
- Selecting appropriate equipment or devices
- Assembling the ATD or AT system when delivered
- Customizing, adjusting, and modifying the ATD or AT system for the consumer
- Training the consumer and caregiver(s) in the use and maintenance of the AT
- Being available to answer questions and providing follow-up about the AT and its use
- Gathering information from consumers and professionals on the improvement of ATD
- Providing assistance in locating funding sources to pay for the ATD or AT system
- Providing training or referrals when repairs and maintenance are needed[3,4]

These services may be provided by multidisciplinary teams in which each member does an evaluation separately, then shares the findings with other team members and provides the specified services that have been identified. Members of an interdisciplinary team will meet and formulate an integrated intervention plan using a team-based solution when problems arise. Another type of team is a transdisciplinary team in which two or more professionals jointly assess a consumer, after which the team meets to develop an intervention plan. During the intervention phase, professional roles may be exchanged. For example, an occupational therapist, a physical therapist, and a vendor will jointly evaluate a consumer for positioning and a wheelchair. However, during the intervention phase, an occupational therapist or teacher may use specific therapeutic techniques usually carried out by a physical therapist. The various types of teams that deliver AT services are complex and require skills, knowledge, the cooperation of both professional and nonprofessional members, and the full participation of the consumer.

SERVICE DELIVERY MODELS

The most frequent service delivery models cited in the literature are the Rehabilitation Engineering and Assistive Technology Society of North America (RESNA) models: (1) the medical model in rehabilitation or university settings, (2) the education models in schools and universities, (3) the community-based developmental disability/independent living model, (4) vocational rehabilitation models in state agencies, (5) employer models influenced by the Americans with Disabilities Act,[5] and (6) the consumer/customer model.[3,6,7] Church and Glennen[8] classified AT models as indirect and direct. Indirect service delivery systems focus on staff training, information dissemination, and public awareness, whereas direct systems provide service delivery such as assessment, selection of AT, and implementation of technology with consumers. They classify models according to centers (e.g., information and demonstration centers, short-term evaluation centers, long-term evaluation and training centers, and long-term centers). Furthermore, they recognize that each model varies in the proportion of services allocated to indirect and direct services. In this chapter, a composite of the RESNA models and the center models is cited and summarized in Table 21-1.

All the models share some common themes. These include the following questions that must be answered: why is the service needed, why is it expected to be successful, what are the expected outcomes, what are the consequences if the service is not provided, what factors interfere with the outcome, and what are the follow-up plans.[7] AT services are needed by persons of all ages with various degrees of function to enhance their capabilities, encourage their independence, increase their participation in school, work, and the community, and live productive lives. AT has been successful as noted throughout this book; however, there is limited outcome research to validate the cost-effectiveness and efficiency of AT service delivery. In a study conducted by the National Council on Disability,[9] it was reported that 75 percent of children who received AT were able to remain in regular classrooms. About 62 percent of working-aged persons were able to reduce their dependency on their families (58 percent were able to reduce their dependence on paid assistance). Eighty percent of older persons were able to reduce their dependency on others, about half were able to avoid entering a nursing home, and 67 percent reported that AT had helped them to obtain employment.

The numerous factors that interfere with outcomes include the lack of consumer involvement in their needs assessment, development of equipment, and ability to acquire ATDs. Another primary factor is the lack of professionally trained personnel in this encompassing and recently developed specialty area. Perhaps the major determining factor is the lack of coordination among service delivery providers.[4,8,10–13] Few centers provide follow-up, as noted in the survey cited in Chapter 3 and in the rehabilitation literature.[15]

Table 21-1 Models of Assistive Technology Service Delivery

Model	Purpose	Population	Funding
Medical			
Rehabilitation setting Multidisciplinary team	Support other rehabilitation services	Spinal cord injuries, cerebrovascular accidents, head injuries, amputees	Third-party Insurance payees
Education			
University and school-based transdisciplinary or multidisciplinary team	Research Direct service to consumer Education and training of school-age children and professionals	Varies School age, college age professionals	Contracts and grants Mandated by law Third-party payees
Community-based			
Local or national nonprofit disability organizations United Cerebral Palsy, American Foundation for the Blind, Easter Seals) Team vary	Serve individual with particular disability Provide and loan equipment	According to disability group	Fund-raising events Grants Contracts Donation
Vocational			
Rehabilitation dept. Interdisciplinary team	Assist individuals who are seeking or maintaining employment	≥ 16 years	Mandated by state and federal laws
Veterans			
Multidisciplinary team	Service to veterans Research	Veterans with service-related disabilities	Federal
Durable medical			
Supplies (durable medical equipment) For-profit agencies	Provide and maintain equipment	Varies	Third-party Medicare
Private practice			
For profit Small business	Consultation to agencies, schools Direct service	Varies depending on professional background	Fees for service

(Data from Galvin[4] and Smith.[3])

Some of the service delivery problems are being addressed by recent legislation (presented in Chapter 1) and by organizations such as RESNA, the American Occupational Therapy Association, and the International Society for Augmentative and Alternative Communication. Various educational groups (e.g., the Council for Exceptional Children) are involved in upgrading AT service delivery. In addition, consumers are becoming more knowledgeable and are advocating for ATDs and effective AT service delivery.

SERVICE DELIVERY IN EUROPE

In 1993 to 1994, the Horizontal European Activities in Rehabilitation Technology (HEART) carried out an AT study by a consortium of 21 institutions, organizations, and companies of the European Union under the leadership of the Swedish Handicap Institute.[15] The purpose of the study was to improve the quality of life for persons with disabilities and elderly persons by creating a single European market in AT.

The study indicated that service delivery in Europe varies in basic principles, procedures, and coverage because of the geographic, cultural, and political differences. Some countries have a medically based system, whereas others have a socially based system that affects how persons obtain AT and the extent to which ATDs are considered an essential part of rehabilitation. Referrals are made by medical specialists, and authorization is mainly done by persons working for the health, social services, employment, education, and/or public/private insurance systems. Some common trends they noted were the lack of international cooperation, limited professional and financial resources, and poor user information and networking systems. They identified that a good service delivery system should be accessible, flexible, coordinated, and efficient, with adequate competence and user influence.

The major conclusions of the study are that there is a need for national policy and legislation to ensure the rights of persons with disabilities who need AT and to ensure coordination within the delivery system. The United Nations Standard Rules on the Equalization of Opportunities for Persons with Disabilities and the European Commission White Paper, known as "European Social Policy: A Way Forward for the Union," were recently adopted and are similar to the results and recommendations of the HEART study. Furthermore, persons with disabilities and the elderly should have the right to appeal. Another conclusion was the need for continuing education for professionals and for user involvement. The need for a coherent taxonomy regarding AT and service delivery with common terminology and definitions was another study conclusion.

The three main service delivery recommendations of the HEART study were

1. To stimulate networking and information exchange by establishing a European network for coordination, dissemination of information, and exchange of AT research and service delivery

2. To develop procedures in service delivery systems for systematic collection and processing of user feedback

3. To continue the work started by this study in updating the description of service delivery, developing quality criteria, and furthering the international discussion

For further information on European AT service delivery and a list of 16 national contacts, see the HEART report.[16]

SUMMARY

If AT service delivery is to be efficient and effective, the following should take place:

1. Consumers will need to become active participants in the assessment, selection, development, and procurement of appropriate ATDs and AT services. They must become advocates and appeal when the system is not effective. Rather than abandoning costly equipment, they should work to improve it.

2. Professionals will need to become knowledgeable about holistic assessment, selection of low- and high-technology devices, and laws and public policies governing AT services. They should conduct outcome studies and research, develop quality assurance methods, and work with consumers to promote device development and effective service delivery systems including funding.

3. Society will need to become aware of the improved quality of life for both persons with disabilities and their families when AT services are delivered. In addition, ATDs and AT services can be cost-effective when persons with disabilities are educated, employed, and able to live independently in their own homes as part of the community.

REFERENCES

1. Technology-Related Assistance for Individuals with Disabilities Act of 1988. PL 100-407, Title 29, U.S.C. 2201 et seq: U.S. Statutes at Large, 102, 1044–1065, August 19, 1988

2. Technology-Related Assistance for Individuals with Disabilities Act of 1994. PL 103-218, Title 29, U.S.C. 2201 et seq: U.S. Statutes at Large, 108, 50–97, March 9, 1994

3. Smith R: Models of service delivery in rehabilitation technology. pp. 7–25. In Perlman L, Enders A (eds): Rehabilitation Technology Service Delivery: A Practical Guide. RESNA, Washington, DC, 1987

4. Galvin J: Professional Conduct. Module 9. Assistive Technology Credentialing Review Course. RESNA, Arlington, VA, 1996

5. Americans with Disabilities Act (ADA) of 1990. PL 101-336, Title 42 U.S.C. 12101 et seq: U.S. Statutes at Large, 104, 327–378, July 26, 1990

6. Cook A, Hussey S: Assistive Technologies: Principles and Practice. Mosby, New York, 1995

7. Warren CG: Cost effectiveness and efficiency in assistive technology service delivery. Assist Technol 5:61–65, 1993

8. Church G, Glennen S: Assistive technology program development. pp. 1–26. In: The Handbook of Assistive Technology. Singular Publishing Group Inc., San Diego, CA, 1992

9. National Council on Disabilities: Study on the Financing of Assistive Technology Devices and Services for Individuals with Disabilities. NCD, Washington, DC, 1993

10. Nochajski: S, Oddo C: Technology in the Workplace. pp. 197–261. In: Mann W, Lane J (eds): Assistive Technology for Person with Disabilities. 2nd Ed. American Occupational Therapy Association, Rockville, MD, 1995

11. Flippo K, Inge K, Barcus JM: Assistive Technology: A Resource for School, Work, and Community. Paul HJ Brookes Publishing Co., Baltimore, MD, 1995

12. O'Day B, Corcoran P: Assistive technology: problems and policy alternatives. Arch Phys Med Rehabil 75:1165–1169, 1994

13. Phillips B: Technology abandonment from the consumer point of view. NARIC Q 3:3–11, 1992

14. Bain BK, Block L, Strehlow A: Survey report on the assessment of individuals with spinal cord injuries for assistive technology. Technol Disability 5 (3/4): 289–294, 1996

15. Lane P, Usiak D, Moffatt M: Consumer criteria for assistive devices: operationalizing generic criteria for specific AbleData categories, pp. 146–148. In: Proceedings of RESNA 1996. RESNA Press, Arlington, VA, 1996

16. Fagerberg G, Lagerwall T: Horizontal European Activities in Rehabilitation Technology, Tide Study 309. Annex 22–26. Swedish Handicap Institute, Wallingby, Sweden, 1995

Assistive
Technology:
An
Interdisciplinary
Approach

Transition

Transition has been characterized as the bridge between the security and structure offered by the school and the opportunities and risks of adult life.[1] The U.S. Department of Education, Office of Special Education and Rehabilitative Services, in 1983 introduced transition as a priority for students with disabilities. This national effort was directed at providing transition planning and services that would enable youth with disabilities to successfully live, learn, and work in the community. The intent of the legislation in this past decade, particularly the Americans with Disabilities Act, the Individuals with Disabilities Education Act, the administration's Goals 2000: Educate America Act, and the recent School to Work Initiative have broadened and synchronized public policy and national efforts that focus on a collaborative service delivery system. As a result, transition planning and services for young people with disabilities have received greater emphasis. The challenge of collaboration in this effort impacts all segments of the community: parents, consumers, educators, employees, health professionals, and rehabilitation service providers.

The unemployment rate in 1993 for persons with disabilities was 70 percent, according to the President's Committee on Employment of People with Disabilities. One reason frequently cited is that people with disabilities may have a low level of education and training. Another equally important concern may result from inadequate work behaviors including a sense of time and responsibility, personal hygiene, the ability to accept and use supervision, and the ability to make friends and cooperate with coworkers.

Despite the fact that in the past decades there have been numerous programs developed that emphasize a business-education-rehabilitation partnership to provide transition services, there is much more to be done to improve the postschool success of youth with disabilities. The application of assistive technology (AT) is expected to be an integral factor in the future success of transition planning service delivery for young people with disabilities.

One such program is the Upward Bound Program, in the Metro Center of New York University. This program uses a postsecondary preparation model already in existence for minority, disadvantaged, and first-generation youth and incorporates key transition components and AT to better serve young people with disabilities. This year-round program, funded by the U.S. Department of Education, serves 50 high school students with disabilities enrolled in New York City public schools. Students are recruited as early as ninth grade, although most enter in the tenth grade. The program is conducted on campus at New York University. Students attend activities on Saturdays during the school term and a full-time, 6-week component during the summer. On an average, students participate for 3 years until they complete high school and transfer into their selected postsecondary environments. The program provides ongoing follow-up services for its graduates.

263

Transition

The primary focus of the program is to provide individualized assessment and planning needed to facilitate each student's successful post-school transition. The model focuses on a collaborative effort involving all aspects of the community.

Upward Bound provides a variety of academic services including tutoring, basic skills remediation, precollege courses, computer studies (word processing, graphics), study skills, and high school and college courses for credit. Career and college planning services emphasize a life-long access to opportunities. Students participate in career exploration activities including job preparation, job shadowing, job seeking skills, workshops, volunteer internships, and paid employment experiences. These opportunities are available through a comprehensive collaboration with local agencies, employers, schools, and community service centers. Decision-making skills, social skill development, and self-advocacy are incorporated in group counseling activities and independent living skills workshops that are provided by various community agencies and local independent living centers. College planning services include structured workshops, visits to colleges, financial aid workshops, and individualized college counseling that addresses needs related to choosing, applying to, and getting accepted to a college. College survival courses focus on the skills needed to enter and succeed in postsecondary education and include activities from living independently, managing time, test taking, writing a term paper, negotiating services, and resource development for job and career preparation.

Upward Bound services are provided not only to students but also to their families. The involvement of the student, the family, the school staff, agency staff, employer, educators, and rehabilitation providers together in a cooperative effort is essential in helping the student with the exposure to and experiences in dealing with the demands and expectations of ordinary environments.

ASSISTIVE TECHNOLOGY

Transition to employment is a process through formal and informal education and using many forms of AT that begins at birth and extends over a person's entire life. With AT, many children with physical and mental disabilities can learn to use augmentative and alternative communication devices to make their needs known and increase their social interaction skills. Some adolescents with disabilities use powered wheelchairs to increase their ability to move about in the community and outside their homes in residential custodial environments; others are learning to use computers in the first grade, which gives them a sense of accomplishment and can lead to a variety of future job possibilities. To become a productive worker, the child or adolescent with a disability may need to improve physical coordination, strength, and endurance. They also need to learn cooperative behavior and time management, which should be fostered in the home and encouraged in school environments.

A transition program at New York University uses AT for students in a variety of ways. It can be as simple as providing a piece of adaptive equipment that enables a student to be mainstreamed into a vocational education course at the high school or providing special touch-sensitive keyboards for the microcomputer that help students to participate fully in a computer applications class. It can be as complex as providing an on-loan microcomputer system to a student with a learning disability to help the student improve academic skills and complete homework assignments more successfully or introducing power mobility to a student to provide access to a work experience or the ability to travel independently to and from school. The program emphasizes the use of the microcomputer as a cognitive and effective tool to facilitate learning in all areas. The potential to motivate and to improve self-confidence may be the microcomputer's greatest contribution to education and career exploration. The integration of the computer in all aspects of Upward Bound (career exploration, academic skills, college information searches, and employment participation) serves as a vehicle to provide knowledge and skills within an environment that is controlled by the student. The introduction of AT early in the transition planning process is becoming more viable. AT can expand the options available to young people during their early school years and initial career exploration endeavors, thereby increasing the likelihood of success in postsecondary outcomes such as college, vocational training, or employment.

REFERENCES

1. Wills M: Programming for the Transition of Youth with Disabilities: Bridges from School to Working Life. U.S. Department of Education (OSERS), Washington, DC, 1983

SUGGESTED READINGS

Bailey T, Merrit D: The School-to-Work Transition and Youth Apprenticeship: Lessons from the U.S. Experience. Manpower Demonstration Research Corporation, New York, 1993

D'Amico R, Morder C: The Early Work Experiences of Youth with Disabilities: Trends in Employment Rates and Job Characteristics. SRI Executive Summary, Menlo Park, CA, 1990

Hasazi S, Gordon L, Roe C: Factors associated with the employment status of handicapped youth existing high schools from 1979 to 1983. Exceptional Children 51:6, 1985

The University of the State of New York and the State Education Department: Opportunity and Independence Meeting the Needs of New Yorkers with Disabilities. The Final Report of the Regents Select Commission on Disability. State Education Department, New York, 1993

U.S. Department of Education, National Center for Educational Statistics, Office of Educational Research and Improvement: Profile of Handicapped Students in Postsecondary Education, 1987. U.S. Department of Education (OSERS), Washington, DC, 1989

U.S. Department of Education, Office of Special Education and Rehabilitation Services: News in Print. U.S. Department of Education (OSERS), Washington, DC, 1993

Wagner M: The Transition Experiences of Youth from the National Longitudinal Transition Study. SRI International, Menlo Park, CA, 1990

CHAPTER 23

GAIL TISHCOFF
BEVERLY K. BAIN

Independent Living Centers

Independence is a concept, a state of mind, and an attitude. In this country, independence is a driving force—a theme since our national inception. For persons with disabilities, independence means achieving and controlling decisions regarding everyday activities. It is this attitude and driving force that forms the basis for the independent living movement; a philosophic stance articulated by advocates for the disabled that has had tremendous political impact.

Independent living as defined by this movement involves the fullest state of self-determination possible. It involves options to use the least degree of reliance on others while maintaining the highest degree of control over decisions regarding everyday activities. It adheres to a commitment to fulfilling social roles within the family and in the community.[1] According to the Texas Institute for Rehabilitation Research Independent Living Research Utilization Project,[2] *independence* is defined as

Control over one's life based on the choice of acceptable options that minimize reliance on others in making decisions and in performing everyday activities. This includes managing one's own affairs; participating in day-to-day life in the community; fulfilling a range of social roles; and making decisions that lead to self-determination and the minimization of psychological or physical dependence upon others. Independence is a relative concept, which may be defined personally by each individual.

Independent living centers (ILCs) are community-based programs with consumer involvement that provide advocacy information and independent living rehabilitation services for persons with disabilities. ILCs also provide information and referral services on housing, benefits, transportation, personal care services, independent living skills training, peer counseling, and a variety of additional services specific to that center. According to the Rehabilitation Act of 1973 as amended in 1978, 1986, and 1992, there are four core services that each center should provide: individual and systems advocacy, peer counseling, information and referral, and independent living skills in the community.

The concept of ILCs grew out of the independent living movement in the late 1960s and early 1970s because persons with disabilities wanted to take active roles in shaping the decisions that affected their lives. They wanted self-determination. The earliest ILC was formed in 1972 in Berkeley, California. To date, there are 421 nonresidential, nonmedical service centers throughout North America. See the resource list at the end of this section for information on the location of centers.

Funding for the centers includes grants from the Department of Education, Rehabilitation Services Administration, National Institute on Disability and Rehabilitation Research, and foundations such as the Robert J. Johnson Foundation, the Dole Foundation, and the Milbank Foundation (personal communication with ILRU, November 1994). Some centers receive funding from special fund-raising events and private membership; however, services are generally offered free of charge to all persons with disabilities.

HISTORY OF THE INDEPENDENT LIVING MOVEMENT

The concept of ILCs has evolved from the civil rights movement of the 1960s, which inspired the independent living movement to search for sources of the attitudes and behaviors of the public toward persons with disabilities. In 1972, a bill was passed by Congress (HR 8395) that included comprehensive rehabilitation services and independent living provisions. It was vetoed by the President who felt that independent living would dilute the funding resources and impair the potential achievement of the vocational program. In 1978, an amendment to the Rehabilitation Act, Title VII, Comprehensive Services for Independent Living, authorized states to "establish programs, similar to state vocational rehabilitation programs, to provide comprehensive independent-living programs" that "must have substantial involvement of disabled individuals in policy direction, management, and employment within the programs."[3] The 1992 amendments to the Rehabilitation Act address both independent living and assistive technology (AT).

The basic principles of most ILCs today are that people with disabilities can live independent lives with the proper resources, that the best judge of the person's needs is that individual, and that outdated social attitudes toward the disabled are the greatest handicap for citizens who happen to have a disability.

ILCs, RESIDENTIAL PROGRAMS, AND TRANSITIONAL PROGRAMS

An ILC is defined as being based in the community, not-for-profit, and nonresidential. A majority of disabled consumers must be in positions of control with the mission "to increase personal self-determination and to minimize unnecessary dependence upon others."[4]

Distinct from ILCs are those programs that offer long-term or transitional residential services. These are called independent living residential programs and independent living transitional programs. Transitional programs are typically goal based and time limited, with a primary focus on skills training, with professionals teaching individuals with disabilities how to cope with various social, vocational, and medical issues.[5] Residential programs typically pool attendant and transportation services, providing an accessible living environment for small groups of disabled individuals but not necessarily managed by them.

The 1978 and 1986 amendments to the Rehabilitation Act specifies ILC operational criteria as including the following: 51 percent of the governing board members are to be disabled individuals, at least one disabled person should be employed in a managerial position and at least one disabled person should be employed in a nonmanagerial position. It is argued that many residential independent living programs do not meet these criteria, and even though they facilitate independent living styles for those they serve, they are by nature segregational and contrary to the movement's goal to integrate disabled individuals into the community. Others within the movement's leadership, however, argue that independent living programs are "separate yet parallel" manifestations of the independent living movement's philosophies.[5]

EXAMPLE OF AN ILC

This center was established in 1970 and provides services and support to individuals with all types of disabilities, assisting them in independence within their communities. The services offered include information and referral on housing, home care, benefit advisement and advocacy, counseling services (peer and professional), independent living skills training, and transportation. The ILC also works cooperatively with the Client Assistance Program (CAP), which provides information and advocacy relating to vocational rehabilitation.

The director described the center's role as the advocacy and information center for persons with disabilities and the focus on educating consumers about independent living options. Funded by state and private sources, it serves more than 1,200 consumers annually. When fully staffed, the office of 13 employees includes a benefits/independent living skills counselor, a deafness counselor, and a housing counselor. They have two adapted vans to service transportation needs for consumers who require it (private communication with Director, July 1989).

TECHNOLOGY AND ILCs

As centers for education and advocacy, ILCs fulfill an important role for consumers regarding information about the availability of and funding sources for technological devices.

A good example of this was provided by the coordinator of a CAP working with an ILC. She described her role in the case of a consumer with cerebral palsy who required an updated augmentative and alternative communication (AAC) device to function vocationally. This individual had been using an old manual board that he felt had severe limitations. His request for funding from his vocational counselor had been rejected, based in part on letters in his file from previous professionals stating that his manual board was serving his needs sufficiently. The coordinator explained that every consumer has the right to an appeal and a fair hearing on rejection from the State Vocational Agency (OVR). CAP looked into the consumer's file, gathered the necessary data, and even represented the consumer at the fair hearing. In this case, the coordinator followed up by contacting the professionals involved to determine how they had decided the person's needs were being served by an outdated device, when other professionals had recommended that he was a fine candidate for an AAC device. She was very optimistic about the chances of a reversal in OVR's decision and the possibility of obtaining the assistive technology device (ATD) for this consumer.

On request, ILCs will provide information on conferences regarding technology and the workplace, para-transit services, updates on ATD, and the government grants available for those interested in AT and the needs of the disabled. Some centers have adaptive equipment banks including ATDs for loan to consumers on a trial or permanent basis.

We have found the ILCs to be of value in the three major areas: as an information resource center in AT and service; as assistants in housing; and as peer counselors. Frequently, when there is question on the best selection of one ATD over another, the authors will discuss it with an ILC-referred user. For example, the best judge of a powered wheelchair is a long-term user, and ILCs usually can refer questions to a long-time user. Furthermore, some centers have lists of places where wheelchairs can best be serviced in their geographic area.

Another example of the valuable ILC referral services is in the case of a wheelchair user who was offered a job and needed information on the most efficient public transportation. He called the ILC nearest him and was given several possibilities and local transit telephone numbers.

Housing for persons with disabilities can include public or private residential facilities, group homes owned cooperatively by residents, or privately managed supervised apartments. The most effective residential options to foster independent living may include renting and purchasing a residence of choice with unrestricted access to community activities. ILCs are most helpful in assisting persons with disabilities to make decisions on where they want to live, to help with financial planning, to identify support agencies or groups within communities, and to assist in finding accessible housing. Many centers have referrals of places that they have personally surveyed where other consumers have found accessible housing with conveniently located public transportation and shopping.

In another case, an ILC was asked to recommend a contractor to make necessary home modifications. The center suggested two local contractors that had successfully modified three apartments and a home for a reasonable charge.

We have found ILCs to be most beneficial in the area of peer counseling, for a person who has experience with the numerous government agencies can best assist another person to find their way through the maze. In addition, peer counseling can provide a support group, a mentor, and friends for a person who may accomplish goals in a different manner.

In the future, consumers and professionals must be advocates in any health care reform legislation to ensure that the independent living movement focuses on abilities, independence, inclusion, and empowerment to improve the quality of life for all persons with disabilities.

As one director said, "You can have all the equipment in the world, but if you lack the knowledge to use the equipment, or the money to fund the equipment, it's no good. And many people don't know they can get funding for some assistive technology. The center is here to make sure that people know what they need and how to go about getting it" (private communication with Director, July 1989).

ACKNOWLEDGMENT

The authors acknowledge Lynne Luxton, Ed.D., CRC, Deputy Director, Center for Independence of Disabled in New York, for her comments and review of this section.

REFERENCES

1. Frieden L, Cole JA: Independence: the ultimate goal of rehabilitation for spinal cord-injured persons. Am J Occup Ther 39:734–739, 1985

2. Texas Institute for Rehabilitation Research Independent Living Research Utilization Project, 1978

3. Dalrymple L, Richards L, Freiden L: Independent living: an update for the mid-eighties. Annu Rev Rehabil 4:241–264, 1985

4. Nosek MA, Jones SD, Znu Y: Levels of compliance with federal requirements in independent living centers. J Rehabil 2:31–37, 1989

5. Frieden L: Independent living models. Rehabil Literature 41:169–173, 1980

RITA MARIE LEVEY
BEVERLY K. BAIN

CHAPTER 24

Assistive Technology in Postsecondary Education

The Rehabilitation Act of 1992 has a great impact on the growing use of assistive technology (AT) in the postsecondary educational setting. It allows students with documented disabilities to request auxiliary aids that will enable them to benefit from all programs and activities. Postsecondary educational institutions that receive federal financial assistance must make accommodations to ensure that academic programs are accessible to the greatest extent possible. Some colleges and universities have established wheelchair-accessible computer stations, adapted computers for the visually impaired, telecommunication systems for the deaf, and other accommodations to provide technological assistive devices and services. As amended, this act mandates that each state's division of vocational rehabilitation financially assist individuals with disabilities as they pursue postsecondary education. This assistance has enabled students to purchase adaptations for computers provided that the rehabilitation professional recommending this equipment for postsecondary education can document its impact on the individual's future vocational potential. In addition, the division of vocational rehabilitation may also be responsible for the evaluation of a person for specific technological devices or educational programs.

The following is a list of organizations that have been found by rehabilitation professionals and consumers to be excellent resources regarding the application of AT in postsecondary educational institutions.

ASSOCIATION ON HIGHER EDUCATION AND DISABILITY

The Association on Higher Education and Disability (AHEAD) is an international organization, founded in 1978, that addresses the need and concern for improving the quality of services available to persons with disabilities in postsecondary education. The Association promotes excellence through education, communication, and training. AHEAD sponsors training programs, workshops, publications, and conferences. Members of AHEAD have access to the latest developments in the field of disability support services. The association has established many special interest groups. The most relevant to this book are in the areas of community college, independent colleges and universities, blindness/visual impairments, deafness/hard of hearing, and disabilities studies. Conferences provide an atmosphere for networking and professional interaction and collaboration. AHEAD is also responsible for the publication of the *Journal of Postsecondary Education and Disability*. Other relevant publications available through AHEAD include *Testing Accommodations for Students with Disabilities, Faculty In-service Education Kit,* and *How to Choose a College: A Guide for the Student with a Disability*. Also available are two video tapes: "College: A Viable Option" and "In Their Own Words," which includes a study guide.

HIGHER EDUCATION AND ADULT TRAINING FOR PEOPLE WITH HANDICAPS

The Higher Education and Adult Training for People with Handicaps (HEATH) Resource Center is a national clearinghouse that provides information about disability issues and postsecondary education. HEATH is funded by the American Council on Education of the United States Department of Education. The purpose of the HEATH Resource Center is to identify educational and training opportunities and to promote accommodations, thereby enabling individuals with disabilities to fully participate in postsecondary programs. The use and application of AT is a topic that is frequently addressed by the clearinghouse. A newsletter is published three times a year and is distributed nationally, free-of-charge to subscribers. HEATH provides resource papers, guides, fact sheets, and directories focusing on disability-related issues as they arise on college campuses or in vocational-technical training schools. HEATH also publishes a 40-page resource directory each year. All materials disseminated by HEATH may be reproduced.

REHABILITATION ENGINEERING AND ASSISTIVE TECHNOLOGY SOCIETY OF NORTH AMERICA

The Rehabilitation Engineering and Assistive Technology Society of North America (RESNA) is an interdisciplinary association for the advancement of rehabilitation and AT. RESNA provides a forum in which rehabilitation professionals, providers, and consumers can interact to better serve the needs of individuals who may benefit from AT. Members of RESNA receive the semiannual journal *Assistive Technology,* a special interest group newsletter, and numerous other publications available from RESNA, including the annual conference proceedings and the *Assistive Technology Source Book (1990),* a valuable book with a section on postsecondary education with resources, edited by Ender and Hall. Recently, RESNA has produced a series of AT videos. RESNA has established many special interest groups that are relevant to the use of AT in the postsecondary educational environment, including groups on service delivery and public policy issues, personal transportation, computer applications, job accommodation, and employment.

TRACE RESEARCH AND DEVELOPMENT CENTER FOR COMMUNICATION, CONTROL, AND COMPUTER ACCESS FOR HANDICAPPED INDIVIDUALS

The Trace Research and Development Center for Communication, Control, and Computer Access for Handicapped Individuals is an excellent resource for information on augmentative and alternative communication aids and other AT devices that can enhance the abilities of students with disabilities. The Trace resource books are a cross-referenced registry of communication aids, switches, environmental control systems, and modified computer software and hardware. These books may be exceptionally useful to universities and colleges that are interested in improving and/or providing equal access to postsecondary programs using the most appropriate AT available. These books contain photographs as well as descriptions of products, names and addresses of vendors, and cost.

CLOSING THE GAP

Closing the Gap (CTG) hosts an annual national conference on computer technology for the handicapped. CTG publishes a bimonthly newsletter focusing on computer applications for individuals with disabilities in special education and rehabilitation professionals. It also has a database.

Resources

ORGANIZATIONS

AHEAD (Association on Higher Education
  and Disability)
P.O. Box 21192
Columbus, OH 43221–0192
(614) 488-4972 TDD/Voice

Higher Education and Adult Training for
  People with Handicaps (HEATH)
American Council on Education
One Dupont Circle, Suite 800
Washington, DC 20036-1193
(202) 939-9320/ (800) 544-3284
  (Voice and Typed Text, TDD)
(202) 833-4760 Fax

Rehabilitation Engineering and Assistive Technology
  Society of North America (RESNA)
Suite 1540
1700 North Moore Street
Arlington, VA 22209-1903
(703) 524-6686
(703) 524-6630 Fax

Trace Research & Development Center
  for Communication, Control, and Computer
  Access for Handicapped Individuals
Waisman Center
1500 Highland Avenue
Madison, WI 53705
(608) 262-6966 (voice)
(608) 263-5408 (TDD)

Closing the Gap (CTG)
P.O. Box 68
Henderson, MN 56044
(612) 248-3294

Lift, Inc.

Lift, Inc. is a nonprofit corporation that recruits, trains, hires, and places computer programmer analysts who have substantial physical disabilities. Since its incorporation in 1975, the firm has worked with more than 70 of the country's largest corporations. Its corporate clients have come from major industry sectors, including insurance, finance, manufacturing, and consumer goods, and include such companies as New York Life Insurance, Marine Midland Bank, AT&T, Kraft General Foods, TRW, Baker & Taylor Books, and Pepsico.

In recent years, some college guidance counselors have begun to refer to Lift as "the Harvard of Rehab," not only because Lift has a rigorous screening process but also because Lift trainees have excellent head starts in their careers. Many graduates move quickly into management or onto highly technical career paths.

Successful applicants have a high degree of analytical ability and ambition, enjoy intellectual challenges, and enjoy working in teams. Graduates have had disabilities such as spinal cord injuries, muscular dystrophy, neurologic impairments, and blindness and typically use some form of assistive technology (AT) to access computers, to communicate with users, or to participate in staff meetings. Often, the technology needed is as simple as a speakerphone, although the requirements can be much more complex.

The "Lift process" is a five-stage comprehensive approach:

1. Corporate planning
2. Recruitment
3. Training
4. Contract employment
5. Direct placement

During the corporate planning stage, Lift works with prospective client corporations to determine where they are most likely to have a need for systems professionals and what precise skills will be needed for immediate and future placements. This can be critical because many of today's data processing environments are in transition.

During the recruitment stage, Lift screens candidates who are referred by a very broad network of individuals and organizations, including vocational rehabilitation agencies, universities, independent living centers, rehabilitation hospitals, and insurance companies. Many successful applicants are self-referred. Candidates participate in sophisticated aptitude testing and in-depth interviewing. A prior background in computer programming is not a requirement, although special placements are often available for experienced programmers.

The training phase usually takes 6 months. Each trainee follows an intensive, individually tailored curriculum in a study environment that emulates the actual intended working environment; that is, the trainee uses the same hardware, software, and AT that he or she is expected to use on the job. In this way, any problems in the environment (e.g., a computer system that does not respond, or a delay in receiving custom-ordered devices, or an inaccessible door) will be smoothed out long before they have a chance to slow or hinder a programmer who is trying to get a job done.

Many Lift programmers do some if not most of their work from home. Lift was a pioneer in the field of telecommuting, applying advanced technology and business practices to encourage programming work from home at a time, in the mid-1970s, when few others were even dreaming of home offices. Telecommuting can be a practical, even sometimes a necessary, accommodation, and it typically results in higher productivity (whether the employee has a disability or not). I (the president of Lift) believe that part of the reason for the frequently superior performance of computer professionals who graduate from the program is that they work where, when, and how they will be most productive.

Telecommuting trainees study at home but have weekly mentoring sessions on-site so that they can establish rapport with the informal organization of associates and managers with whom they will be interacting on a regular basis. Trainees who intend to work on-site will often complete all their training on-site.

The fourth stage of the Lift process is contract employment. Graduates of the training program are hired by Lift and begin working full-time for their corporate sponsors. Starting salaries are excellent. Lift management carefully monitors the performance of the programmer/analysts as well as the flow of work and communication from the corporate site to the professional. Lift staff provide corporate clients with awareness training for their employees as well as with individualized consultation concerning management and appraisal of telecommuting employees, management and appraisal of employees with disabilities, and integration of AT into a changing workplace.

At the end of a year of contract employment, Lift invites the corporate clients to hire the Lift-trained computer professionals as their own employees, which is the fifth, and final, stage of the process, direct placement. Although no longer the employer, Lift remains available for as-needed consultations with both corporate clients and former employees. An annual survey of former employees helps Lift track the success of its graduates.

And a very successful group they are! Their job titles, salaries, and employer evaluations testify to the value of the unique Lift process. And the richness of their lives testifies daily to the importance of work, career, and financial independence in contemporary society.

Resources

ORGANIZATIONS

Lift
P.O. Box 1072
Mountainside, NS 07092
(908) 789-2443

Independent Living Research
    Utilization (ILRU)
2323 South Shepard, Suite 1000
Houston, Texas 77019
(713) 520-0232
(713) 520-5136 (TDD)

Provision of Assistive Technology

A MODEL FOR SERVICE DELIVERY

281

Provision of
Assistive
Technology:
A Model for
Service Delivery

A successful integration/reintegration of persons with severe physical disabilities into productive and independent living situations, specifically educationally and vocationally related, is frequently overwhelmingly difficult. Although assistive technology (AT) is being developed at a rapid rate and in an increasingly wide variety, there continues to be great difficulty in the delivery of sophisticated technology to the consumer in a comprehensive manner.

The volume and range of assistive technology devices (ATDs) developed after World War II have been extensive. There are currently some 25 clearly identified areas of technology categories in which there is research and service delivery (e.g., biofeedback, computer applications, accessibility, transportation, mobility, augmentative and alternative communication [AAC], environmental control units [ECU], robotics, job accommodation, and virtual reality, to name just a few). During that period of time, the consumer-device interface and integration have become more of an organized process in some selective centers. However, some of those approaches to service delivery have often been unable to address the need to integrate electronic solutions used to manipulate information and communications, with mechanical solutions required to manipulate the physical components of the work site.

Three primary problems are frequently identified with respect to current technology service delivery approaches:

- Fragmentation between the provider of the sophisticated AT and the classic vocational rehabilitation professional
- Fragmentation between the providers of electronic technology and the providers of mechanical technology
- The consumer is not included in the process, either from an educational point of view or by the attitudes of the service providers

The goals of this chapter will be threefold:

1. To present a current model of comprehensive step-by-step service delivery
2. To provide a framework for the process of assessment of the consumer and evaluation of the equipment
3. To provide resources available to both consumers and technology service providers

Before outlining the service delivery process, it would be helpful to provide some descriptive information about the Technology and Education at Mount Sinai (TEAMS) Laboratory.

ASSISTIVE TECHNOLOGY SERVICES— TEAMS LABORATORY

The TEAMS Laboratory at Mount Sinai Medical Center in New York City provides a multidisciplinary functional approach to the application of AT to consumers with physical, sensory, cognitive, and/or perceptual disabilities.

The program is tailored to individual needs, with the goal of increasing independence at home, in school, and/or on the job. The laboratory is equipped with state-of-the-art technology. Solutions can range from simple modifications, such as adjusting work surfaces or providing single-function devices, to the sophisticated use of technology that may require alternate access to computer systems or the integration of several systems such as AAC, computer access, and/or powered mobility. The technology may be used in a variety of ways, for

- Prevention
- Remediation
- Energy conservation and work simplification
- Substitution for loss or limitation of function
- Hands-on evaluation and equipment selection
- User training
- Finding solutions for multiple needs requiring the integration of systems and ATDs

SCOPE OF TECHNOLOGY OFFERED

The laboratory is equipped with state-of-the-art devices and equipment in the areas discussed below. Although this service is delivered primarily on an outpatient basis, inpatient services are provided as needed. For example, environmental controls are provided at the bedside for functions such as nurse call, telephone, television, lights, and bed controls. Education about current technology is provided in group sessions for persons with disabilities to begin the process of becoming well-informed consumers. Other technology interventions may be appropriate during the treatment program or for functional independence and planning to return to work and/or school.

DEVICE CATEGORIES FOR SERVICE DELIVERY

SEATING AND POSITIONING

Most of the consumers referred for equipment access have inadequate seating and positioning for the proposed intervention (e.g., access to a work station, computer access, and access to and mounting for an augmentative communication system). These usually require evaluation for and provision of seating, positioning, and mobility needs using both commercially available and customized options.

POWERED MOBILITY

Specialized powered mobility systems and alternate access controls and switches are provided, as well as integration of the mobility systems with other electronic devices.

COMPUTER ACCESS

Consumers are provided with alternative means of computer access other than standard keyboard input. Solutions include hardware and software alternatives along with work station design and modification.

ENVIRONMENTAL CONTROL

Environmental control is provided via single function devices, multi-function units, or systems and services that allow the user to control electrical appliances, emergency and alarm systems, and telecommunications devices. Both commercially available off-the-shelf devices as well as units that have been designed to meet the needs of special populations of consumers with disabilities can be provided.

AUGMENTATIVE AND ALTERNATIVE COMMUNICATION

Services and devices are provided for individuals who are unable to meet all their communication needs through speech and/or writing. Specialized services use both low- and high-technology solutions. Those solutions include special techniques, strategies, skills, and devices or combinations of those options.

WORK STATION MODIFICATION

Interventions cover a variety of solutions from simple single-function devices (e.g., keyboard or telephone access/selection) to detailed task and system analysis that would require new work stations and work area modifications including strategies for the integration and installation of high-technology solutions.

OFF-SITE EVALUATION OF WORK SITE/HOME/SCHOOL

Services are available when necessary and are provided more often around work site needs.

REHABILITATION ENGINEERING SOLUTIONS

Technology services involving integration of devices and systems are included. For example, solutions could mean the use of a powered wheelchair controller to operate a computer or environmental control unit or modifying and mounting an electronic system in a work station. The solu-

283

Provision of
Assistive
Technology:
A Model for
Service Delivery

tions usually require understanding the electronics of several systems and finding if and how they can be operated for a particular consumer and/or solution. The availability of our integration of ATDs and systems is a major advantage for persons with very severe physical disabilities who need more than one category of equipment but have very little physical control for access to those ATDs and systems.

TEAM BASED SERVICES

Because of the comprehensive nature of the scope of services and available categories of equipment/devices available, an overwhelming majority of the consumers are provided services by a team of people, both professional and nonprofessional, who are involved with the consumer and may include any of the following during all or portions of the process:

- Consumer, caregiver, and significant others
- Referral source representative: typically a vocational rehabilitation counselor or insurance company case manager
- Physician
- Occupational therapist
- Speech-language pathologist
- Rehabilitation technologist/rehabilitation engineer
- Vocational counselor
- Educator
- Employer
- Psychologist
- Physical therapist
- Social worker
- Vendor
- Special consultants: neuro-ophthalmologist, orthotist, prosthetist, dentist, reading specialist

The most important consideration should always be that the appropriate members of the team include those people needed to help make the best decisions possible around the issues for this consumer.

STAFF COMPETENCY AND EXPERIENCE

The quality of both the process and the practitioners delivering the service is crucial for providing the most advantageous situation for successful outcomes. The TEAMS Laboratory primary staff professionals consist of clinical specialists in occupational therapy, speech-language pathology, and rehabilitation technology. Along with other members of the team, the staff is able to provide service for consumers who have more complicated situations and/or disabilities.

It is important to briefly consider the scope of health care technology in relation to providers of service delivery and the consumer. Health care technology is both medical technology and rehabilitation technology. Medical technology is generally applied by professionals in an institutional setting such as hospitals and other facilities. That technology is more related to diagnostic testing, treatment, monitoring, life support, and surgical applications. Because it is institutionally based, there is less volume and it is easier to follow from an equipment evaluation point of view. Rehabilitation technology, however, is used to facilitate independence for consumers, and most of its use is outside the institution in living situations such as home, school, and work. The successful delivery of this technology then requires a framework of service providers who can adequately address the following five parallel components:

- **Products:** specific ATDs and systems
- **Services:** includes evaluation and analysis; equipment access methods, equipment selection; prescription preparation; product and environmental adaptation; technical consultation and customizing
- **Information:** availability of products; product features; what is available for demonstration, simulation, and hands-on trials and training; what kinds of networks exist as sources and means of referral and funding
- **Labor:** practitioners who are trained to provide adequate service delivery, particularly in the areas of consumer evaluation, methods of task and site analysis, have the ability to integrate multiple technologies, can locate and coordinate varieties of sources in such areas as materials management, customizing, funding, training, and technical service providers
- **Materials and management methods**

EDUCATION, TRAINING, AND RESOURCE SERVICES

Because of the specialized nature of the service and the experience and skill of the staff, the program is able to provide a broad range of education and training workshops and seminars that are directed to health care professionals, students in health care curriculums (e.g., occupational therapists, speech-language pathology students, vocational counseling students), vocational counselors, educators, employers and other business community sources, insurance companies, and other third-party funding agents. Having access to a broad range of technology and using our special knowledge to incorporate technological advances into the lives of people with disabilities have put us in an excellent position to educate the third-party payor groups with special benefit to vocational rehabilitation counselors. We have also been able to educate the business community to increase awareness and foster a positive attitude in that community, to encourage integrating people with disabilities into the mainstream. We are also a frequently used local, national, and international resource on technology. TEAMS Laboratory staff has presented some educational seminars

285

Provision of
Assistive
Technology:
A Model for
Service Delivery

to business groups interested in the Americans with Disabilities Act (ADA) as it relates to technology.

CONSUMER-BASED SERVICE

From its inception in 1988, the service has been consumer driven. We approach the service delivery of AT goods and services by providing consumers with the tools they need to seek out and acquire that technology. This has been our approach long before the Technology-Related Assistance for Individuals with Disabilities Act (Tech Act) of 1988,[1] which was the first legislation to use the term *consumer responsive* in defining how services should be provided. The Tech Act and the passage of the ADA[2] in 1990 have brought emphasis to the concept of independence for all persons with disabilities. The ability to live independently means that individuals theoretically will have the means to control their lives and therefore the ability to participate in all aspects of society.

Most consumers acquire their initial technology, as well as subsequent technology, through recommendations by knowledgeable professionals who select equipment for the "good of the consumer." To have a consumer-oriented market, our service delivery must more closely fit the general consumer model. The professionals and others in the service delivery process must develop standards and must become truly knowledgeable consults to the consumer. Services, products, and information must meet consumer needs, and the process must be approached with attitudes that support this concept.[3–5]

PROCESS OF COMPREHENSIVE SERVICE DELIVERY

The following process was developed by the TEAMS Laboratory to address the problems identified at the onset of this chapter.[6,7] This process is generic and can be used for the assessment of all kinds of AT. We have discovered in using this process that to achieve more successful outcomes, the following guidelines are useful:

- Appropriate seating and positioning that includes prevention of deformity, relief of pressure, comfort, adequate respiration, a good body image, and maximum independence for functional activity must be available.
- Each step of the process must be included and in sequence so that the evaluation and analysis move from global to detailed problem solving and are inclusive of all information needed to formulate appropriate goals and include the necessary consumer-oriented education and information.
- Early goal identification should be made.
- Case coordination should be done by the team doing the actual technology service delivery.

- Interdisciplinary team-oriented service delivery must be available.
- Analytical and detailed problem-solving process should be provided.
- A high degree of consumer participation and responsibility should be encouraged.
- Informed consumer decision-making should be ensured by providing appropriate consumer education. The role of the team in the service delivery process is that of consultant and can be provided most effectively by this process.
- Hands-on evaluation and training of all equipment as well as access systems and methods of operation being considered and eventually selected should be provided. There are NO exceptions to this guideline. Until the consumer has actual functional experience with the equipment, there is no way that he or she can make an informed decision.
- Technical support should be ensured.

Introduction and integration of the technology into the consumer's environment include the following 13-step process. This is particularly important when the consumer requires intervention and subsequent integration of technologies in more than one area.

287

Provision of
Assistive
Technology:
A Model for
Service Delivery

STEP 1

PRESCREENING

▶ Prescreening is necessary to determine the appropriateness of service. Any documentation concerning the referral should be requested and reviewed. The information generated should include the consumer's

- **History,** including consideration of diagnostic information that would have an effect on the provision of equipment, such as progressive diseases, lifelong conditions, and traumatic injuries
- **Funding source(s)**
- **Goals**—There must be an identified goal for the use of the technology as a tool (e.g., the consumer must have specific need for the technology to do course work in school or a job that has specific tasks that can be accomplished with technology solutions)
- **Motivation**

STEP 2

FUNDING APPROVAL

▶ Funding approval for evaluation and potential equipment acquisition.

STEP 3

PHYSICIAN REFERRAL

STEP 4

INITIAL NEEDS ASSESSMENT

▶ Initial needs assessment (INA) is a comprehensive assessment of the consumer's need for technology intervention; it is based on the assessment of a wide variety of aspects of the environment, including medical history; physical function; orthopaedic conditions; sensory modalities; vision, hearing, cognition, perception; activity of daily living status, positioning, and mobility needs; communication, educational/vocational history; environmental control and accessibility needs; and history of device use. At the conclusion of the INA, a summary must include

- Readdressing the consumer's self-assessed goals
- A summary of present status and indications for success
- Recommendations for any further testing that should be done
- Recommendations for the preliminary preparation of skills to be addressed before equipment evaluation is undertaken
- Identification of long-term and short-term goals and recommendations as to the length of time for the services to be rendered, including consideration for training needs

STEP 5
CONSUMER EVALUATION
▶ Consumer evaluation is an in-depth evaluation of the most effective physical means of ATD access as well as the best strategies for access based on the capabilities of the consumer. Frequently referred to as an access evaluation, this evaluation is performed by the occupational therapist and takes into consideration all the devices/systems that need to be operated. It is a hands-on process of locating all the consumer's available control movements, their anatomic locations, and the quality of the motions. Functional and comfortable positioning should be established before or in tandem with this step.

STEP 6
TASK ANALYSIS
▶ Task analysis is a careful look at the consumer's activities with a focus on their type, nature, patterns, goals, and interaction with the environment. On the job, this requires that the tasks be analyzed as to primary and secondary activities, those things that are essential functions as well as secondary or peripheral functions that may be done either less frequently or at peripheral locations (away from the main work station). Tasks may fall into categories such as information management, communication, and item manipulation. All tasks need to be evaluated for frequency, duration, adaptability, and physical requirements for execution.

STEP 7
SITE EVALUATION
▶ Site evaluation is a detailed look at the consumer's environment(s) with a focus of how it has an effect on the accomplishment of functional tasks. This includes (1) where the work is to be accomplished: primary, secondary, or tertiary (e.g., off-site); (2) the nature of the site (e.g., stress, attitudes, security, available support); (3) physical characteristics and layout (floor plan); and (4) consideration of all existing equipment.

STEP 8
SOLUTION EXPLORATION
▶ Solution exploration includes hands-on access to products and methods of operation, which means to present solutions and experiment with a loop of variables that interact and influence each other to create a design for the best solution(s). Those variables include the consumer, task, site, the equipment, and the strategies that involve

- **Equipment evaluation:** device operation, performance, construction, and installation; technical complexity; competition; compatibility/flexibility; available consumer evaluation; engineering evaluation; availability; maintenance and repair issues; and training needs
- **Simulated tasks:** hands-on evaluation, TEAMS Laboratory research, analysis of results, and comparison of potential solutions
- **Consumer education**

It is important to keep in mind that there is a hierarchy of solution selection when the solution is based on using AT and that those solutions vary from simple to complex and range from very inexpensive to several thousand dollars. Federal government studies have shown that only 22 percent of employees with disabilities may need accommodations of some kind at the work site.[8] The cost to employers for those accommodations indicated that for 31 percent there is no cost, for 57 percent the cost is between $1 and $1,000, for 11 percent between $1,000 and $5,000, and for 1 percent more than $5,000. The solution hierarchy includes the following:

- *Re-arrange* existing materials
- Look for commercially available *"off-the-shelf" products* that have the desired features needed by the user. This frequently turns out to be single function/stand alone devices such as telephones or door openers
- *Unorthodox placement,* mounting, or modification of devices
- *Special products* with special features that can be set up to meet the unique needs of the user. Usually the solution is a product designed for persons with disabilities and the products are systems that do multifunctional tasks, such as computer applications, or they are integrated systems that have a single controller with multiple inputs that can access a powered wheelchair, a computer, and an augmentative communication system or ECU
- *Customized* "one-of-a-kind" solutions
- The final solution is more often a *combination* of all or some of the above, in which the consumer uses both mechanical, electronic, and manipulated work site arrangements

ABBREVIATED SOLUTION EXAMPLE

- **Consumer:** 47-year-old man with a genetic degeneration disability. He is quadriparetic with only partial functional motion with decreased range and strength available bilaterally in the upper extremities when positioned in balance forearm orthotics (BFO). Mobility is achieved via a powered wheelchair in which he requires complicated and extensive positioning. The wheelchair is controlled by a centrally positioned and adapted digital joystick (Fig. 26-1).
- **Employment status:** receptionist and intake worker in city government office. Work environment and supervisor are unsupportive. Equipment requires excessive space. He has some secretarial help.
- **Equipment:** INA and site evaluation are done on initial visit. This man worked at several locations that had multiple single-function adaptations:

289

Provision of
Assistive
Technology:
A Model for
Service Delivery

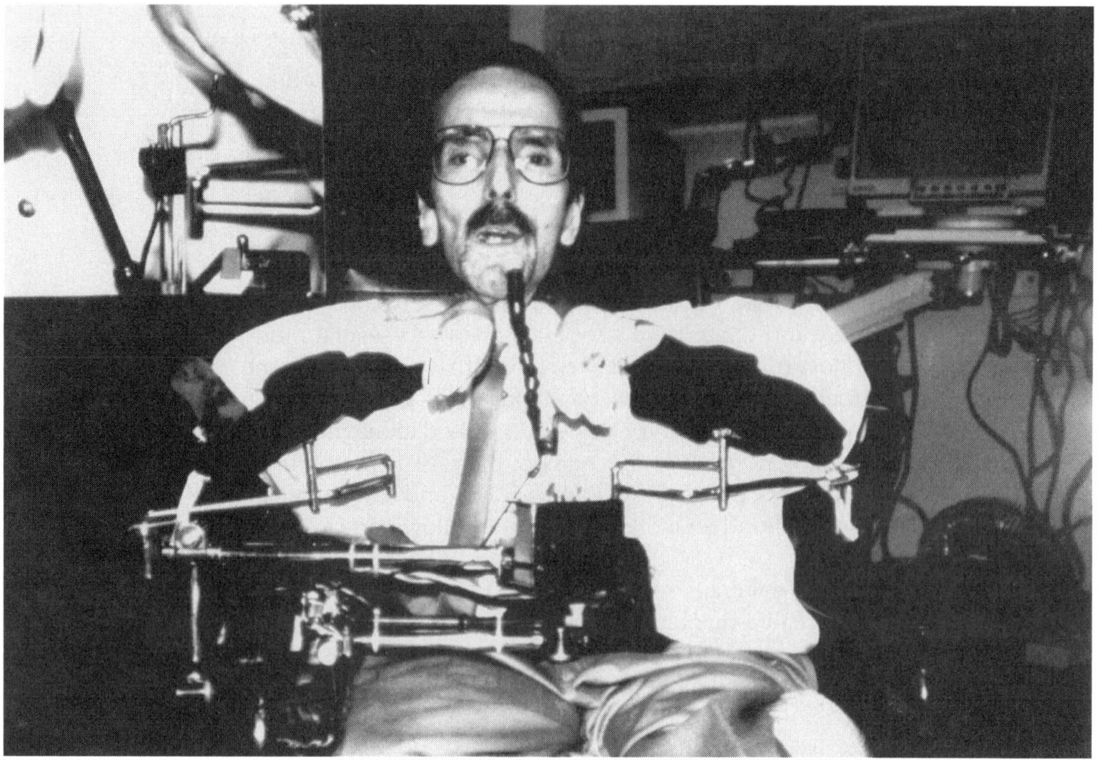

Figure 26-1. The client positioned in ballbearing forearm orthosis with a joystick at midline. Inset is a closeup of the adapted joystick that the client used both before and after intervention.

Telephone adapted with wired weighted flipper and handset on
a gooseneck
Tape recorder set to record with stop watch
Carousel with rotary files and book stands
Telephone directory, battery operated
Heater on desk
Home computer with repositioned keyboard linked to a central
office computer

All equipment was accessed by repositioning the wheelchair to reach each device via the BFOs (Fig. 26-2).

- **Main problems**
  Underuse of skills
  Unable to access information
  All single-function devices hard and time-consuming and difficult
  to access
  Decreased voice volume
  Seating and positioning becoming inadequate and outdated for
  physical condition
  Limited funding

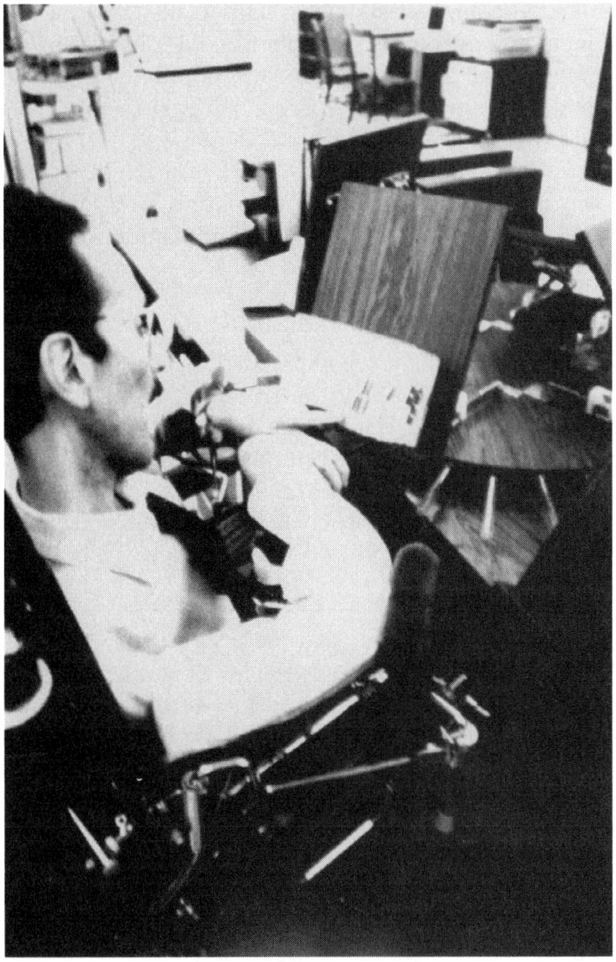

Figure 26-2. Before intervention, each functional task required a separate location on a large table and a special work area for the telephone necessitating frequent repositioning of the powered wheelchair. This figure shows a bookrest holding a Rolodex mounted on a lazy Susan. Projections at 3-in. intervals allowed the client to turn the base with the left index finger.

291

Provision of
Assistive
Technology:
A Model for
Service Delivery

- **Goals**
    Provide adequate seating, positioning, and powered mobility
    Decrease reliance on secretary
    Work with supervisor and employer
    Establish independent access to telephone, note taking, document generation, and information
    Increase voice volume through positioning and equipment
    Find funding
- **Final solution**
    Powered wheelchair with adequate seating and positioning for pressure relief, functional tasks, energy conservation, and respiratory needs: tilt-in-space, customized, molded seating

Integrated computer system to handle all communication needs including telephone (Ideaphone), with handset on goose-neck. Small foot-print keyboard mounted on an extended arm and access with upper extremities in BFOs (Fig. 26-3)

X-10 powerhouse ECU for appliances

Laser printer and page turner

Voice amplification through a telephone headset as an amplifier

- **Follow-up:** on-going technical support and clinical intervention

STEP 9

EQUIPMENT SPECIFICATIONS

▶ A detailed list of equipment recommendations leading to prescription is important. With the completion of the solution exploration, there should be a summary of the findings of the evaluation process and a readdressing of questions, such as (1) were the priorities addressed? (2) were worker/employer issues addressed? (3) are the solutions feasible from cost and management points of view? (4) are all parties aware of the advantages/

Figure 26-3. The final solution was a computer work station incorporating all the individual single function areas. The small keyboard is positioned on a magic arm with a superclamp mounted from the desktop. The access to the telephone is via the Ideaphone from Ideatech, consisting of a card that plugs into the computer. A standard handset is mounted on a Luxo arm. The lower right inset shows the telephone selections on the monitor. The upper left inset depicts a back view of the keyboard and telephone handset mount.

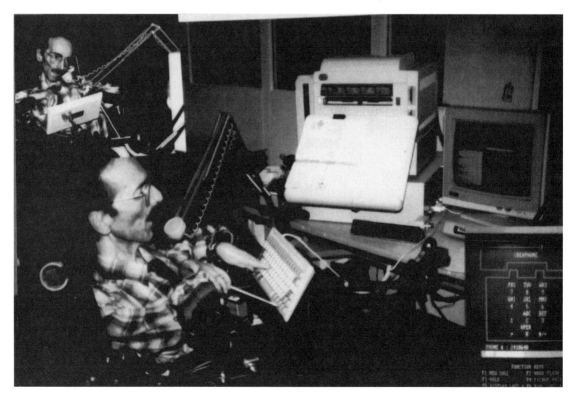

disadvantages of the solution(s)? and (5) is follow-up support available and is there a way to monitor for change?

STEP 10

PRESCRIPTION AND JUSTIFICATION

▶ Prescription and justification leading to equipment delivery must be prepared.

STEP 11

INSTALLATION/ASSEMBLY/EQUIPMENT INTEGRATION

STEP 12

USE TRAINING

▶ Use training consists of use of actual equipment solutions, implementation of strategies, problem solving, evaluation of potential for change. A great deal of training has been accomplished during the evaluation process for the consumer to understand basic operation of the ATDs and systems, particularly if there is an alternate access system necessary. Frequently, that is the only training that is done during this process, and more detailed training is almost always necessary and should be considered as part of the initial plan of service delivery back at the time of the INA. After installation and set-up of the equipment, operational use of all aspects of the systems should be done along with practical applications of situations to be encountered by the user. For example, the user may be aware of how to use the access system to a computer such as with a head mouse but not be really computer literate. That basic operation should be addressed in the training sessions. The missing of this step results in lack of full device use or at best only limited potential for the consumer and frequent frustration for the consumer and the employer.

293

Provision of
Assistive
Technology:
A Model for
Service Delivery

STEP 13

FOLLOW-UP/SUPPORT

▶ Follow-up should be done by all parties involved in the preceding process to identify areas of both success and failure.

CONCLUSION

Technology cannot substitute for or provide clear goals, train the user, operate efficiently without maintenance and repair, eliminate barriers of acceptance, substitute for social interaction, or overcome poor work habits or attitudes. However, technology can substitute for loss or limitation of physical function, conserve energy, provide ways to simplify processes and tasks, help compensate for cognitive and sensory disabilities, and provide access to almost any kind of device or system.[9]

This chapter outlines the need and provides guidelines for more successful outcomes in the process of the selection of AT. We must be ever mindful that AT is a tool and that it must be provided within the context of the consumer's whole environment. It must take into consideration all their needs: physical, psychosocial, environmental, and educational/vocational.

The service delivery must be done with the consumer as an active responsible member of the team. Service delivery personnel must provide honest realistic services concentrating on the consumer's abilities and emphasizing specific and targeted goals. That service delivery is most successful if it is team oriented and provided by knowledgeable and skillful practitioners. Successful outcomes will allow persons with even the most severe disabilities to be included in the mainstream of whatever activities they pursue.

REFERENCES

1. Technology-Related Assistance for Individuals with Disabilities Act of 1988. PL 100-407, Title 29, U.S.C. 2201 et seq: U.S. Statutes at Large, 102, 1044–1065, August 19, 1988

2. Americans with Disabilities Act (ADA) of 1990. PL 101-336, Title 42 U.S.C. 12101 et seq: U.S. Statutes at Large, 104, 327–378, July 26, 1990

3. Post KM: Consumer-oriented service delivery. Am J Occup Ther 47(11):1046–1047, 1993

4. Shaver MS: Retrospective study of electronic technical aid use among high-level quadriplegic males. In Dickey RE (ed): Electronic Technical Aids for Persons with Severe Physical Disabilities. Rusk Institute of Rehabilitation Medicine, New York, 1985

5. Batavia DI, Hammer GS: Toward the development of consumer-based criteria for the evaluation of assistive devices. J Rehabil Res Dev 27(4,19):425, 1990

6. Dickey RE: Work station simulation laboratory for persons with severe physical disabilities (Summary Report, RSA Grant H128A91022). Rehabilitation Services Administration, Washington, DC, 1992

7. Dickey RE, Loeser A, Specht E: Environmental control for persons with disabilities. pp. 257–283. In Redford JB, Basmajian J, Trautman P (eds): Orthotics: Clinical Practice and Rehabilitation Technology. Churchill Livingstone, New York, 1995

8. Eastern Paralyzed Veterans Association: Understanding the Americans with Disabilities Act. EVPA, New York, 1991

9. Specht E: Rehabilitation Technology Services and Solutions. Paper presented at the Hunter College Vocational Counselor Technology Workshop, Mount Sinai Medical Center, New York, 1994

SUGGESTED READINGS

Dickey RE: High technology at home. p. 415. In Portnow J (ed): Physical Medicine and Rehabilitation, Home Health Care and Rehabilitation. Vol. 2. Hanley & Belfus, Inc., Philadelphia, 1988

Lazzaro JL: Adaptive Technologies for Learning and Work Environments. American Library Association, Chicago, 1993

Lee KS, Thomas DJ: Control of Computer-based Technology for People with Physical Disabilities: An Assessment Manual. University of Toronto Press, Toronto, 1990

Mann WC, Lane JP: Assistive Technology for Persons with Disabilities: The Role of Occupational Therapy. 2nd Ed. American Occupational Therapy Association, Rockville, MD, 1995

Mueller J: The Workplace Workbook: An Illustrated Guide to Job Accommodation and Assistive Technology. The Dole Foundation, Washington, DC, 1990

Somerville NJ, Wilson DJ, Shanfield KJ, Mack W: A survey of the assistive technology training needs of occupational therapists. Assist Technol 2(2):41, 1990

Trace Research and Development Center: Assistive Technologies for Communication, Control and Computer Access. 1996–1997 Ed. Madison, WI Trace Research and Development Center, 1995

295

Provision of
Assistive
Technology:
A Model for
Service Delivery

Resources

ORGANIZATIONS

Centre de Réadaptation
Professionnelle et Fonctionnelle de
    Nanteau-sur-Lunain
B.P 34
F-77 792 Nemours Cedex
France
+33 1 64451515 (phone)
+33 1 64290517 (fax)

Centro Estatal De Autonomia Personal y
    Ayudas Technicas
Los Extremeños, 1
28038 Madrid
Spain
+34 1 778 90 61 (phone)
+34 1 778 41 17 (fax)

Danish Centre for Technical Aids for
    Rehabilitation and Education
Gregersensvej
DK-2630 TAASTRUP
Denmark
+45 43 99 33 22 (phone)
+45 43 52 70 72 (fax)

DPI-Europe
Lönnrotsgatan 9D-14
SF-00120 Helsinki
Finland
+358 0 680-1591 (phone)
+358 0 680 1569 (fax)

ECRS
Danske Döves Landsförbund
Box 704
DK-2200 Köpenhamn N
Denmark
+45 3536 1588 (phone)
+45 3536 0155 (fax)

ECRS Office
110, Rue Franklin
B-1040 Bruxelles
Belgium
+32 2735 7218 (phone)
+32 2735 5354 (fax)

Escuela Universitaria de Informática
Universidad Politecnica de Madrid
Ctra. de Valencia Km. 7
28031 Madrid
Spain
+34 1 331 17 10 (phone)
+34 1 331 17 67 (fax)

Eurolink Age
1 Place du Luxembourg
B-1040 Brussels
Belgium
+32 2 512 9946
+32 2 512 6673

European Blind Union
c/o Dansk Blindeförbund
Thoravej 35
DK-2400 Kobenhagen
Denmark
+45 31 198 844 (phone)
+45 38 331 137 (fax)

International League of Societies for
    Persons with Mental Handicap
European Association
Avenue Louise 248, bte 17
B-1050 Bruxelles
Belgium
+32 2 647 2969 (fax)

Richter Reha Design GmbH
Hutschdorfer Strasse 2
D-95349 Thurnau
Germany
+49 9228 686 (phone)
+49 92285633 (fax)

GENERAL ORGANIZATIONS

American Association for the
    Advancement of Science
Project on Science Technology
    and Disability
1333 H Street NW
Washington, DC 20005
(202) 326-6645

American Foundation for the Blind
15 West 16th Street
New York, NY 10011
(212) 620-2000

American Occupational Therapy
   Association (AOTA)
1383 Piccard Drive
Rockville, MD 20850
(301) 948-9626
(800) 843-2682 (members only)

American Rehabilitation Association
1910 Association Drive, Suite 200
Reston, VA 22091
(703) 648-9300
(800) 368-3513

American Speech-Language-Hearing
   Association (ASHA)
10801 Rockville Pike
Rockville, MD 20852
(800) 638-8255 or 6868

Closing the Gap, Inc.
P.O. Box 68
Henderson, MN 56044
(612) 248-3294

EASI: Equal Access to Software
   and Information
c/o American Association for
   Higher Education
One Dupont Circle, Suite 360
Washington, DC 20036

International Society for Augmentative and
   Alternative Communications (ISAAC)
428 East Preston Street
Baltimore, MD 21202-3993

Job Accommodation Network (JAN)
809 Allen Hall
West Virginia University
Morgantown, WV 26506
(800) 526-7234

National Easter Seal Society
70 East Lake Street
Chicago, IL 60601
(312) 726-6200 (voice)
(312) 726-4258 (TDD)

National Information Center on Deafness
Gallaudet University
800 Florida Avenue NE
Washington, DC 20002
(202) 651-5051 (voice)
(202) 651-5052 (TDD)

National Institute on Disability and
    Rehabilitation Research (NIDRR)
US Department of Education
400 Maryland Avenue SW
Washington, DC 20202
(202) 732-1134

Office of Special Education and
    Rehabilitation Services (OSERS)
US Department of Education
Switzer Building, Room 3129
330 C Street SW
Washington, DC 20202

Rehabilitation Engineering and Assistive Technology
    Society of North America (RESNA)
Technical Assistance Project
1700 North Moore Street, Suite 1540
Arlington, VA 22209
(703) 524-6686
(703) 524-6630 (fax)

Technical Aids and Assistance for
    the Disabled
1950 West Roosevelt Road
Chicago, IL 60608
(313) 421-3373
(800) 346-2959

United Cerebral Palsy Association
1522 K Street NW, Suite 1112
Washington, DC 20005
(202) 842-1266
(800) 872-5827

AUGMENTATIVE COMMUNICATION RESOURCES

American Speech-Language-Hearing
    Association (ASHA)
10801 Rockville Pike
Rockville, MD 20852

Blissymbolics Communication International
250 Ferrand Drive, Suite 200
Don Mills, Ontario M3C 3P2, Canada

International Society for Augmentative and
   Alternative Communication (ISAAC)
P.O. Box 1762, Station R
Toronto, Ontario Canada L8N 3K7

Trace Research and Development Center on
   Communication Control and Computer Access
University of Wisconsin–Madison
S-151 Waisman Center
1500 Highland Avenue
Madison, WI 53705

US Society for Augmentative and Alternative
   Communication (USSAAC) Newsletter
1850 Sand Hill Road, Apartment 10
Palo Alto, CA 94304

DRIVER EDUCATION RESOURCES

American Automobile Association
Traffic Safety-Disabled Driver Programs
1000 AAA Drive
Heathrow, FL 32746
(407) 444-7962

Association of Driver Educators
   for the Disabled
P.O. Box 49
109 West Street
Edgerton, WI 53534
(608) 884-8833

As-Tech Inc.
8 Shovel Shop Square
North Easton, MA 02356-1445

The Braun Corporation
1014 South Monticello
P.O. Box 310
Winamac, IN 46996

Bruno Independent Living Aids, Inc.
1780 Executive Drive
P.O. Box 84
Oconomowoc, WI 53066

Crow River Industries, Inc.
14800 28th Avenue N
Minneapolis, MN 55447

Doron Precision Systems, Inc.
P.O. Box 400
Binghamton, NY 13902-0400

EMC, Inc.
2001 Wooddale Boulevard
Baton Rouge, LA 70806

Mobile Tech Corporation
P.O. Box 2326
Hutchinson, KS 67504-2326

National Mobility Equipment Dealers
　Association (NMEDA)
909 East Skagway Avenue
Tampa, FL 33604
(813) 932-8566

Society of Automotive Engineers
400 Commonwealth Drive
Warrendale, PA 15096
(412) 776-4841

HIGHER EDUCATION RESOURCES

AHEAD (Association on Higher Education
　and Disability)
P.O. Box 21192
Columbus, OH 43221-0192
(614) 488-4972 (TDD/voice)

Higher Education and Adult Training for People
　with Handicaps (HEATH)
American Council on Education
One Dupont Circle, Suite 800
Washington, DC 20036-1193
(202) 939-9320 / (800) 544-3284 (voice and
　typed text, TDD)
(202) 833-4760 (fax)

INDEPENDENT LIVING RESOURCES

Independent Living Research Utilization (ILRU)
2323 South Shepard, Suite 1000
Houston, Texas 77019
(713) 520-0232
(713) 520-5136 (TDD)

MOBILITY EQUIPMENT

European Conference on the Advancement of
　Rehabilitation Technology (ECART)
Uallingby
Sweden
+46 86201700

National Registry of Rehabilitation
  Technology Suppliers
Lubbock, TX
(806) 797-7299

National Association of Medical Equipment
  Suppliers (NAMES)
Atlanta, GA
(703) 836-6363
Annual show of medical equipment

VISUAL IMPAIRMENTS

Baruch College Computer Center for the
  Visually Impaired
The City University of New York
17 Lexington Avenue, Box 515
New York, NY 10010

US RESEARCH CENTERS

Apple Computers, Inc.
20525 Mariani Avenue
Cupertino, CA 95014
(408) 996-1010

Lucent Technologies Accessible Communication
(formerly AT&T Special Needs Center)
2001 Route 46, Suite 310
Parsippany, NJ 07054
(800) 233-1222
(800) 833-3232 (TDD)

Breaking New Ground Resource Center
Purdue University
1146 Agricultural Engineering Building
West Lafayette, IN 47907-1146
(317) 494-5088 (mail or TDD)

Center for Rehabilitation Technology
College of Architecture
Georgia Institute of Technology
Atlanta, GA 30332-0156

Center for Therapeutic Applications
  of Technology
University of Buffalo
Buffalo, NY

HEATH Resource Center
American Council on Education
1 Dupont Circle, Suite 80
Washington, DC 20036-1193

IBM National Support Center for Persons
  with Disabilities
P.O. Box 1328
Boca Raton, FL 33429-1328
(800) 436-4832 Independent Series

National Clearinghouse on Technology and Aging
University Center on Aging
University of Massachusetts Medical Center
55 Lake Avenue N
Worchester, MA 01655
(508) 856-3662

Rehabilitation Engineering Center
National Rehabilitation Hospital
120 Irving Street NW
Washington, DC 20010-2949

Rochester Institute of Technology
National Technical Institute for the Deaf
National Center for Employment of the Deaf
Lyndon Baines Johnson Building
P.O. Box 9887
Rochester, NY 14623-0087
(716) 475-6834 (voice)
(716) 475-6205 (TDD)

TECH REACH
National Center for Disability Services
201 IU Willets Road
Albertson, NY 11507-1599
(800) 487-2805

Trace Research and Development Center
S-151 Waisman Center
1500 Highland Avenue
Madison, WI 53705
(608) 262-6966 (voice)
(608) 263-5408 (TDD)

West Virginia Rehabilitation Research and
  Training Center
5088 Washington Street W, Suite 200
Cross Lanes, WV 25313
(304) 759-0716

DATABASES

AbleData
8455 Colesville Road, Suite 935
Silver Springs, MD 20910-3319

AbleInform
(301) 589-3563

America On-Line
8619 Westwood Center Drive
Vienna, VA 22182
(800) 827-6364

AOTA—The Reliable Source
1383 Piccard Drive
P.O. Box 1725
Rockville, MD 20849-1725
(301) 948-9626

BRS Information Technologies
1200 Route 7
Latham, NY 12110
(800) 345-4BRS
(800) 468-0908
(518) 783-7251

Combined Health Information Database
National Institutes of Health (NIH)
Box NDTC-CHID
Bethesda, MD 20205
(301) 468-6555
(800) 346-2742

CompuServe
CompuServe Information Service
5000 Arlington Center Boulevard
Columbia, OH 43220
(800) 848-8199 or 8990 (helpline)
(614) 457-8600

Co-Net (Cooperative Database Distribution
   Network for Assistive Technology)
Trace Research and Development Center
S-151 Waisman Center, UW-Madison
1500 Highland Avenue
Madison, WI 53705
(608) 262-6966
(608) 263-5408 (TDD)
info@trace.waisman.wisc.edu

CTG Solutions
Closing the Gap, Inc.
P.O. Box 68
Henderson, MN 56044
(612) 248-3294

Development Disabilities Library
Association for Retarded Citizens of the US
2501 Avenue J
Arlington, TX 76006
(817) 261-6003 (voice)
(817) 277-6989 (computer)

ERIC (Educational Resources
   Information Center)
Council for Exceptional Children
1920 Association Drive
Reston, VA 22091
(701) 620-3660

GTE Educational Resources
8505 Freeport Parkway
Irving, TX 75063
(800) 634-5644

IBM Database
Building 904, 9448
11400 Burnet Road
Austin, TX 78758
(800) 426-4832

Job Accommodation Network
   (JAN) Bulletin Board
(800) 342-5526

MEDLINE
NIH-MEDLARS
8600 Rockville Pike
Bethesda, MD 20894
(301) 496-6193

National Technology Database
American Federation for the Blind
National Technology Center
15 West 16th Street
New York, NY 10011
(212) 620-2080
(800) AFB-LIND

Project Enable
Rehabilitation Technology Associates
West Virginia Research and Training Center
One Dunbar Plaza, Suite E
Dunbar, WV 25064–3098

REHABDATA
National Rehabilitation Information Center
   (NARIC)
8455 Colesville Road, Suite 935
Silver Springs, MD 20910–3319
(800) 346-2742
(301) 588-9284

SpecialNet
GTE Education Services
GTE Place
West Airfield Drive
P.O. Box 619810
DFW Airport, TX 75261–9810
(800) 927-3000

TECH.LINE
Center for Special Education Technology
The Council for Exceptional Children
1920 Association Drive
Reston, VA 22091
(703) 620-3660
(800) 873-8255

Technology Resource Center of Manhattan
(212) 979-9700

VA Rehabilitation Database
Office of Technology Transfer
VA Prosthetics, R&D Center
103 South Gay Street
Baltimore, MD 21202
(301) 962-1800

US GOVERNMENT AGENCIES

ADA RESOURCES

Architectural and Transportation Barriers Compliance Board
1331 F Street NW
Washington, DC 20004-1111
(800) USA-ABLE
(202) 272-5434 (voice)
(202) 272-5449 (TDD)
(202) 272-5447 (fax)

Accessible design in new construction and alterations

Department of Justice
Office on the ADA; Civil Rights Division
P.O. Box 66118
Washington, DC 20035-6118
(202) 514-0301
(202) 514-0318

Public accommodation; state and local government services

Department of Transportation
400 Seventh Street SW
Washington, DC 20590
(202) 366-9305
(202) 755-7687 (TTD)

Transportation issues

Equal Employment Opportunity Commission
1801 L Street NW
Washington, DC 20507
(202) 663-4900
(800) 800-3302 (TTD)
Employment issues

Federal Communications Commission
1919 M Street NW
Washington, DC 20554
(202) 632-7260
(202) 632-6999 (TTD)
Telecommunications issues

Internal Revenue Service
Department of the Treasury
1111 Constitution Avenue NW
Washington, DC 20044
(202) 566-2000
Tax credits and deductions for business

US STATE AGENCIES

Alabama Statewide Technology Access and
  Response Project (STAR)
2125 East South Boulevard
P.O. Box 20752
Birmingham, AL 36120-0752
(205) 281-2276

Assistive Technologies of Alaska
400 "D" Street, Suite 230
Anchorage, AK 99501
(907) 272-9547

Arkansas Increasing Capabilities Access Network
2201 Brookwood, Suite 117
Little Rock, AR 72202
(501) 666-8868

California Assistive Technology System
CA Department of Rehabilitation
830 K Street, Room 307
Sacramento, CA 95814
(916) 323-0595

Colorado Assistive Technology Project
Rocky Mountain Resource and Training Institute
6355 Ward Road, Suite 310
Arvada, CO 80004
(303) 420-2942

Connecticut Assistive Technology Project
Bureau of Rehabilitation Services
10 Griffin Road N
Windsor, CT 06095
(203) 298-2018

D.C. Partnership for Assistive Technology
National Rehabilitation Hospital
102 Riving Street NW
Washington, DC 20010
(202) 877-1932

Delaware Assistive Technology Initiative
University of Delaware/duPont Institute
1600 Rockland Road, Room 154
Wilmington, DE 19899
(302) 651-4000

Florida Assistive Technology Project
Department of Labor and Employment,
    Division of Vocational Rehabilitation
Bureau of Client Services, Rehabilitation
    Engineering Technology
1709–A Mahan Drive
Tallahassee, FL 32399-0696
(904) 487-3423

Georgia Tools for Life
Division of Rehabilitation Services
2 Peachtree Street NW, Suite 23-411
Atlanta, GA 30303
(800) 726-9119

Hawaii Assistive Technology Training and
    Service Project
677 Ala Moana Boulevard, Suite 403
Honolulu, HI 96813
(800) 532-7110

Idaho Assistive Technology Project
129 West 3rd Street
Moscow, ID 83843
(208) 885-9429

Illinois Assistive Technology Project
110 Iles Park Place
Springfield, IL 62718
(217) 522-7985

Indiana Attain (Accessing Technology Through
   Awareness in Indiana) Project
P.O. Box 7083
402 West Washington Street
Room W453
Indianapolis, IN 46207–7083
(812) 855-9396

Iowa Program Assistive Technology
Iowa University Affiliated Program
University Hospital School
Iowa City, IA 52242
(800) 331-3027

Assistive Technology for Kansas Project
2501 Gabriel
P.O. Box 738
Parons, KS 67357
(316) 421-8367

Kentucky Assistive Technology
   Services Network
Coordinating Center
427 Versailles Road
Frankfort, KY 40601
(502) 573-4665

Louisiana Technology Assistive Network
P.O. Box 3455, Bin 14
Baton Rouge, LA 70821-3455
(800) 922-DIAL

Maine Consumer Information and Technology
   Training Exchange (Main Cite)
Maine CITE Coordinating Center
University of Maine at Augusta
46 University Drive
Augusta, ME 04330
(207) 621-3195

Maryland Technology Assistive Program
Governor's Office for Individuals
   with Disabilities
300 West Lexington Street, Box 10
Baltimore, MD 21201
(800) 832-4827

Massachusetts Assistive Technology
   Partnership Center
Children's Hospital
300 Longwood Avenue
Boston, MA 02115
(617) 727-5540

Michigan Tech 2000
Michigan Department of Education
Rehabilitation Services
P.O. Box 30010
Lansing, MI 48909
(517) 373-4056

Minnesota Star Program
300-Centennial Building
658 Cedar Street
St. Paul, MN 55155
(800) 331-3027

Mississippi Project Start
P.O. Box 1698
300-Capers Avenue, Building 3
Jackson, MS 39215-1698
(601) 987-4872

Missouri Assistive Technology Project
4731 South Cochise, Suite 114
Independence, MO 64055-6975
(800) 647-8558

MonTECH
The University of Montana, MUARID, MonTECH
634 Eddy Avenue
Missoula, MT 59812
(406) 243-5676

Nebraska Assistive Technology Project
301 Centennial Mall South
P.O. Box 94987
Lincoln, NE 68509-4987
(702) 687-4452

Nevada Assistive Technology Project
Rehabilitation Division
Community-based Services Development
711 South Stewart Street
Carson City, NV 89710
(702) 687-4452

New Hampshire Technology Partnership Project
Institute on Disability UAP
14 Ten Ferry Street
The Concord Center
Concord, NH 03301
(603) 224-0630

New Jersey Technology Assistive Resource Program
135 East State Street
CN 398
Trenton, NJ 08625
(609) 292-7496

New Mexico Technology Assistance Program
435 St. Michael's Drive, Building D
Santa Fe, NM 87503
(800) 866-2253

New York State Triad Project
Office of Advocate for the Disabled
One Empire State Plaza, Tenth Floor
Albany, NY 12223-0001
(518) 474-2625

North Carolina Assistive Technology Project
Department of Human Resources
Division of Vocational Rehabilitation Services
1110 Navaho Drive, Suite 101
Raleigh, NC 27609
(800) 852-0042

North Dakota Interagency Program for Assistive
    Technology (IPAT)
P.O. Box 743
Cavalier, ND 58220
(701) 265-4807

Ohio Train
400 East Campus View Boulevard, SW5F
Columbus, OH 43235-4604
(614) 438-1450

Oregon Technology Access for Life Needs
    Project (TALN)
Chemeketa Community College
P.O. Box 14007
Salem, OR 97309-7070
(503) 945-6265

Pennsylvania's Initiative on Assistive Technology
Institute on Disability/UAP
Ritter Hall Annex 433 (004-00)
Philadelphia, PA 19122
(610) 204-1356

Puerto Rico Assistive Technology Project
Box 22484, University of Puerto Rico Station
Rio Piedras, PR 00931
(809) 758-2525

Rhode Island Assistive Technology Access Project
Office of Rehabilitation Services
40 Fountain Street
Province, RI 02903-1898
(401) 421-7005

South Carolina Assistive Technology Program
Vocational Rehabilitation Department
P.O. Box 15, 1410-C Boston Avenue
West Columbia, SC 29171-0015
(803) 822-5404

Dakota Link
1925 Plaza Boulevard
Rapid City, SD 57702
(800) 645-0673

Tennessee Technology Access Project
710 James Robertson Parkway
Gateway Plaza, 11th Floor
Nashville, TN 3723-0675
(615) 532-6530

Texas Assistive Technology Project
University of Texas at Austin
UAP of Texas
Department of Special Education, EDB 306
Austin, Texas 78712
(512) 471-7621

Utah Assistive Technology Program
Center for Persons with Disabilities
UMC 6855
Logan, UT 84322-6855
(800) 333-UTAH

Vermont Assistive Technology Project
103 South Main Street, Weeks 1
Waterbury, VT 05671-2305
(802) 241-2620

Virginia Assistive Technology System
8004 Franklin Farms Drive
P.O. Box K300
Richmond, VA 23288–0300
(804) 662-9993

Washington Assistive Technology Alliance DSHS/DVR
P.O. Box 45340
Olympia, WA 98504-5340
(206) 438-8049

West Virginia Assistive Technology System
Division of Rehabilitation Services
Capital Complex
Charleston, WV 25305-0890
(800) 841-8436

Wistech
Division of Vocational Rehabilitation
P.O. Box 7852
1 West Wilson Street, Room 950
Madison, WI 53707-7852
(608) 266-5395

Wyoming's New Options in Technology (WYNOT)
Division of Vocational Rehabilitation
1100 Herschler Building
Cheyenne, WY 82002
(307) 777-6947

American Samoa Assistive Technology Project
Division of Vocational Rehabilitation
Department of Human Resources
Pago Pago, American Somoa 96799
(684) 633-2336

PUBLICATIONS

JOURNALS AND NEWSLETTERS

Accent on Living
Bloomington, IL
(309) 378-2961
Quarterly

American Journal of Occupational Therapy (AJOT)
American Occupational Therapy Association
Monthly

Augmentative Communication News
One Surf Way, Suite 215
Monterey, CA 93940
(408) 649-3050
Bimonthly

Assistive Technology
1700 N. Moore Street, Suite 1540
Arlington, VA 22209
Published by RESNA twice a year (1989-)

Beginner's Guide to Personal Computers for the Blind
  and Visually Impaired
National Braille Press
88 Stephen Street
Boston, MA 02115
(617) 266-6160

Careers and the Disabled
Equal Opportunity Publications, Inc.
150 Motor Parkway, Suite 420
Happauge, NY 11788
Published 3 times a year

Closing the Gap (newsletter)
P.O. Box 68
Henderson, MN 56044
(612) 248-3294

Computer Resources for People with Disabilities
The Alliance for Technology Access
Hunter House Publishing, 1994
CRT News Update
Center for Rehabilitation Technology
Georgia Institute of Technology
Atlanta, GA 30332-0156

Exceptional Parent: Parenting Your Child with
  a Disability
P.O. Box 3000, Department EP
Denville, NJ 07834

The Guide to Augmentative and Alternative
  Communication Devices (1996 Edition)
Rehabilitation Engineering Research Center on
  AAC Applied Science and Engineering Labs
University of Delaware/A.I. duPont Institute
P.O. Box 269, 1600 Rockland Road
Wilmington, DE 19899

IEEE Transactions in Rehabilitation Engineering
IEEE Headquarters
345 East 47th Street
New York, NY 10017-2394
Quarterly

Independent Living
Equal Opportunity Publications, Inc.
150 Motor Parkway, Suite 420
Happauge, NY 11788
Published 3 times a year

International Journal of Rehabilitation Research
Schindale (publishers)
Heidelberg, Germany
Quarterly (March 1991-)

Journal of Rehabilitation Research and Development
Rehabilitation Research and Development Services
Department of Veterans Affairs
103 South Gay Street
Baltimore, MD 21202-4051
(301) 962-0850
Quarterly (Spring 1990-)

Occupational Therapy Journal of Research
Slack, Inc.
6900 Grove Road
Thorofare, NJ 08086-9447
Quarterly (1981-)

OT Newsletter Special Interest Sections
Technology, Physical Dysfunction,
    Developmental Disabilities
American Occupational Therapy Association
Quarterly

Paraplegia News
Paralyzed Veterans of America (PVA)
5201 North 19th Avenue, Suite 111
Phoenix, AZ 85015
(602) 246-9426

Proceedings, RESNA Annual Conferences
RESNA
1700 N. Moore Street, Suite 1540
Arlington, VA 22209
(703) 524-6686
(703) 524-6630 (fax)
Annual (1980-)

Team Rehab Report for Professionals in
    Assistive Technology
P.O. Box 8987
23815 Stuart Ranch Road
Malibu, CA 90265
(310) 317-4522
Monthly

Technology and Disabilities
Elsevier Science Ireland Ltd.
Bay 15
Shannon Industrial Estate Co.
Claire, Ireland
(35) 361-471944

BOOKS

Access to Information: Materials, Technologies, and
    Services for Print-Impaired Readers
Tom McNulty and Dawn M. Suvino
American Library Association, Chicago, IL 1993

The Accessible Housing Design File:
    Barrier Free Environments
Ronald L. Mace
New York: Van Nostrand Reinhold, 1991

Assistive Technologies: Principles and Practice
Albert M. Cook and Susan M. Hussey
St. Louis, MO: Mosby, 1995

Assistive Technology: A Resource for School, Work,
    and Community
Karen F. Flippo, Katherine J. Inge, and
    J. Michael Barcus (eds)
Baltimore, MD: Paul H Brookes, 1995

Assistive Technology for Persons with Disabilities
    (2nd Ed)
William C. Mann and Joseph P. Lane
Rockville, MD: American Occupational Therapy
    Association, Inc, 1995

Assistive Technology for Rehabilitation Therapists
Jennifer Angelo
Philadelphia: FA Davis Co, 1997

Assistive Technology Sourcebook
Alexandra Enders and Marian Hall (eds)
Arlington, VA: RESNA Press, 1990

Control of Computer-Based Technology for People
    with Physical Disabilities: An Assessment Manual
K. Lee and D. Thomas
Toronto: University of Toronto Press, 1990

Disabled Village Children
David Werner
Palo Alto, CA: The Hesperian Foundation, 1988

Electronic Devices for Rehabilitation
J. Webster, A. Cook, W. Tompkins, and
    G. Vanderheiden (eds)
New York: John Wiley, 1985

Evaluating, Selecting, and Using Appropriate
    Assistive Technology
Jan C. Galvin and Marcia J. Scherer
Gaithersburg, MD: Aspen Publishers, 1996

From Toys to Computers: Access for the Physically
    Disabled Child
Christian Wright and Marie Nomura
San Jose, CA, 1991

The Handbook of Assistive Technology
Gregory Church and Sharon Glennen
San Diego, CA: Singular Publishing Group, 1992

Living in the State of Stuck (2nd Ed)
Marcia J. Scherer
Webster, NY: Brookline Books, 1996

Lifespace Access Profile: Assistive Technology
    Planning for Individuals with Severe or
    Multiple Disabilities
W. Williams, G. Stemach, S. Wolfe, and C. Stanger
Sebastopol, CA: Lifespace Access, 1993

Orthotics: Clinical Practice and
    Rehabilitation Technology
John B. Redford, John V. Basmajian, and
    Paul Trautman (eds)
New York: Churchill Livingstone, 1995

The Resource Guide for the Disabled
Gayle Backstrom
Dallas, TX: Taylor Publishing Co, 1994

Trace Resource Book: Assistive Technologies for
    Communication, Control, and Computer Access
    (1996-1997 Ed)
Trace Research and Development Center
Madison, WI: University of Wisconsin, 1996

Selected Readings on Powered Mobility for Children
    and Adults with Severe Physical Disabilities
RESNA
Arlington, VA: RESNA Press, 1986

Selection and Use of Simple Technology in Home,
    School, Work, and Community
J. Lewin and L. Scherfenberg
Minneapolis, MN: Ablenet, 1990

Technology and Aging in America
Congress of the United States
Office of Technology Assessment
Washington, DC: U.S. Government Printing Office,
    1985

The Workplace Workbook
James Mueller
Washington, DC: The Dole Foundation, 1992

Selected Resources for Computer Use in Schools

Alliance for Technology Access: Computer Resources
  for People with Disabilities (2nd ed)
Alameda, CA: Hunter House, Inc, 1996

*Written for parents, consumers, and professionals, this
guide presents a process for readers to follow in selecting
the assistive technology tools that will meet their specific
needs. Informative section on selecting access methods*

Closing the Gap: Annual Resource Directory
Henderson, MN: Closing the gap

*A comprehensive and up-to-date listing of numerous
products—hardware, software, peripherals, and augmentative and alternative communication aids—with brief
descriptions, prices, and vendor information*

Exceptional Parent. 13th Annual Technology Issue
25(11), November 1995

*Each Annual Technology Issue is filled with helpful
resources and personal stories about how assistive technology is changing the lives of children with disabilities*

Learning and Leading with Technology The Journal
  of the International Society for Technology in
  Education (ISTE)

*This journal for technology-using educators publishes
successful uses of computers in schools, often arranged
by subject area*

Male M: Technology for Inclusion: Meeting the
  Special Needs of All Students. Boston, MA: Allyn
  and Bacon, 1994

*With a third edition about to be published, this is the best
text available on integrating computers into the curriculum in schools*

ATD MANUFACTURERS
AUGMENTATIVE AND ALTERNATIVE COMMUNICATION DEVICES

Don Johnston Development Equipment, Inc.
P.O. Box 639
Wauconda, IL 60084

Mayer-Johnson Co.
P.O. Box 1579
Solana Beach, CA 92075

Prentke Romich Co.
1022 Heyl Road
Wooster, OH 44691
Sentient Systems Technology, Inc.
2100 Wharton Street
Pittsburgh, Pa 15203

Technical Aids and Systems for the Handicapped, Inc.
   (TASH)
Unit 1, 91 Station Street
Ajax, Ontario L1S 3H2 Canada

Words +, Inc.
P.O. Box 1229
Lancaster, CA 93535

Zygo Industries, Inc.
P.O. Box 1008
Portland, OR 97207

ENVIRONMENTAL CONTROL UNITS

ACS Technologies, Inc.
(800) 227-2922

APT Technology Inc. (formerly Du-It)
Shreve, OH
(216) 567-2001

Crestwood Co.
Milwaukee, WI
(414) 352-5678

Don Johnston, Inc.
Wauconda, IL
(800) 999-4660

Prentke Romich Co.
Wooster, OH
(800) 642-8255

Quartet Technology, Inc.
Tyngsboro, MA
(508) 692-9313

Radio Shack (Tandy)
Fort Worth, TX
(817) 390-3011

TASH, Inc.
Ajax, Ontario, Canada
(800) 463-5685

Teledyne Brown Engineering
(800) 944-8002

X–10 (USA), Inc.
Closter, NJ
(201) 784-9700

X-10 LTD
Hong Kong
(852) 344-6848

COMPUTERS

Apple Computer Resources in Special Education
    and Rehabilitation
DLM Teaching Resources, Inc.
Allen, TX 75002

Beginner's Guide to Personal Computers for the Blind
    and Visually Impaired
National Braille Press
Boston, MA 02115

COMPUTER TRAINING AND JOB PLACEMENT PROGRAM

Lift, Inc.
P.O. Box 1072
Mountainside, New Jersey 07092
(908) 789-2443

MAJOR COMPUTER MANUFACTURERS

Apple Macintosh Special Needs
(408) 974-7910

Don Johnston, Inc.
(800) 999-4660

Dragon (Dictate) Systems Inc.
(617) 965-5200

IBM Special Needs Center
(800) 426-4832

IntelliTools, Inc.
(800) 899-6687

Madenta Communications, Inc.
(403) 450-8926

Microsystems Software, Inc.
(800) 828-2600

Words+, Inc.
(800) 869-8521

SOFTWARE PUBLISHERS AND ASSISTIVE DEVICE MANUFACTURERS

Apple/Macintosh
(800) 600-7808 or (408) 974-7910
Educational and special needs programs

Broderbund Software
(800) 521-6263
Living Books Series. School editions include helpful
    teacher's guides

Claris Corporation
(800) 325-2747
ClarisWorks

Davidson and Associates, Inc.
(800) 545-7677
Spell It 3, Math Blaster Plus

Don Johnston Developmental Equipment,
(800) 999-4660
Ke:nx, Co:Writer, Write: OutLoud, and other easy-to-
    use access products and special software

Dragon Systems
(617) 965-5200
DragonDictate

Edmark Corporation
(800) 426-0856
The Imagination Express series; Destinations:
    Rain Forest, Neighborhood, Ocean, Pyramids,
    Time Trip USA
Early Learning series: Millie's Math House, Bailey's
    Book House, Sammy's Science House, Thinkin'
    Things 1, Trudi's Time and Place House, Stanley's
    Sticker Stories
School editions include helpful teacher's guides

Educational Resources
(800) 624-2926
Excellent selection and discount prices on
    educational software

IBM; Independence Series Products
(800) 426-2133
Speech Viewer II—speech modification/therapy program
Thinkable/DOS—attention and memory program
Screen Reader—text-to-speech conversion

Inspiration Software (available from Educational
    Resources)
(800) 624-2926
Inspiration—a "brain storming" and project planning
    program

IntelliTools
(800) 899-6687
IntelliKeys, customizing software for all platforms,
    and special software. Overlay packages for popular
    Edmark and Broderbund software programs

In Touch Systems
(914) 354-7431
Magic Wand mini keyboard

Laureate Learning Systems
(800) 562-6801
Software for language development

The Learning Company
(800) 852-2255
The Writing Center, The Reader Rabbit series

McIntyre Computer Systems,
(810) 645-5090
Wordwriter (on-screen keyboard)

MECC
(612) 569-1500
Storybook Weaver Deluxe, a popular story writing
    program
"Trail" series: Oregon Trail, Yukon Trail, Amazon Trail,
    Africa Trail
Many innovative educational software programs,
    especially learning adventures, problem-solving
    journeys, and creative writing tools

Prentke Romich
(800) 262-1984
HeadMaster

Roger Wagner Publishing
(800) 421-6526
HyperStudio—multimedia presentation software

MAJOR MANUFACTURERS OF POWERED WHEELCHAIRS

Everest and Jennings
St. Louis, MO
(800) 235-4661

Invacare
Elyria, OH
(800) 333-6900

LA BAC System
Lakewood, CO
(303) 914-9914

Permobil
Woburn, MA
(617) 932-9009

Quickie
Fresno, CA
(800) 456-8165

ROBOTICS

Kinetic Rehabilitation Instruments, Inc.
155 Webster Street, Suite J
Hanover, MA 02339
(800) 244-8882
The "Helping Hand" Robotic Arm

Glossary

Abbreviation expansion: a computer short-hand feature.

AccessDOS: includes StickyKeys, MouseKeys, ToggleKeys (which indicates the on/off status of CAPS LOCK, NUM LOCK, and SCROLL LOCK).

AC/DC: abbreviation for alternating current/direct current; equipment able to operate on either type of current supply: either AC power lines using a transformer or low-voltage DC (e.g., car battery).

Adjustable keyboard responses: enhancements that can adjust the response of the keyboard, timing, accept time of a key press, adjustments, a program until pressure is released.

Alternate keyboards: displayed on a separate monitor usually do not resemble the standard QWERTY keyboard but are arranged for efficiency when using the intended input device. Alternate keyboards usually require the use of a separate hardware unit to interface between the keyboard and the serial port, but newer models are capable of direct attachment to the keyboard port.

Alternate mouse emulators: alternative methods for achieving mouse emulation functions.

Alternating current (AC): electricity that flows in a circuit, first in one direction and then in reverse at regularly recurring intervals, many times per second at a constant rate. AC is used to denote the current supplied via power lines.

Ampere: measure of strength of electric current indicating the rate of electron flow.

Anode: the positive pole of an electron tube or battery (+) that attracts negatively charged (–) ions.

Arm supports: table-mounted devices that offer an articulated resting surface for the forearm. Similar to wrist supports.

Assessment: the instrument or means of gathering data from specific testing procedures.

Assistive technology device: any item, piece of equipment, or product system, whether acquired commercially off-the-shelf, modified, or customized, that is used to increase, maintain, or improve functional capabilities of individuals with disabilities (from the Technology Related Assistance Act of 1988).

Atom: the smallest particle of an element containing a positively charged nucleus made up of protons and neutrons and negatively charged electrons in their surrounding orbits.

Battery: a device that converts chemical energy into electrical energy composed of two or more electrical cells connected together. It is used as a source of portable power to operate electrical/electronic devices.

Baud: unit of the rate of serial transmission of digital signals along a pair of wires.

Cable: an insulated wire or set of insulated wires bound together in an overall covering.

Caretaker or careprovider or assistant: Any person(s) who assist the consumer in any or all activities of daily living.

Cathode: the negative pole (–) of an electron tube or battery that attracts positively charged (+) ions.

Cathode-ray tube (CRT): an electron beam display device used in instrument tubes (e.g., oscilloscopes) and picture tubes (e.g., television and radar).

Cell: any device that has an electric output, often joined to make batteries for supplying higher voltages. A photocell is a light-sensitive cell that provides voltage output when illuminated.

Charge: particles of the atom carry electric charge. Protons inside the nucleus carry a positive charge; electrons are negatively charged. When electrons balance protons, the atom itself has no overall charge. If any electrons (negative charge) move away from the atom, the atom is left positively charged. If more electrons are gained by the atom, it becomes negatively charged. Positive and negative charges attract each other, but like charges repel.

Chip: small slice from a semiconductor wafer on which a transistor or integrated circuit is fabricated.

Circuit: circular path through which electric current moves from the source through wires and appliances and back again to the source (generator or battery). A complete circuit contains (1) conductors, (2) switch, (3) load, and (4) electrical source. An open circuit is one with a physical break in the path (caused by opening a switch, disconnecting a wire, or burning out a fuse), through which no current can flow.

Circuit breaker: a form of overload switch that interrupts or breaks the circuit when excessive current is flowing or when a voltage surge occurs. An electromagnetic or thermal device interrupts the circuit when current exceeds a predetermined amount. It is akin to the fuse but reusable (e.g., manually reset).

Computer-based augmentative communication systems: software programs that can be loaded into fixed or portable laptop computers. Computer-based programs provide the user with the flexibility to use the same system for multiple uses, including communication, word processing/desktop publishing, environmental control, and information gathering on the internet. The use of a computer-based augmentative system permits both augmented verbal and written communication.

Conduction: transmission of energy by particle movement. Electrical conduction in metal is usually the result of the movement of free electrons. Conduction in gases and liquids is by movement of ions.

Conductor: a low-resistance material that allows electric current to travel easily. Copper and silver are good carriers of electricity.

Consumer or client or user: any individual who uses technology to increase, maintain, or improve their function.

Contoured: a surface that has a generic contour.

Control site: the body part that is used to activate a switch.

Cumulative trauma disorders (CTD): disorders of the muscles, tendons, peripheral nerves, or vascular system that are the result of mechanical factors such as excessive force, repeated or sustained exertions, vibration, or cold, among others. Also known as repetitive motion injuries, repetitive stress injuries, or overuse injuries.

Current: the movement or flow of electrons through a circuit, measured in amperes.

Dedicated communication device: assistive technology device designed for the single purpose of substituting for verbal speech production. Dedicated communication devices can range from simple, providing just a few choices with limited vocabulary, to complex programmable devices with liquid crystal displays and multiple connecting levels with access to a vast stored dictionary of vocabulary.

Direct current (DC): electricity that flows through a conductor or circuit in only one direction, such as in a battery.

Direct selection: a method of accessing an augmentative and alternative communication aid by activating a single space or individual key on either a membrane or computer keyboard. Direct selection can also be accomplished by touching a defined area on the surface of a liquid crystal display or on a touch-sensitive window mounted directly over a computer screen. Automatic repeat feature of individual keys is available. Computer-based augmentative system users may also take advantage of alternative keyboards. These include enlarged keyboard designs, miniature keyboards for users with adequate pointing skills within a decreased range of mobility, numeric keyboards, and modified keyboard arrangements in an alphabetical or frequency of occurrence organization instead of a standard QWERTY pattern.

Directional crossovers and extensions: when a driver is unable to access the directional signal with the left upper extremity secondary to decreased function, adaptation must be provided for actuation. The unit is attached to the existing activator, extends over the steering column and relocates the directional to the right. If function is present in the left and access is marginally denied, an extension can be added to the existing actuator. This type of unit can also be used in cases in which the left knee will activate the directional. When a person is unable to access the gear selector secondary to decreased function in the right upper extremity, a crossover or extension can be incorporated with the existing actuator.

Driver rehabilitation programs: medically oriented programs based on the medical requirement and necessity to remain independent in mobility. Referral into a program is done by prescription of a physician of any specialty. A program can consist of several progressions including predriver or clinical assessment, simulation, behind-the-wheel training, driver rehabilitation/training, licensure issues, prescription development, transportation alternatives, and follow-up services.

Dry cell: a combination of different metals in a chemical solution that produces electricity that is stored in a leakproof container; a type of battery.

Electricity: an invisible force that can produce heat, light, motion, and other physical effects. The force is due to an attraction or repulsion between electric charges.

Electrolyte: a solution that conducts (through which electricity can flow) due to the presence of charged particles or ions (e.g., water).

Electromagnetic: fields formed by the interaction of electric and magnetic fields. These are part of the spectrum that furnishes the basis for radio, television, radar, X-rays, infrared and ultraviolet frequencies, etc.

Electromagnetism: magnetic field caused by electric currents; commonly by passage of electric current through a coil of insulated wire wrapped around a soft iron core.

Electron: part of an atom having a negative charge (–) that orbits the nucleus.

Electronic mail (e-mail): messages are typed into a computer and sent to a receiving monitor by telephone lines.

Electronics: the science or study of controlling electrons in motion, or applications of the electron. Generally refers to complex devices such as radio, television, and computers; the circuits and devices of a piece of electronic equipment.

Electrostatic force: the push and pull of electrical charges of particles that tend to hold electrons in orbit around the nucleus.

Emulators: external devices and/or software programs that provide an alternate method for input of character selection.

Encoding methods: use of code or shorthand commands to send signal to the computer (e.g., Morse code or voice recognition technology).

Enhancements: usually software programs that provide a special function making character entry and/or the use of a computer easier and/or more efficient.

Enlarged character imagery: the size of text presented on the monitor can be magnified from 2 to 12 times normal size through specialized programs sold separately or as a feature of other specialized applications.

Enlarged keyboards: a large keyboard, of up to 24 × 18 in., that is used to enable easier access for individuals with visual or motor control deficits.

Environment: physical, sensory, and psychological surroundings in which the consumer may use assistive devices including bed, home, school, workplace, and community. The physical environment also refers to levels conditions of terrain, weather conditions, distances, etc. The sensory environment refers to light, temperature, and noise. The psychological environment refers to the atmosphere or mood such as pleasant or hostile, cooperative, organized or disorganized, etc.

Evaluation: a composite picture of the technology system; the sum of all assessment procedures.

Facsimile (fax): instant delivery of a document over phone lines. An individual inserts a paper, form, or document into a machine and a copy of that item goes to the chosen destination over telephone lines. No one needs to be on the receiving end while transmitting the fax; the copy can be picked up at a later time.

Feedback or display: the response to the input-throughput-output that reports to the user that the assistive technology device is activated by a light, sound, motion, etc. Sometimes, the feedback may also be the output (e.g., motion of the wheelchair or the light going on/off of an environmental control unit or the monitor of a computer).

Fixed deficits: structural limitations or deformities in joint range or over a bony area that limit the client's ability to achieve a posture or interface with a standard support surface.

Fuse: a protective device that acts as a safety factor. It consists of a metal wire with a low melting point. Excessive current (e.g., that exceeds the ampere rating of the fuse) flowing through the fuse will melt the metal and break the circuit.

Generator: a machine or dynamo that produces electricity from mechanical energy. A generator consists of a rotating coil (rotor) and a magnetic field (stator).

Graphic-based augmentative communication programs: all-purpose graphic program that allows a direct selection user to type text and have it synthetically voiced. Many programs also contain a menu of preprogrammed words and phrases that can be "quick voiced" with a single keystroke even as additional text is being typed. Additional "quick voice" phrases can be customized to suit the needs of an individual user. Graphic-based programs are also accessible via scanning.

Grasp enhancers: a grasp enhancer such as a keybar has been designed to assist those unable to manipulate a control due to lack of reliable grip, decreased active range of motion, or impaired fine motor coordination. These devices can be made of many different materials with the most common being wood, metals, and plastics. They include off-the-shelf and devices customized to meet the needs of a consumer. Many devices are modified and/or created in the occupational therapy clinic or by a rehabilitation engineer. In relation to driving, these devices are most often used to facilitate key manipulation. This can include unlocking and locking doors, key box control centers, or in ignition activation. The devices can eliminate the need for costly high-tech adaptations for both cars and vans.

Ground: an electrical connection between a circuit and the earth, or between a circuit and some metal object that substitutes for the earth.

Hand controls: automobile adaptations used to provide access to automobile controls for drivers with disabilities. These include spinner knob (most commonly used); single post grip; V-grip, bi-pin, or quad yoke; tri-pin; Sierra driving ring; palm-grip; splints; and orthotics. Mechanical hand controls are used when a person is not able to use either lower extremity for efficient acceleration and braking function. Different types of hand controls are push/pull hand controls; push/pull right angle controls; push/twist controls; push/lever pull down controls; and floor mount push/pull controls.

Hard drive system: the internal data storage capability of a computer.

Iconic augmentative and alternative communications systems: picture representations used on communication systems with both picture-producing (e.g., apple, bed, sun) and non-picture-producing vocabulary (e.g., happy, gentle). The ability to recognize a picture symbol and assign meaning to it requires life and social experience within a culture, familiarity with signs and symbols, cognitive skill including the ability to make within-class associations, a learning process, and the absence of any significant visual impairment.

Identifier: the person or persons who notice that a person is having a problem with a task and believes that assistive technology might provide a solution.

Inhibit: to stop or circumvent an activity.

Input or control interface or switch or signal or transducer: a device or process that activates any electronic instrument/device such as assistive technology devices: details in switch section (e.g., light switch, joystick, pneumatic transducer [sip and puff], a keyboard of a computer).

Insulator: any material that does not allow electricity to pass freely; a poor conductor of electricity also known as a nonconductor. Used to separate conductors and prevent electric flow between them, such as the rubber coating on a cable.

Integrated circuit (IC): a circuit constructed on a silicon chip that has high reliability and low cost.

Integration: a single input device that can interface with and control several assistive technology devices.

Ion: a particle with a charge (negative or positive) that results from an electron being added to or lost from a neutral atom.

Key latching/locking: a mechanical keyboard assist that works to block an individual key (usually shift).

Keyboard assists: usually hardware additions to the computer system that will make the process of character entry easier for the individual.

Keyboard holding devices: adjustable platforms that have been designed to maintain a keyboard in an alternate static position when the height or angle of the table surface is not adequate for the user.

Keyguards: a lightweight plastic cutout overlay that fits over a computer or membrane keyboard isolating each individual key. This can help to increase the precision of direct selection and eliminate accidental keystrokes to neighboring keys adjacent to the target.

Kilowatt: the measure of large quantities of electric power; 1 kW = 1,000 W.

Latching switch: a method of maintaining the activation of a device in which it remains on until it is activated again (e.g., a wall light switch).

Light pen: alternative method of interfacing with the computer using a light pen to direct the movements of the cursor. Photocell mounted on a pen holder used in conjunction with a computer program to write or select on the monitor screen; an input device.

Lines of force: electric or magnetic field direction; invisible lines of force running from one pole of a magnet to the other forming the magnetic field.

Load: the device in a circuit that is operated by the current through the circuit (e.g., light bulb, radio).

Lodestone: a naturally magnetic iron ore also known as magnetite.

Macro: computer application program that automates a sequence of commands or phrases that are frequently used in the smallest number of keystrokes.

Magnet: a substance, either natural or synthetic, that has the power to attract materials such as iron, nickel, steel, or cobalt.

Magnetism: a property or phenomenon involving attraction and repulsion.

Mechanical key locking/latching devices: hardware devices that through a lever or spring-loading mechanism will hold down a specific key (usually the shift key) until released.

Mini keyboards: small keyboards, accessed by finger, mouthstick, or wand. They have an average "foot-print" of approximately 8 × 8 in., and are useful for people with a small functional "work-window" or constrained work space.

Modem: acronym for modulator-demodulator. A device used to convert digital signals into form for long-distance transmission and to reconvert transmitted signals. It is widely used for linking computers over telephone lines.

Molded: a surface that has been created from an exact image of the person's surface contours.

Molecule: two or more atoms that have bonded together; the smallest part of a compound or mixture that can be identified as that compound.

Momentary switch: the device is activated as long as pressure is applied, when the pressure is released, the device is no longer activated (e.g., a car horn).

Monitor: the video display terminal or "screen" of the computer.

Mouse emulators: devices that assist keyboard access by imitating the drag and click functions of a mouse (e.g., trackballs and rollerballs).

Mouse keys: mouse functions can be controlled through the keys of the numeric keypad.

Neutron: A part of the nucleus of an atom that has no electrical charge.

Nicad: a nickel-cadmium cell or battery (rechargeable form of alkaline electrolyte cell) used as a power source in portable equipment.

Normalize: to bring into conformity with an established norm or standard.

Nucleus: the center of an atom composed of neutrons and protons.

Ohm: a measure of resistance in an electrical circuit. One ohm of resistance is present when 1 V of electromotive force causes 1 A of current to flow in an electric circuit.

Optical character reader (OCR): a device that scans printed characters and provides digital output to a computer.

Output or peripheral: a device that receives and processes a command from the throughput and produces a product or response. Some examples might include the movement of a powered wheelchair when activated by a joystick; a light being turned on by environmental control unit activation that sends a signal to a lamp; printing hard copy by selecting the print option on the computer screen.

Overload: current demand exceeding the suggested limits of the circuit or equipment.

Parallel circuit: a circuit for which two or more components are directly connected to the source of electricity. There is more than one path for electrons to pass through the circuit.

Peripheral keyboards: alternate keyboards that may have different types of input devices. These include row-column and step scan methods that can be operated with a variety of switches, including sip-and-puff or light pointers.

Planar: flat surface, or surface that appears flat.

Plug: a male connector for linking signals or power (e.g., a device on a flexible cord inserted into a receptacle). A polarized plug has prongs that are designed to enter the receptacle in only one orientation.

Pop-up utilities: software applications, commercial and/or specialized, that permit the user to access and dial telephone numbers, use a calculator, take messages and notes in a separate window.

Postural support: cushioning devices used to establish proper posture and optimal control for an individual to perform a task.

Power-assisted driving controls (PAC): digital controls used to access an automobile.

Predicted words: a feature in which the computer seems to anticipate the user's next word.

Proportional switch: the device is gradually activated and responds according to the amount of pressure applied to the switch; e.g., slow starting motor of a powered wheelchair.

Proton: a stable, positively charged particle in the nucleus of an atom.

Receptacle: an outlet set into a wall or baseboard used to connect appliances to the wiring system. It contains a live lead wire from a fuse box or circuit breaker and a return wire.

Rectifier: a device that allows alternating current to flow in only one direction; in electron tubes or solid state devices, rectifiers change AC to DC.

Relay: an electromechanical switch. Current flowing through coils causes a magnetic field, which in turn attracts an armature. The movement of the armature opens or closes the switch contacts.

Resistance: the tendency of a conductor to inhibit the flow of current or the degree of opposition to electron conduction of any wire or circuit measured in units called ohms. Conductors, such as copper and aluminum, offer little resistance. Glass, wood, and other poor conductors offer more resistance.

Rollerballs: alternate graphical interface for the computer, similar to a trackball that is manipulated to move the cursor on a computer screen.

Scanning: for physically challenged individuals, scanning is the optimal mode for access to either a dedicated or nondedicated augmentative system. A single switch activated by a reliable body movement (i.e., head, hand, foot, elbow, knee, eye gaze, eyebrow or facial movement, etc.) is connected to the corresponding port of a dedicated device or via interface to a computer-based system. Scanning may be manual or automatic. In automatic scanning, a light (dedicated device) or cursor (computer-based system) typically moves in a row-column display. Switch activation stops the scanner and identifies the selection. Scanning speed and patterns can often be modified to fit the needs of an individual user. Manual scanning involves user control of the scanning light or cursor. Each switch activation moves the scanner toward the intended target. Manual scanning extends response time even more significantly than in automatic scanning but is often optimal for younger consumers with cognitive impairments and/or multiple disabilities.

Scanning assistive technology for drivers: devices used to increase the visual field for a driver. The strategic placement of auxiliary mirrors can allow the operator visual access to blind spots to the front, rear, and sides of the vehicle.

Schematic diagram: a drawing of an electrical or electronic device that uses symbols for each component.

Semiconductor: a material, such as silicon or germanium, whose conductivity can be controlled by the presence of impurities. These materials may act as good conductors under certain conditions and poor conductors under others.

Sensor: a device that detects changes (e.g., in light, temperature, strain, or rotation) and transmits change as an electrical signal.

Series circuit: a circuit in which current flows through all parts and back to its source via one path.

Short circuit: an event that occurs when two wires make contact (either bare or lacking insulation). The result is an overload on the circuit (delivering too much current).

Silicon: a nonmetallic element in crystal form that is a semiconductor; used in the manufacture of transistors and integrated circuits.

Socket: a device that holds a light bulb and connects it to the household wiring or electrical current; a female connector.

Software compatibility: ensuring that different types of computer programs (word processing, spread sheet, etc.) or specific application programs will work together in a single or linked computer system.

Solar cell: an electric generator made of silicon; a device that uses radiant energy from the sun to produce electric current.

Solid state: a device that has no moving parts or tubes; the term used to describe transistors and integrated circuits.

Spark: an electric discharge.

Spectrum: a range of frequencies or wavelengths; consists of all electromagnetic waves.

Static electricity: when certain materials are rubbed together, electrons move from one material to the other. The substance losing electrons becomes positively charged while the substance gaining electrons gets a negative charge. As opposite charges attract, the materials "stick" together. Once the electrons have built up on one material, they do not flow and therefore become "static." If the buildup of electrons is great enough, they may leap across to the positively charged material as a spark. Static electricity is then discharged. It is a form of electricity in which electrons are at rest or not flowing as a current.

Steering assistive devices: devices to ensure adequate steering function for individuals with singular upper extremity impairment. These devices, operated by using the unaffected limb, allow for the completion of steering sequences without a break from contact with the steering wheel. Positioning the device on the wheel will be determined by the limb to be used and comfort zone of the individual. Steering devices are quite often used in conjunction with hand controls.

Supine: lying on the back with the face up.

Switch: a component used to either open or close the path for electron flow in a circuit. When the switch is off, an open circuit exists and the current will not flow. Conversely, a switch in the "on" position will close the circuit and permit current flow. A method for making, breaking, or changing electrical connections.

Synthesized speech: sounds artificially generated by a voice synthesizer.

Technological devices or assistive technology devices or technological aids: in this manual, refers to powered mobility aids such as powered wheelchairs, augmentative communication devices such as a speech synthesizer, environmental control systems such as a remote control to turn on a light, adapted/modified computers. Not included are electronic devices such as pacemakers, diaphragm pacers, and ventilators.

Telecommunication device for the deaf (TDD):   TDDs type out messages on an illuminated light-emitting diode (LED) display screen. They operate in Baudot code. Baudot code operates in a slow transmission and receiving rate. TDDs cannot communicate directly with computers which communicate in ASCII code. These codes are not compatible. To operate the TDD, the user places the handset of a phone on the acoustic modem cups (no special telephone is necessary). Once the individual gets a steady glowing light (which is the dial tone), he or she may then dial the desired telephone number. The visual light indicator will blink for each ring or blink rapidly in succession for a busy signal. Once the desired party answers the phone, the caller and callee may have a conversation using the TDD keyboard to type in the messages. The user can see what the other person is saying/typing on his or her LED display screen. This device enables a deaf or severely hearing-impaired individual to hold a phone conversation with another deaf or hearing individual.

Throughput or processor: receives a signal from the input and processes the command, which activates the assistive technology device (e.g., the central processing unit of a computer or the battery of the powered wheelchair or the house current of an environmental control unit).

Touch screens: alternate graphic interface for the computer in which the screen is touched to activate and manipulate a software program.

Tone: the normal degree of tension and vigor in muscle, the slight continuous contraction of muscle, which in skeletal muscles aids in the maintenance of posture and the return of blood to the heart.

Trackballs: alternate graphic interfaces similar to a mouse in which a ball is rotated to position the cursor on the computer screen. They may take different shapes, and the click and drag button(s) may be located in different positions.

Transformer: an electrical device that changes voltage of electrical alternating current (e.g., raises or lowers the current).

Transistor: a small, solid-state device designed to replace the electron tube. This semiconductor amplifies electrical signals.

Turbine: a fanlike device or engine operates by steam or water power used to turn electrical generators.

Underwriter's label (UL label):   a label applied to manufactured devices that have been tested for safety and approved by the Underwriters' Laboratories.

Unilever driving systems: commonly known as joystick-operated systems, acceleration, braking, and steering functions are all accessed through the activation of one lever or, in one system, small-diameter wheel. Left and right movement controls steering, forward acceleration, and backward braking in most applications.

Unmouse: a graphic tablet through which the user can control the selection pointer on the monitor with the movement of a finger or metal pen.

Video conferencing: simultaneous transmission of video and audio signals between two offices, corporations, or businesses for communication purposes. The users see and hear the person/people they are conducting business with as if they were actually holding a meeting or conference in person instead of at a distance.

Visual cues for "warning beeps":   for individuals with hearing impairments, several companies offer visual cues (a flashing symbol or screen flashing) to substitute for the normal warning beeps of the computer.

Voice recognition: technology that uses the voice to access a computer and make commands for the operation of software and hardware.

Voltage: the measure of electrical pressure (electromagnetic force [EMF] measured in the unit, volt) or the potential difference between two points in an electrical circuit or electricity-producing device.

Voltage drop: the loss of electric current caused by overloading wires, usually indicated by the dimming of lights and the slowing of motors.

Watt: a measurement unit of electrical power (or wattage); volts times amperes equals watts of electric energy used.

Wet cell: a device that produces electricity from the reaction of liquid chemicals; a type of battery.

Windows: window types of applications require the use of mouse emulating functions to access different computer software.

Word prediction: artificial intelligence in which the computer anticipates the next word choice to reduce the number of required keystrokes. The word prediction software dictionary can be customized over time to be the most responsive to an individual user. Abbreviation/expansion programs allow a user to type in a standardized or customized abbreviation for frequently used vocabulary. The computer recognizes the abbreviation and types in the complete word.

Wrist rests: positioning devices, usually static, that support the wrist during typing.

Index

Page numbers followed by *f* indicate figures; page numbers followed by *t* indicate tables.

Graphic-based augmentative communication programs
    compared to iconic representations, 103–104
    definition of, 103–104
Graphic tablets, 153
Grasp enhancers, 155, 212, 329
Grounding, electrical, 54–55, 329

H

Hand controls
    advantages of, 219
    definition of, 330
    floor mount push/pull, 218–219
    push/level pull down, 218
    push/pull, 217
    push/pull right-angle, 217, 218f
    push/twist, 217–218
    types of, 192
    vehicle requirements with, 216–217
Hand tools, ergonomic, 245
Handwritten communications
    skills needed for, 77t
    word processing programs and, 169
Hard drive system, 143–144, 330
Hardware
    alternatives to mouse emulation, 153
    described, 142–143
    in evaluation of computer access technology, 151
    off-the-shelf, 153–154
Head-righting control, switches in, 65, 65f
Headsets, 93, 93f
Head switch, 63
Health care technology, service delivery and, 285
Health insurance, 114, 204
Hearing aid-compatible handsets, 90
Hearing impairments
    assistive devices for
      in schools, 172, 173
      sign language-enhanced storybooks, 173
      speech viewers, 172
      in telephone communication, 90–91
      in workplace, 80t–81t, 82t
    communication problems with, 76t–77t
    telecommunication devices for, 91, 92, 335
    telecommunications relay services for, 74, 91
    visual cues for, 158, 336
    visual impairments and, 82t
    workplace accommodations for, 74
HEART (Horizontal European Activities in Rehabilitation Technology), 260
HEATH (Higher Education and Adult Training for People with Handicaps), 255, 274, 276
Higher Education and Adult Training for People with Handicaps (HEATH), 255, 274, 276

High technology devices
    in AAC systems, 100, 109–112
    definition of, 6
    in vehicle modifications, 219–222
Home
    assistive technology in, 12–13, 131, 133
    telephone communication in, 89–99
Horizontal European Activities in Rehabilitation Technology (HEART), 260
House wiring
    compared to alternative ECU transmitters, 122t–123t, 131, 131f
    transmission distance of, 126
Housing resources, independent living centers and, 270
House of Representatives 8395, 268
Human factors, 231
Human work system, 232

I

IBM personal computer (PC), 144, 159
IBM Speech Viewer II, 172
IC (integrated circuit), 330
Iconic augmentative and alternative communication systems
    for children, 107–109, 108f
    compared to graphic representations, 103–104
    definition of, 330
    examples of, 103
    picture symbol vocabulary in, 107–108, 108f
IDEA. *See* Individuals with Disabilities Education Act (IDEA)
Identifier, 38, 330
IEP (individualized education plan), 114, 178
Immersion approach, in learning AAC systems, 108, 111–112
Independence
    definition of, 267
    impact of assistive technology on, 11–12
    integration of AAC systems and ECUs and, 112–113
    robotic assistance for, 133–134
Independent living centers, 267–271
    example of, 269
    funding of, 268
    history of, 267–268
    operational criteria for, 268–269
    residential programs offered by, 269
    resources for
      information, 267, 269–270
      organizations, 279, 302
    services provided by, 267, 269–271
    technology and, 269–271
    transitional programs offered by, 268–269
Indirect selection, switches and, 63
Individualized education plan (IEP), 114, 178
Individuals with Disabilities Education Act (IDEA)
    AT funding requirements in, 114, 178
    purpose of, 3, 3t